Moving Imagination

Advances in Consciousness Research (AiCR)

Provides a forum for scholars from different scientific disciplines and fields of knowledge who study consciousness in its multifaceted aspects. Thus the Series includes (but is not limited to) the various areas of cognitive science, including cognitive psychology, brain science, philosophy and linguistics. The orientation of the series is toward developing new interdisciplinary and integrative approaches for the investigation, description and theory of consciousness, as well as the practical consequences of this research for the individual in society.
From 1999 the Series consists of two subseries that cover the most important types of contributions to consciousness studies:
Series A: Theory and Method. Contributions to the development of theory and method in the study of consciousness; Series B: Research in Progress. Experimental, descriptive and clinical research in consciousness.
This book is a contribution to Series B.

For an overview of all books published in this series, please see
http://benjamins.com/catalog/aicr

Volume 89

Moving Imagination. Explorations of gesture and inner movement
Edited by Helena De Preester

Moving Imagination

Explorations of gesture and inner movement

Edited by

Helena De Preester
University College Ghent and Ghent University

John Benjamins Publishing Company
Amsterdam / Philadelphia

∞[TM] The paper used in this publication meets the minimum requirements of the American National Standard for Information Sciences – Permanence of Paper for Printed Library Materials, ANSI Z39.48-1984.

Acknowledgements
Research for this project was financially supported by the Research Fund of University College Ghent.

Library of Congress Cataloging-in-Publication Data

Moving imagination : explorations of gesture and inner movement / Edited by Helena De Preester.
p. cm. (Advances in Consciousness Research, ISSN 1381-589X ; v. 89)
Includes bibliographical references and index.
1. Mind and body. 2. Human beings--Attitude and movement. 3. Arts--Psychological aspects. 4. Arts audiences--Psychology. I. Preester, Helena de.
BF171.M68 2013
700.1'9--dc22 2013005329
ISBN 978 90 272 1356 3 (Hb ; alk. paper)
ISBN 978 90 272 7200 3 (Eb)

John Benjamins Publishing Co. · P.O. Box 36224 · 1020 ME Amsterdam · The Netherlands
John Benjamins North America · P.O. Box 27519 · Philadelphia PA 19118-0519 · USA

Table of Contents

Moving imagination

Headlines and themes

Helena De Preester
University College Ghent and Ghent University

This collective volume brings together contributions from different disciplines and perspectives, focussing on the way the moving body functions in artistic imagination, ranging from the drawing and painting hand, over embodied perception of sculpture and performing arts such as drama and dance, to embodied listening to sound in film. The contributions share a point of view that takes inspiration from the phenomenological tradition and theories of embodied cognition. The disciplinary backgrounds of the contributors, however, are deliberately chosen from divergent disciplines and fields. Not only art historians and philosophers, but also artists were invited to reflect on the topic of the motor dimension of imagination and to report insights and experiences from their specific field of expertise. The result is a rich collection of ideas about the way in which the moving body and the faculties of imagination and perception are intertwined. Although embodied perception has received a lot of attention both in phenomenology and contemporary cognitive science, the relation between the motor body and imagination is still underexposed in the current literature. We could not imagine a better domain than the domain of visual and performing arts in order to take up the burgeoning interest in 'moving imagination'. In recent years, attention both for visual perception of the performing artist's gestures and movements, and for static traces of gestures and movement, has grown rapidly, but results from this relatively new field of interest have remained scattered until now.

This volume therefore explores the role of the moving and gesturing body in the imaginative perception of works of art. Bodily resonance with the way a work of art is performed or has been created is an essential part of much of our aesthetic experience and appreciation. A guiding notion in the majority of chapters is the notion of "inner movement", referring to the bodily resonance involved in both the perception and the creation of works of art. "Inner movement" is part of our experience of a whole range of works of art, from an implicit tracing of the draughtsman's hand in drawings to an embodied listening to audiovisual works or an explicit feeling of co-embodiment in dance or theatre performances. As such, the notion of "inner movement" does not refer to the representation of movement in works of art, but to the constitutive and creative dimension of the motor body in the perception of works of art, and more generally, to the motor dimension of imagination.

The shared background of this volume is the phenomenological tradition, broadly conceived and ranging from key figures in phenomenological theory such as Edmund Husserl and Maurice Merleau-Ponty to so-called practical phenomenologists like Marcel Jousse or post-phenomenologists like Don Ihde. A second and equally important source of inspiration shared by the authors is the empirical perspective. This empirical perspective is twofold, referring to empirical data from scientific research on the one hand, and to art practices on the other hand.

In the last two decades, phenomenology and cognitive science have explored phenomena of embodiment along parallel lines and sometimes in cooperation. The mutual "enlightenment" between phenomenology and cognitive science is visible in many of the contributions, which employ a phenomenological perspective while taking into account suggestions from the field of the cognitive science.

Yet thinking about imagination and the perception of works of art is greatly advanced by paying attention to the concrete experience of both the creator and the beholder of works of art, and a detailed study of the phenomena of embodiment related to the arts reveals a complex and fascinating involvement of the moving body in art practice and in the perception of works of art. Specialists who have both a phenomenological and a practical background in dance, theatre, sculpture, sound creation, or who are closely affiliated to artistic practice offer detailed analyses and descriptions of several art practices and disciplines, with a focus on the motor dimension of the body. Although the shared background is phenomenological, the volume includes not only contributions by philosophers, but also from specialists or practitioners in the domain of art history, dance, sound, acting, cultural studies, the clinical field, sculpture, or even human anatomy.

This interdisciplinary perspective, often combining phenomenology and cognitive sciences, but also theory and art practice show in what sense the motor body is active in the coming about and the perception of works of art and how a wide variety of artistic activities leaves marks that are intersubjectively perceived as the traces of a fellow human being. The reader is not only introduced into more general issues regarding the motor perception of works of art, but also into the particular domains of drawing and painting, acting and dancing, and into the less evident role of the moving body in the perception of sculpture or sound in film. Several contributions focus on the imagining hand, and analyse and sometimes critically question how we cope with the static traces of gestures of others in works of art. Other contributions pay attention to the meaning and expression of the moving body in recent digital film techniques, taking into account recent findings in cognitive science, or they open up the field of the hearable, and offer a number of rare analyses of hearing and sound, with a focus on embodiment and sound in film.

The opening chapter by Maxine Sheets-Johnstone discusses our appreciation of works of art, starting from the observation that we have a native capacity to think in movement. Sheets-Johnstone was a professor of dance, choreographer, performer, and dance scholar for a number of years prior to her professorship in philosophy. From this combined background, she introduces us into what will be the guiding principle of the present volume: our appreciation of works of art is anchored in the very creation of these works, i.e. the various forms of art embody the kinetic dynamics of their creation, and these kinetic dynamics constitute the basis of the aesthetic appreciation we have of works of art. The notion of "inner movement" proves to be useful for referring to the constitutive and creative dimension of a *moving* body, inhabited by a *moving* dimension of imagination. Artistic realities, be they temporally or spatially defined, depend on the living movement dynamics of the artists creating or performing the work, embodied in the work itself and giving a work of art a certain qualitative character.

This implies that an art work cannot be separated from the artist's forming of the work and the compositional, dynamic process or making of it, informed by the process of thinking in movement and the imaginative consciousness of movement. Moving lines of force, imaginatively traced or drawn and kinaesthetically or kinetically constituted, experienced as linear designs of our own moving bodies or as linear patterns created by movement in art or in everyday life are spatio-temporal-energic entities. These dynamics enter into our perception of works of art.

This brings us to mirror neurons in present-day human brain research, an issue entered by many other contributors to the present volume. According to Sheets-Johnstone, while exclusively referring to the brain, insights from mirror neuron research bypasses the experienced, kinaesthetically realized dynamics of real-life, real-time movement, also in the specification of embodied simulation in art appreciation. Sheets-Johnstone takes an alternative view of such "bodily resonance", coupling our being kinaesthetically "moved" by works of art to affective bodily experiences. The dynamics of the work resonate both affectively and kinetically, a phenomenon on which both our appreciation and understanding of works of art rest. Distant from a reflective awareness, it is our faculty to think in movement and our imaginative consciousness of movement that are fundamental to the creation and appreciation of art.

Xavier Escribano, specialised in the phenomenology of Maurice Merleau-Ponty, joins this perspective by focussing on the active and expressive body which gives rise to works of art, in particular in the context of drama. Drawing on the work of Maurice Merleau-Ponty, Jacques Lecoq and Marcel Jousse, Escribano goes into our capacity to take and recreate in our own flesh the forms and beings of the world, developing a bodily understanding of it. The main theses of Merleau-Ponty's phenomenology of the lived body can be used for exploring dance and drama. Focussing on the phenomenon of motor intentionality, Escribano shows how the pedagogy of dramatic expression of Jacques Lecoq, based on Jousses' fundamental distinction between *mimicry* (a representation of the form) and *mimism* (a dynamic search for sense), requires a dramatic exploration of the cosmos on the basis of the resonance of the elements, forms and movements of nature produced in the actor. The so far underexplored parallels between Merleau-Ponty, Jousse and Lecoq point to an understanding of the world on the basis of a pre-thematic relationship to the world and a physical-bodily recreation of it in expressive action. Reality is gesturally internalised and recreated, allowing us to rediscover the world *in statu nascendi* – a task attributed to art by Merleau-Ponty, but elaborated in Lecoq's pedagogy of drama.

William Seeley, in his contribution, takes up dance and discusses the growing field of the neuroscience of dance, focussing on the underlying sensorimotor processes that underwrite our ordinary perceptual engagement with the environment. From a background in experimental philosophy and neuroscience of art, Seeley examines this research with an eye to the potential contribution neuroscience can make to our understanding of choreographed movements as artworks. What we need is a story that links explanations of how artworks work as perceptual stimuli to explanations of how we recognise and understand their *artistic* salience. Seeley therefore rehearses a range of objections which demonstrate that neuroscience of dance does not succeed as an *aesthetic* theory of art. One objection is that it is not clear that kinaesthetic empathy is sufficient to provide viewers access to the range of artistic conventions necessary to recognise and understand choreographed movements as works of dance. Based on a distinction by Arthur Danto, artistic salience would be a function of what is *shown*, not what is *seen*, such that a spectator would have to tease out the relationship between what is seen and what is shown in order to understand its artistic salience. This distinction is essential for delineating artistically salient features and for connecting them to the range of formal features and compositional relations present in a work. In the vast majority of cases, a tacit understanding of the general practices that define common categories of art, and the stylistic conventions and productive practices that define them, suffice. Applied to dance, this would mean that awareness of the expressive qualities of movement does not suffice to explain their artistic salience. The challenge for neuroscience of dance is, therefore, to understand how choreographers and dancers use kinaesthetic empathy in the context of artistic conventions to express the content of the work. Seeley sketches out into detail a sensorimotor model for audience engagement with dance that can serve as a framework for understanding how dance can communicate the artistic salience of its formal and compositional features. In his view, objections to the neuroscience of dance, and neuroscience of art more generally, can be overcome by paying closer attention to the full range of variables that contribute to our understanding of artistic salience in ordinary contexts.

Gabriele Sofia, who trained as an actor but also did research on the neurophysiology of the actor and the spectator, also focuses on audience engagement and the difference between neuromotor processes underlying perception of movement in daily life and in the context of drama. Starting from the idea that the work of the actor does not entail any dichotomy between imagination and motion, and that the spectator cooperates in the construction of another reality on stage, Sofia investigates the actor's creativity and its effect on the spectator's experience, emphasising the intersubjective relation between actor and spectator. Sofia's main hypothesis is that the neuromotor processes underlying this intersubjective relation is different from those operating in everyday imaginative activities. The actor should not be considered as someone who is very good at *imitating* reality, since the naturalness of the actor's action is an *effect* made possible by the actor's technique. The actor's action has two different aims, giving rise to a "double intention" or – in Sofia's terms – a *dilated intention* that broadens from the performed action out to the audience. This "dilated" intention concerns a peculiar neuromotor dimension. In order to achieve the *effect of spontaneity* for the spectator, the actor's actions must be *believable*, which does not entail that they necessarily have to be similar to everyday action. Sofia discusses the mirror neurons mechanism and goes into the difference between the motor resonance as occurring in everyday life and at the theatre, showing that preparation for action and anticipating the actions to follow is for the actor a double-edged weapon, since it can help as well as hinder her or his performance. The actor has to elaborate special body-schematic strategies in order to obtain a higher pre-reflexive control, different from our daily pre-reflexive experience of it. This is necessary not only to inhibit the unwished anticipating movements but also to reconstruct the fluency the action requires in order to appear effectively spontaneous. Unlike everyday pre-reflective control, the actor has to broaden out his intention to the spectator, a strategy which also affects the constitution of the world on stage, and therefore also the co-constitutive experience of the spectator. This is exactly when the spectator turns to his imagination, and taking into account the peculiarities of the "dilated" intention of an actor is crucial to study the motor dimension of the imaginative processes that renders the actor-spectator relationship an artistic experience.

Sofia emphasises that the spectator-actor relation is different in the case of theatre and acting in front of a camera, and this issue is taken up by Marco Luceri, who turns to contemporary American cinema and the consequences of the increasing use of digital technology, in particular motion capture and facial performance replacement, both creating a virtual image of the actor's body. Luceri, an art historian specialised in film studies, explains how digital performance is part of a broader transformation of the role of the actor and the representation of the body in American cinema over the last fifteen years. While typical of today's tendency to leave behind the limitations of the body, Luceri connects the digitalisation of the actor's body to the dream of European symbolists of the late 19th and 20th century. Gordon Craig, one of the important "heirs" of the symbolist utopia turned motion into the most important vehicle of theatrical expression, at the same time trying to overcome the physical presence of the actor on scene. Notwithstanding the attempts of Craig and the symbolists to eliminate the actor, the actor's corporeality and kinetic force not only did not disappear, but became an essential condition of the retheatralisation hoped for at the beginning of the 20th century. With the arrival of cinema, the relationship between reality and its representation was renegotiated, turning the physical presence of the actor into an image, such that cinema can be said to have found a certain "equilibrium" between the ideals of the symbolists and the idea of retheatralisation. The use of digital technologies seems to have awakened again the "problem" of the actor due to the attempt to overcome the actor's physicality by replacing it by a digital image. This reawakens the question if contemporary American cinema has been able to realise the dream of the symbolists and which are the consequences for the mechanisms of empathy between spectator and actor. What happens if actors act without being represented? Does this entail an elimination of the bodily dimension of actors or does the corporeal dimension continue to determine the relationship between cinematographic representation and sensible reality? To answer these questions, Luceri not only focuses on the function of the actor and the experience of the spectator, but also on the nature and thus the ontology of the cinematographic image.

Another author focussing on the relation between technology and bodily performance, but now in the domain of music, is post-phenomenologist (and painter) Don Ihde, who takes a broad look at music production and experience, with a focus upon "musical technologies" or instrumentation and the different forms of embodiment which the different music productions take. The electronic and digital explosion of music dissemination and its implications for a deeper understanding of the human experience of music asks for a discussion of what Ihde calls "constructed musics". After some anthropological-archaeological speculation concerning human music origins and some observations related to the history of technologies, Ihde distinguishes between directly bodily expressive musical production and varieties of musical technologies, i.e. instruments, which are first directly incorporated into bodily practices (cf. his notion of *embodiment relations*), requiring highly skilled bodily movement, and evolving into mechanised playing. This development caused arguments concerning the alienation of "pure" hand playing, degraded into "mechanical" playing of music, and objections regarding the loss of expressivity and nuance. Some of the resistance is nonetheless understandable, for musicians had to learn new skills – something which takes time and discipline. Finally, Ihde turns to late modern music and its embeddedness in late modern musical technologies, in particular electric and electronic technologies. These technologies range from minimalist and transparent ones, bringing about changes in the bodily activity of, e.g. singing, to more "active" technologies which are much more *indirectly* related to first-person practices, leading to "constructed" music, e.g. in increasing musical editing. To listen to constructed music may entail a certain blindness to this process, since it entails much more than first-person or bodily-instrumental mediation. The strength of this technological trajectory lies not in traditional bodily skills, but in the development of new bodily skills and the exploration of which new sounds can be produced. Giving numerous concrete examples from the history of music technologies, Ihde ends with "posthuman" music which exceeds ordinary human performance capacities but consistently defends the idea that the human bodily actor always remains involved, although in a continuously changing way. This means that *all* musics involve embodiment and experienced perception in relation to musical sounds. A final variation concerns musics not yet heard, more in particular the translation of ultra- and infra-sound frequencies recently discovered by biologists (e.g. in courting songs by male mice). Whereas the embodied human is here engaged only in the set up of the technology complex, it indicates that the possibilities of recorded musics are far from exhausted, but it also makes us aware of our embodied listening to sound.

A joint chapter by Michael Funk and Mark Coeckelbergh, both interested in technology and phenomenology, tackles the question if gesture is knowledge. They offer a philosophical approach to the epistemology of musical gestures which points to the limits of propositional knowledge and the potentials of implicit knowledge for an epistemology of musical gestures. The increasing interest in the relation between music and gestures caused methodological changes in musical scholarship, from score centred research to body oriented studies. To the interdisciplinary study of musical gestures, Funk and Coeckelberg add a conceptual analysis with respect to the history of philosophical thinking. Although there is no adequate definition of gesture available, it seems that movement (action) and meaning (significance) in relation to sound shape the roots of 21st century research on musical gestures. Clearly, the concept of propositional knowledge with its Platonic implications is not fit for explaining body-movement and knowledge implied in musical gestures. Funk and Coeckelberg show that Plato was in fact aware of the limits of propositional knowledge, but did not succeed in finding the "missing parameter". Pointing to implicit knowledge, it was Michael Polanyi who offered a solution for the epistemological paradox present in Plato's *Meno*. The recognition of the non-propositional basis of human knowing involves the recognition that we know more than we can tell. This means that a musician has knowledge in realising meaningful body movements but that he is not able to explain this knowledge in strict and true words. Funk and Coeckelberg go into the historical antecedents of both epistemological points of view (Plato, Descartes versus Polanyi, Gilbert Ryle, but also Ludwig Wittgenstein), reminding us that the history of philosophy, or its dominant currents, has long been unable to recognise embodied, implicit or tacit knowledge. Accounts of sensorimotor knowledge open up the study of mastering skills and techniques, so central in music, and point to a typically human corporeal understanding of the world, and of music. In line with Don Ihde, technical mediation of gestural body movements is discussed, emphasising that music is a certain kind of embodied technical praxis, and that we need a material, non-linguistic, hermeneutics in order to cope with this phenomenon. Playing music, however, does not only involve sensorimotor knowledge. Explicit, theoretical knowledge (cf. notation scores, theory of harmony etc.) and perceptual knowledge in the interpretation of music are necessary as well, but not sufficient. The involvement of different kinds of knowledge has lead to a split, in Western music, between a "score-part" and a "performance" part, and to a dynamics between processes of disembodiment and re-embodiment. This dynamics and the part played by a propositional or an embodied way of knowing, varies. Indian classical music idealises improvisation, whereas composition is the ideal in European music.

Listening to sound and the recording of sound is discussed in the contribution by Martine Huvenne. Huvenne is a musicologist, but continued her career in dance and specialised in the role of sound in film. This combination of disciplines makes her resist the dominant position of the visual image, and she goes into the crucial role of sound in transmitting an experience in film. From a phenomenological-embodied perspective, she discusses listening to sound in terms of energetic movement, pre-reflective experience and bodily resonance. Two opposite views in studying sound in film are common: the sound theory of Michel Chion, in which sound in film is considered an "added" value to the image, and the film theory by Gilles Deleuze, who considers sound in film as autonomous and equivalent to the visual image. In Huvenne's view on audiovisual perception, inspired by Véronique Campan and Maxine Sheets-Johnstone, sound is neither dependent, nor independent of the image. Explaining different listening strategies from a first-person perspective, Huvenne emphasises that sound is essentially an audible movement and therefore constituted in the course of the act of listening. This emphasis leads to an alternative view on sound in film, in which the perception of visible and audible movements and actions is central, rather than the perception of a visual image on screen. Different strategies of listening are examined on the basis of a film fragment from *A man escaped* by Robert Bresson: listening to the meaning of a sound, listening to the source of sound in combination with the act producing the sound, listening to the position of a sound in space, listening to the relation between the sound recording and the original position of sound in space, an embodied resonating listening to a sound without attending to the meaning or the source of the sound, and listening to sound as a trace throughout the totality of a film. Huvenne examines whether an embodied way of listening necessarily evokes images and what exactly we imagine in listening to the dynamics of sound. She claims that not only visual images, but also motor imagery play a crucial role in experiencing and understanding sound.

With the contribution by Michael Parmenter, professor of dance and internationally recognised choreographer, we continue the discussion of film and movement, but also go back to movement and dance. His contribution makes the reader aware of the importance of physical inscriptions into a medium as traces of the artist's gestures. The idea of dance occupies a central place in the work and writings of Len Lye, who continually referred to his process of creating movement in his sculptures as "choreography". Although representations of the human body are absent in his art works – mostly abstract films of lines, patches and fields of colour, or abstract steel sculptures, and although Lye wanted to free his art from the constraints of the human body, it is the body that played a pivotal role in the creation and the reception of his work. Parmenter focuses on the intimate relation between the movement of the world and kinaesthetic experience in Lye's practice. His work is not concerned with the representation of movement, but with how that movement is experienced in his own body – a concern we also find in Lecoq's pedagogy of drama (cf. the contribution by Escribano). Movement, not as a visual, but as a kinaesthetic phenomenon leads Parmenter to consider Lye not so much as a kinetic, but a *kinaesthetic* artist. Painting and inscribing directly onto the film stock and thus physically involved with the medium, his films can be seen as traces of his bodily gestures. As we will see, the traces of bodily gestures in art works are also the focus of the contributions by David Rosand, Francis Halsall and Rajiv Kaushik. Also, the flickering images replicate the irregular firing of the neuromuscular system, an issue taken up by Jay Hetrick where he discusses the work of Henri Michaux.

Similar to the phenomenologically inspired ideas in Escribano, movement for Lye was the expression of a primordial unity between the living being and the world, and Lye's process of creation was anchored in his bodily experience of movement. Here as well, the question how Lye could convey the felt sense of movement to stationary observers (cf. the contribution by Sofia) is tackled in terms of kinaesthesia and kinaesthetic empathy. Delving into the history of empathy and kinaesthesia in dance theory and later on in aesthetic philosophy, Parmenter explores answers to the question of how dance was supposed to make sense to its audience (see also the contribution by Seeley). Dance critic John Martin's notion of *metakinesis,* which points to the sympathetic participation of the viewer in the actual movements of the performer and connects movement perception and the perception of intentions (cf. also Sofia for an account of this in drama), is an attempt to answer the question how meaning is made available in dance. Modernist dance, however, developed into choreographies that were less about expressive movements than about corporeal possibilities. Although this did not rule out Martin's theory of kinaesthetic empathy, the notion was critiqued for being too dependent on a universalist view on bodily experience. Recently, however, the emergence of the field of mirror neuron theory seems to support again Martin's theory of kinaesthetic sympathy (see also the contributions by Sheets-Johnstone, Sofia and Seeley for comments on the mirror neurons theory). Parmenter argues that the idea of cultural specificity championed by recent dance theorists is reconcialable with the notion of kinaesthetic empathy, since studies suggest that though mirror imaging is identified as a biological given, it finds itself actualised differently in different cultural environments. In light of this, it is telling that Lye chose the name of "body *english*" to name the phenomenon of corporeal empathy in his art, avoiding the generalities of a term such as "body language". In line of the regional dimension of kinaesthetic empathy, Parmenter defends the idea that Lye's filmic images and kinetic sculptural figures, retaining in their movements traces of Lye's kinetic gestures, are perceived (and understood) by a perceptual system that reads and translates movements in the world according to the observer's personal repertoire of movement experiences.

Laura Woodward, an artist making "introverted" kinetic sculptures, starts from a discussion of Lye's 1964 essay *The Art that Moves* and examines in what sense her own work relates to it. Woodward emphasises her field of interest as defined by a focus on motion as a material rather than as subject matter, the creation of systems, and a tendency to create works in a space of co-agency, i.e. where artist and material co-create the work in processes of experimentation. "Introversion" points to the phenomenon that the way the work functions and moves is found only within the sculpture itself, and is not placed upon the artwork by the artist. Instead, it develops during the in-studio making of the work, in a process of co-agency between artist and materials, systems, tools, movements and other factors which together drive the emergence of the work.

Woodward shows that Lye's writing contains considerations that can be seen as precursors to her field of interest and thus opens up a space in which introverted kinetic sculpture could emerge almost fifty years later. Two shifts are discernible. First, whereas Lye considers his motion sculptures as a means of externalising his own bodily experiences, Woodward focuses on the potential of motion as a material, and thus on co-agency within the kinetic sculpture. Second, empathy as a bodily response in the introverted kinetic sculpture is positioned differently in Lye and Woodward's work. For Lye, motion in the artwork was representational of kinaesthetic experience, and empathic response was something that he experienced and then transposed into his work. In the introverted kinetic sculpture, the empathic response does not only occur in the viewer's body, but is co-generated between the body of the artwork and the body of the viewer. Woodward is inspired by Donna Haraway's (1985) cyborg manifesto, which functions for her as a signifier to consider the above shifts, in particular in its discussion of multi-generative, techno-human relationships. Whereas Lye touched on the idea of a cyborg in *The Art that Moves*, discussing similarities between organisms and motorised motion sculptures, Woodward starts from the idea of humans and machines not as opposites, but as co-generative and blurred. This frames the emergence of "twitching" behaviour in her introverted kinetic sculptures, pertaining to sensations that involve deeper layers of the body than the primary sense organs. The recognition of a body by a body is supported here by a deep sense of empathy related to the systemic nature of the work.

Boris Wiseman, researcher in a French Studies department, with a particular interest in the 19th and 20th centuries, and Jonathan Cole, a clinical neurologist, continue the discussion of movement and sculpture. In a joint effort, they try to grasp the specificity of Edgar Degas' way of reconstructing movement and his unprecedented drive to see movement from the inside. Through his work, they explore how we are defined by movement and by our bodies. The leading question is not only what an understanding of movement can tell us about Degas' work, but what Degas can tell us about movement. Using clinical and scientific knowledge to extend and take into new domains the views of art critics, Degas' explorations of movement, its unfolding in time, his representation of bodily mass and weight, and his capturing of the experience of the body in movement and repose is explored. Informed by the phenomenological tradition, a reductionist view as can be found in neuroscientific approached is avoided. Degas' insight that freezing parts of a movement through photography was very different to the experience of holding or stopping a movement, gave rise to an analysis of movement as original in aesthetic terms as it was culturally and historically. Although Degas was inspired in part by Etienne-Jules Marey or Eadweard Muybridge-like sequences and saw the revelatory power of those images, he developed a very different and almost incompatible approach to the decomposition and reconstruction of movement sequences. Wiseman and Cole show that Degas is interested in a single movement and what comes immediately before and after it. Unlike the sequences of Marey, the sequences of Degas are not strictly bound by chronology and do not occur in external, measurable time. As Wiseman and Cole explain, the temporal unity of Degas' work is psychological and neurophysiological. Degas' paintings and sculptures of dancers are not meant to invite us to imagine the dance, but the movements involved in dancing or preparing for dancing. Well aware of the dependence of our consciousness of position and movement on a multitude of bodily sensations, Degas tracks these sensations across the skin surfaces of his models. "Muscular consciousness", as Henri Bergson coined it, is the apprehension of our movements through an inner sense, and this interest in the way in which a moving person apprehends her or his movements is what we find in Degas. His primary interest is in the first-person experience of mobility and each person's way of being in the body and in movement. Wiseman and Cole offer an in-depth analysis of different series of works of Degas, and show that Degas had intuited that proprioception underpins locomotor movement and our ability to imagine it.

With David Rosand, art historian with a predilection for phenomenology, we move to the domain of the phenomenology of drawing, which is explored in several contributions in the present volume. Rosand takes into consideration the time it takes to draw a line and the time it takes to read or respond to that line. Elaborating the idea that we rehearse the artist's gestures internally and follow their rhythms through space and thus through time, Rosand offers an intriguing analysis of a number of ideas set out by many other contributors in this volume, but now focussed on drawing. His object of study is line, i.e. the trace of the movement of the hand, the arm or the full body. The issue he raises is how we factor the temporal dimension into understanding our response to an image made by a moving hand. Giving the reader insight into the appreciation of the purity of line, which runs from antiquity through the Middle Ages and the Renaissance and extends into the modern era, Rosand discusses the distinction between the line as graphic reality and as representational fiction. The qualities of the line, developing in time through the movement of the hand, pertain both to the line as record of the drawing gesture and the depicted object. A long tradition of graphic speculation by artists, testify of their fascination by the transformative power of line. As Rosand explains on the basis of examples, line insists upon its own role as protagonist and on establishing its own reciprocal relationship with its maker. As many artists recognise, the draughtsman finds his attention being commanded by his own line, which is an active participant in the act of drawing and asserts its own creative independence. As viewers following that line, we become aware of this independence and respond to the drawn line and its qualities. Since the line recalls the process of becoming through the act of drawing, it invokes a range of kinaesthetic experiences and makes us participant in the somatic vision through which we can see the world. As Rosand describes, knowing the world only by drawing it, the artist sees with hand and eye, and interpretation involves us in the reconstitution of the act of drawing. We sense the temporal dimension of the act of drawing, such that our response to drawing is a matter of re-enactment of the artist's drawing gesture, involving the viewer in the kinaesthetics of the act of drawing. Once again, it becomes clear that it is through the body that we, both the artist and the viewer, perceive the world in space and time.

Starting from Thierry de Duve's drawing of Robert Morris' *Untitled 3 L-Beams*, Francis Halsall, art historian, philosopher and working in higher art education, uses this drawing to understand Morris' Minimalist sculpture from 1965. Halsall argues that drawings like this reveal that Morris' sculpture can be approached through drawing itself, and that a threedimensional sculptural form can be considered a form of drawing. Morris' work would even promote a style of observation that one would adopt if drawing the sculpture. Emphasising that drawing is first and foremost a process and a practice, and thus not defined by the medium used, it is grounded in a type of observation and tactile action, the particularities of which Halsall describes on the basis of the notion of "style". In sum, drawing is a particular style of observation and action, and this perspective on drawing allows us to uncouple the specificity of the act of drawing from medium specificity. The particular style of observation involved in drawing is difficult to attain – something anyone attempting or learning to draw can acknowledge. However, Halsall explains how Minimalism can help achieve the particular style of close looking, for it draws aesthetic attention to the conditions of looking itself or to the conditions by which it is experienced. It does so by removing any elements that might be extraneous to an aesthetic experience. In other words, the primary meaning of the work lies in the manner by which it is experienced. Similarly, drawing is in the first place a non-mimetic process that translates experience according to the material used in the process of drawing and the bodily procedures used by the drawer. Based on Gombrich's notion of "schemata" of drawing, which frame the way the drawer perceives and inhabits the world, Halsall emphasises drawing as a physical and embodied activity that is culturally situated. If drawing is characterised as a practice or processes of looking and acting with a certain style, we are ready to uncouple drawing from any material or medium specificity and to consider drawings as relative to the conditions of the viewer's embodied subjectivity. Precisely this central place of the embodied subject in the completion of the work of art opens up the possibility of the conflation of sculpture and drawing. Next, Halsall goes into Morris' series of

Blind Time Drawings to show that drawing is an embodied, tactile and temporal process (cf. also the contribution by Rosand) similar to experiencing sculptural forms.

Rajiv Kaushik is specialised in phenomenological philosophy and explores the work of Cy Twombly, in particular his ability to address himself to the smallest expressive units of paintings: the expressive potential of the mark, smudge, line, or dot. Kaushik considers these markings as sites in which the body is opened up into the space around it and instances in which the difference between the interior and the exterior is no longer. In this context, Kaushik also explores how we can understand Twombly's so-called language paintings and argues that these works show us the very origins of language from out of the interplay between the body and its space. More in particular, Kaushik argues that we can witness a body opened up and in response to the very process of marking up the canvas. Maurice Merleau-Ponty's hyper-dialectic is helpful in order to understand Twombly's work since the notion of hyper-dialectic refers to a region of human consciousness that is indifferent to interiority and exteriority. Twombly's language paintings help us think through what it means for signification to emerge from out of the space of sensible bodies. Commenting on Roland Barthes' gestural interpretation of Twombly, Kaushik explains how each marking is self-referential in the sense that, rather than referring to the external world of things, it refers to nothing outside of its own origination, such that each time the brushwork reveals the event of its own production and the artist's bodily intentions. Moreover, Twombly's "writings" reveal a continuity between the symbolic and the real. Whereas language is not normally thought to be about the body, Twombly's "graphic texture" leads us to the question how the sign comes to be from out of the accidental aspects of the material. In a merleau-pontian way, Twombly's language paintings reveal the incarnate place of the origins of language and show that language does not originate purely from out of the intentional and volitional. This is what becomes visible if we are ready to see that the characteristics of Twombly's otherwise non-linguistic gestures apply to his language paintings as well. In it, the artist is given over to an expressive potential of the mark, which precedes him.

In view of the enormously complex integrative apparatus needed to achieve and maintain coordination among the sensors, neurons, and skeleto-motor units that contribute to writing, Jan and Koos Jaap van Zwieten also focus on writing. Whereas Koos Jaap van Zwieten is specialised in comparative and functional anatomy of the hand, Jan van Zwieten is a mediaevalist. Together they check a 11th century handwritten manuscript, which looks most like a love poem, for finger and hand movements related to pre-motor activities due to "movements" of inner organs during emotional states. Since deep brain areas like emotional circuits may influence handwriting, visible traces of emotional states may be found in various historical handwritten texts, as long as the characteristics of quill pen writing and the processes of writing by hand are taken into account. Researchers studying brain activation during rejected love, e.g. noticed typical pre-motor activity patterns, as suggested by irregular writing patterns, due to basal ganglia dysfunction. Many linguists presume an emotional state having been present in the mind of the scribe of the Flemish love poem. Nonetheless, Jan and Koos Jaap van Zwieten conclude that the handwriting does not reveal any irregularities caused by emotion, and that no pre-motor dysfunction was present. Therefore, a number of other hypotheses are explored. The sentence may be a pen test (in the form of a hemi-pangram). Alternatively, and taking into account the historical circumstances in which the text was written, some emotional factors could nevertheless have been present. Possibly, the scribe tried to find some mental rest for an overall unhappy situation, a possibility that not only reintroduces the poetic character of the manuscript but also takes into account the upper left quadrant of the end-leaf, displaying a dozen of musical notes in the Gregorian chant notation, which may have accompanied the words of the manuscript. The singing could have helped to overcome unhappy feelings.

With Jay Hetrick, philosopher of art, we continue the discussion of writing and affectivity, but now the focus is on the domain of the pre-gesture in the work of poet and artist Henri Michaux. Hetrick describes the development of Michaux's artistic practice from his earliest experiments with pictorial writing systems, to his more gestural paintings, to his infamous mescaline drawings. Michaux describes this last stage of his work as expressing the "pre-gestural", a term used to refer to the affective and kinaesthetic inner movements that we might locate along the central nervous system. Hetrick discusses Michaux's claim that the domain of the pre-gestural reveals something fundamental about the human brain and connects this to Oliver Sacks' neuroscientific research on migraine aura. In accord with Francisco Varela's vision for a neurophenomenology that takes equal account of first- and third-person investigations, Hetrick shows how Michaux's and Sacks' findings reinforce each other and help construct a neurophenomenology of gesture.

Michaux's early experiments with creating new hieroglyphic alphabets may be interpreted as shifting attention away from what graphic signs mean towards a more performative understanding of the act of writing or drawing itself, entering a form of expression rooted in the raw kinetic and kinaesthetic body and inspired by cave paintings. Michaux was attracted to cave paintings because they are not only visual and gestural but also visceral and powerful, and he speaks about a kinetic desire, that is explained not in terms of the physical or gestural movements of the brush, but in terms of the kinaesthetic and sensual pleasures of the act of painting itself. Michaux's method should not be seen as an incarnation of spontaneous automatism, but as practice that takes inspiration from East Asian calligraphy and maintains his conscious connection to the pre-gestural movements that coursed through his interior. With his mescaline drawings, the search to express the pre-gestural was over and the last two decades of his artistic output can be seen as a recapitulation and refinement of the various techniques he had already experimented with. Michaux had finally discovered a way to transcribe the inner movements of psychic life. Michaux believed that his mescaline drawings render visually the type of vibratory waves that might appear on the encephalogram of a subject under the influence of mescaline. Hetrick emphasises that the context in which we should attempt to understand this phase of Michaux's work is thus not only poetic and artistic, but also a context that utilises, interrogates, and responds to properly neuroscientific problems. Michaux's mescaline drawings should be understood as "pre-gestural" in the sense that they attempt to directly express inner neural movements and vibrations onto the canvas rather than trace the outer movements of twitching muscles of the arm or hand. Hetrick finds in Oliver Sacks' tracing of a lineage of research on hallucination from the early nineteenth century support for Michaux's claim that geometric patterns perceived in hallucinatory experience are the result of the wavelike diffusion and interference of nerve impulses in the brain. Furthermore, he reminds us of Francisco Varela's idea of neurophenomenology, implying that neuroscience must be expanded to include methodologically rigorous first-person investigations of experience. Retrospectively, we can say that Michaux's mescaline drawings and writings present with as much objective distance as possible the domain of the pre-gestural. After ten years of almost meditative investigation, Michaux comes to describe this as a domain of inner neural movements that has a significance beyond mere personal hallucination and, in fact, "reveals" something fundamental about the workings of the human brain.

Natalie Depraz, phenomenologist and specialist in the living body, elaborates a number of Francisco Varela's ideas and methodological suggestions and reflects on the question what it means to move in imagination or to move *inward*? Whereas moving involves a bodily behaviour, which is external and visible for others, inner movement implies that I might move while remaining motionless seen from the outside. Starting from Aristotle's identification of four kinds of movement, Depraz explains that the challenge for phenomenology is to understand *kinesis* as both lived and worldly. Phenomenology's emphasis on the twofold dimension of movement, however, opens the question to what extent it is phenomenologically possible to "move without moving". Depraz explains the account by Maurice Merleau-Ponty, who focusses on the ontological and expressive-gestural nature of inner movement, and the one by Michel Henry, for whom inner movement is affective and self-generating. Both accounts are diametrically opposed, but can nonetheless be considered, in a broadened sense, as third-person approaches. Therefore, Depraz distinguishes within phenomenology between the "pheno-philosophical" accounts by Merleau-Ponty and Henry, and a first-person experiential phenomenology, which is more fitting in order to describe the kind of inner movement at play in two different kinds of practices: sitting meditation and manual fasciatherapy. In these practical frameworks, the experience of "moving inward" is clearly identified because of its structural dissociation from any external move. In other words, both settings are structured by the externally motionless posture of the subject and imply a thematic exploration of what is going on within my lived body while remaining still. Applying the method of *épochè* to movement, i.e. bracketing any external move and redirecting attention to the observation of inner movement, Depraz re-reads the descriptions of her own experiences in the setting of sitting meditation and manual fasciatherapy. Whereas in the first experience, inner movement points to the dynamic and tangible experience of numerous thoughts permeating each other in the mind as an inner mobile space, in the second experience, an exploration of the materiality of the body is guided by a fasciatherapist. By means of hand-pressure at different parts of the body, one feels one's material body from within, in a way that is usually not accessible to experience. As Depraz reports: it is as if the fasciatherapist was touching her from within and she experienced within herself genuine moves while remaining objectively motionless. Depraz offers a detailed phenomenological and first-person account of her experience in these two practical settings, and offers a schematic table in which both the a priori categorical results of Merleau-Ponty and Henry are presented and compared to the a posteriori experiential categories from both first-person practices. The aim is to show that both may generate and constrain each other and may help in establishing more refined accounts of the (plurality of) bodily experience of inner movement.

With Erica Harris, whose main areas of research are psychoanalysis and French phenomenology, we continue the exploration of a deeper and pre-personal bodily layer when she explores the tension between the way one perceives a work of art and habitual objects. Harris comments on painting from the point of view of bodily movement in aesthetic space and suggests that the aura of strangeness that characterizes a painting is a function of the body's relation to it. She argues that the body cannot engage with a painting in the same way that it does with everyday objects, since the painting is a purely visual object that does not offer itself as something that can be explored by the body as a synaesthetic whole. This does not entail that we should give up the separation between perception and imagination that Merleau-Ponty wanted to avoid, but it necessitates a shift from the "I can" of the sensorimotor subject to the "it can" of anonymous movement. The question is if the body that participates in painting is the same as the lived body that inhabits the world in ordinary perception. The painting depicts a place where I cannot go, objects that I can only see, and in general is present to me only as a spectacle. The purely visual space of the painting is radically different from the perceptual space that is polarised by the body schema. But this does not imply that the body has no motor-engagement with the artwork whatsoever. Commenting on the mirror neurons theory, Harris notices that their account leaves aside the difficult phenomenon of the body's response to an aesthetic object that is not recognised as "manipulable" (cf. the "I can"). Our inability to inhabit aesthetic space is essential rather than contingent. The painted space, unlike what Merleau-Ponty's discussion of imagination suggests, is not simply a horizon like others, since it is not open to exploration by the body as a whole. Harris describes the different relation of the body to painting in terms of transitivity, a notion borrowed from Merleau-Ponty. The transitive body is always beneath the surface of the practical body and interpreted as a body that is organized in the same way as its object: a body "in the making". The anonymous bodily experiences pertaining to this transitive body precede and exceed one's sense of *I can*, and is characterised not by "I can", but by "it can". As such the experience of the *it can* is a reversion to a more primordial, unified sense of the body, and it is the body that perceives the painting. Harris argues that the artistic product (at least in its non-representational form) is the visual depiction of the pre-objective world to which the "it can" corresponds.

Interdisciplinary approaches are always a risky undertaking. Not only because they require combined expertise, but also – and particularly in this case – theoretical approaches to practice-based disciplines such as the arts always risk to misunderstand the specifics of the artistic endeavour. Phenomenology, although highly theoretical in nature, might nonetheless be an exceptional and appropriate perspective that is able to capture some of the essential features of what is a stake in the arts. Focussing on the motor dimension of imagination in the arts from a broadly conceived phenomenological perspective, the present volume hopes to respect the particular nature of art practice when it probes into the role of the motor body and imagination in art perception and production. Although it is impossible to avoid generalisations, the phenomenological tradition has always taken the trouble to enable abstract thinking on the basis of research and careful description of what is essential to the phenomena, rather than to inductively generalise away what is particular. We hope that this volume does honour to that phenomenological legacy.

Bodily resonance

Maxine Sheets-Johnstone
Department of Philosophy, University of Oregon

1. Introduction

When we duly reflect on 'the movement we are constantly giving things' in our everyday lives,[1] we realise straightaway not just the reality but the pervasiveness of our native capacity to think in movement. We pick up keys, forks, books, glasses – both reading and drinking kinds – clothes, hangers, bags of groceries, and so on; we open doors, letters, windows, jars, candy wrappers, car trunks, drawers, and so on; we "put" in a number of ways: put on clothes, put things away, put down a pen, put up a wash; and so on. In the course of picking up, opening, putting, and much, much more, we are thinking in movement, thinking in terms of doing something and thereby accomplishing something. We know not just *how* to move in such ways – *how* to do such things; we know *that* moving in such ways fulfils certain desires or aims, or *that* moving in such ways accomplishes or brings about certain results. Thinking in movement comes naturally in the course of learning our bodies and learning to move ourselves. No one gives us instruction in this learning and neither do we come into the world with an owner's manual. Because we have an inborn capacity to think in movement, we have learned our bodies and learned to move ourselves effectively and efficiently in the world, and because we have learned our bodies and learned to move ourselves effectively and efficiently in the world, the movement we are constantly giving things is effective and efficient. We know just how much effort is needed to open a jar, just how far we must stretch our arm and torso to grasp something otherwise out of reach, just how quickly we must move in order to catch a ball or just how stealthily we must move in order to surprise someone from behind. Thinking in movement, we are indeed able to

1. Single quotes are placed around the phrase for I have been unable to determine its origin. I do not think it a phrase of my own making. The closest approximation is in Husserl's observation that "We, as living in wakeful world-consciousness, are constantly active on the basis of our passive having of the world" and in his follow-up observation that "we deal actively in different ways with" "thematic objects" (Husserl 1970, pp. 108–109).

snatch a piece of paper breezily off a desk and run off with it; we are able to grasp a heavy suitcase assuredly and carry it downstairs without a hitch; we are able to balance peas on a fork as we raise the fork to our opening mouth. It is not surprising that we are able to think in movement: movement is our mother tongue. Though we come into the world as strangers, our native ability to move and to think in movement provides us a ready relationship to that world, a direct and immediate kinetic relationship through which meanings are forged. Many of those relationships and meanings are functional in Jakob von Uexküll's notion of "functional tone" (von Uexküll 1957 [1934]); that is, objects in the world come to have a certain useful meaning for us such as something to push, something to pull, something to eat, something to open, and so on.

Brushing, stirring, turning on, turning off, washing, drying – an array and gamut of verbs, not to mention clicking, tweeting, pressing, and so on – attest to the movement we are constantly giving things in our everyday lives, and by that very fact, *attest to our thinking in movement*. Lacking the capacity to think in movement, we would be unable to carry out the movement we are constantly giving things: we would be at a loss to move effectively and efficiently in the object-laden world we inhabit. Present-day talk in cognitive research of "an extended mind", as in philosopher Mark Rowlands' *The New Science of the Mind* (Rowlands 2011) passes over this native capacity, a capacity that comes with learning our bodies and learning to move ourselves to begin with, a learning in infancy that is anchored in our native capacity to think in movement.

These introductory observations are a *natural* point of departure for inquiring into the appreciation of works of art for our appreciation is anchored in the very creation of the works of art themselves. More finely put, what the observations lead us to consider are the distinctive kinds of movement by which the various forms of art are created, and in turn, both the various forms of art themselves that embody the kinetic dynamics of their creation and the way in which those kinetic dynamics constitute the basis of their aesthetic appreciation. The notion of "inner movement" here will refer to the constitutive and creative dimension of a *moving* body, and find among other faculties in that moving body a *moving* dimension of imagination.[2]

2. For validations of the distinction between "motor" (as in motor intentionality, sensorimotor, motor imagery, and so on) and movement (or "kinetic," as in sensory-kinetic), see, for example, Sheets-Johnstone 1990, Chapter 6; Sheets-Johnstone 2012a, 2012b, and expanded second edition 2011 of *The Primacy of Movement*, pp. 470–71.

2. Thinking in movement[3]

As intimated above, however focal our concern with movement in relation to objects, whether in terms of the movement we are constantly giving things in everyday life or in the context of artistic creation, we cannot reasonably discount the movement of our own bodies. Indeed, the dynamics of our own movement are critical to what we accomplish or do not accomplish with respect to "things" or "creations." Through an attentiveness to these dynamics we learn to control our movement and thus assure ourselves of positive practical results. In a deeper epistemological – and aesthetic – sense, we have the possibility of becoming more keenly kinaesthetically informed and astute. To attend in this deeper sense to the dynamics of our own movement is to be attuned to the qualitative character of our movement: its smoothness, its abruptness, its arcing trajectory, its swiftness, its constrictedness, its jaggedness, its intensity, and so on. Certainly in the performance as well as in the creation of art, such awareness is of critical moment. How a musical passage is played, how a monologue is delivered, how a piece of fruit, a tree, or a person is delineated and shaded on canvas, how a dance ensemble spreads apart and gathers together – all such artistic realities depend on the living movement dynamics of the artists creating or performing the work – the composers, painters, choreographers, musicians, playwrights, actors, dancers, sculptors. Those dynamics are *naturally* embodied in the work itself. The crescendo in the music passage, for example, the rising intensity of the monologue, the precision and tonal intensities of the fruit, tree, or person, the attenuated spread and rapid gathering together of the ensemble – all are the result of the movement dynamics of the artists themselves. In short, the literally moving body of an artist instills its kinetic dynamics in the art work being created or performed. These dynamics in turn give the artwork a certain qualitative character. In a qualitative sense, they make the work the work that it is. This relationship is as true in the writing of poetry and novels as it is in the writing and performing of a play. The motif of the poem is dynamically presented in terms of metre, cadence, lines, alliterations, and so on. A poem is not just a string of distinct words, each with its own meaning, but an unfolding of words that has a distinctive dynamic in virtue of the formal relationships that constitute it. In equal measure, the story a novel tells evolves and develops dynamically: it too unfolds and in its unfolding, it may unravel, climax,

3. For the original exposition of thinking in movement with respect to aesthetics, see Sheets-Johnstone 1981. For expanded versions of that article that elucidate the phylogenetic and ontogenetic realities of thinking in movement, see Sheets-Johnstone 1999a/expanded second edition 2011 and Sheets-Johnstone 2010.

explode, attenuate, tighten, and so on. The coherency of a poem and novel alike is anchored in its dynamics, dynamics that poet and novelist constitute in terms of their own felt sense of the motif of the poem and the story the novel tells.

It is relevant to emphasize that thinking in movement is not only foundational to what are commonly categorized as the "temporal arts" – music, dance, theatre, and film, and to poetry and novels as well – it is equally foundational to the "spatial arts". Any artistic composer – whether of a piece of music, a painting, a sculpture, a building, a play, a dance, a film, a poem, a novel – is not just willy-nilly putting this or that together, simply "doing now this, now that". He or she is attentive to the form he or she is creating, intent on its integrity, hence to the way in which it develops, thus we might say, to the way in which it either "hangs together" or not. A work's integrity is thus clearly bound up with its dynamics, both the dynamic relationship of parts themselves and the dynamic relationship of parts to whole. To think in movement is to think in terms of dynamics, to be witness to the qualitative nature of the form one is creating, its waxings and wanings, its now vibrant, now hushed character, the way in which it flows, the way in which it builds, the way in which its parts interconnect – in short, its overall spatio-temporal-energic character. Whatever the art, its creator thinks in dynamic terms, which is to say in movement. We can see this particularly clearly in the performing arts in which musicians, dancers, and actors/actresses are dynamically engaged from head to toe in learning the work they are to perform. They are thinking of their inflections, their tempo, their sustained extensions – in short, they are thoughtfully engaged in the integral flow of the piece they are performing. In their actual performance, they are not moving through a form; the form is moving through them. They know in a bodily felt sense the dynamics of the work from beginning to end and are bringing those dynamics to life.

The same is true of painter, sculptor, and architect: the form they are engaged in creating is a dynamic form that engages them from head to toe. What they are creating is indeed created by their own movement. A painter is not simply choosing colours but choosing how he or she will apply them on canvas; a sculptor is not simply whacking away at a piece of stone but "taking away all that is not David"; an architect is not simply drawing rooms in a house but creating spaces, which, to quote Goethe, involves "the difficult and complicated doctrine of proportions, which gives the building and its various parts their character." (Arnheim 1977, p. 152).[4] Indeed, in the most basic sense, if/then relationships hold sway for all

4. "Man sollte denken, die Baukunst als schöne Kunst arbeite allein für's Auge; allein sie soll vorzüglich, und worauf man am wenigsten Acht hat, für den Sinn der mechanischen Bewegung des menschlichen Körpers arbeiten; wir fühlen eine angenehme Empfindung, wenn

artists; that is, "if I do this, then such and such will result." If I accentuate this redness, for example, or if I accentuate this chord, or if I accentuate this word, or if I accentuate this lift, and so on, then such and such will result. The created form will thus be determined by the qualitative impact of my movement, that is, what I choose to do and thus how I choose to move with respect to the form I am creating.

In sum, whatever the art work, it cannot be separated from the artist, *not* in terms of the artist's intentions, but in terms of the artist's actual forming of the work itself, her or his compositional process or making of the work. That compositional process is a dynamic process, a process that in essential and basic ways is through and through informed by the process of thinking in movement.

3. The imaginative consciousness of movement[5]

As counterintuitive or even startling as it may at first seem, thinking in movement is integrally linked to the imaginative consciousness of movement. The latter is not some murky, occult, or magical incantation but a living reality of everyday human life. When we sit down, stand up, turn around, and so on, the linear design of our body changes. Similarly, when we walk, one leg is always forward, the other always behind; the former is extended the latter is bent and extends as it moves forward. In short, when we move, the linear contours of our body shift: our hips can be

---

wir uns im Tanze nach gewissen Gesetzen bewegen; eine ähnliche Empfindung sollten wir bei jemand erregen können, den wir mit verbundenen Augen durch ein wohlgebautes Haus hindurch führen. Hier tritt die schwere und komplizierte Lehre von den Proportionen ein, wodurch der Charakter des Gebäudes und seiner verschiedenen Teile möglich wird." (Goethe 1998, p. 368.) Another formulation: "Man sollte denken, die Baukunst arbeite allein für's Auge; allein sie arbeitet vorzüglich, und woran am wenigsten gedacht wird, für den einen Sinn der mechanischen Bewegung, der unter keiner anderen gebracht werden kann. Der Körper wie wir im Tanzen sehen, fühlt eine angenehme Empfindung, wenn er im Tanze sich nach gewissen Gesetzen bewegt. Diese Empfindungen sollte ein Blinder haben der durch ein wohlgebautes Haus geführt würde. Die Gesetze der Baukunst sollen aus diesen drei Bedingungen vorzüglich herzuleiten sein. … Hier tritt die schwere und komplizierte Lehre vom Ebenmaß, woraus der Charakter des Gebäudes entspringt, ein" (Goethe 1998, pp. 375–376.)

I am indebted to Mathias Mitteregger, architect and architect theory doctoral student in the Department of Architecture Theory at Vienna Technical University, for the quotation from Goethe and for these references in German.

5. For the original exposition of the imaginative consciousness of movement, see Sheets-Johnstone 1966/ 2nd editions 1979/1980. For an expanded version of the original, see Sheets-Johnstone 2011b.

flexed or extended; our legs can be extended or bent at the knee and ankle; they can be abducted to the side; our arms can be flexed or extended at the elbow and wrist and can be rounded as well as straight; our torsos can be vertical, curved, or twisted. Our bodies as a whole can be tilted diagonally forward as we trudge up a steep hill, twisted in one place and vertically aligned in another as when we turn our head to look behind us, and so on. All of these lines are imaginatively drawn lines; that is, we experience the lines that parts of our moving body form as we move and that our moving body as a whole forms as we move by tracing a line imaginatively from one joint to another, for example, from head to toe, and so on.

In our everyday adult lives, we commonly pay scant if any attention to the linear design of our bodies, unless someone perhaps admonishes us to "stand up straight." Oddly enough, however, we readily *perceive* the linear design of other bodies, as when we see an older person walk with head crooked forward and down, thus breaking the otherwise relatively vertical line of the body as a whole. We in fact readily perceive changing linear designs in a dance performance: we readily *perceive visually* the shifting contours of the dancing bodies. Dancers themselves are exquisitely attuned to the changing linear designs of their moving bodies, but not perceptually except by way of a mirror. When a dancer performs an arabesque, for example, she *feels* the full extension of the leg behind her and is *imaginatively aware* of the straight line formed by that full extension.

How is this imaginative line constituted? It is constituted *kinaesthetically*. While we can visually perceive an extended forward-reaching arm of our own or that of someone else as forming a straight line, we imaginatively constitute the angular line of our bent leg that is behind us in walking. We constitute it on the basis of kinaesthesia, which is to say that, on the basis of neuromuscular pulls and decompressions, we draw imaginative lines from joint to joint and from spinal disc relationships, as well as from head to toe. Accordingly, in virtue of kinaesthesia, we feel the twisted, vertical, or horizontal lines of our bodies as we move, their roundedness, straightness, and so on. Moreover it is not just *the linear design* of our moving bodies that we experience imaginatively; *the linear patterns* of our movement are equally apparent imaginatively in any and all movements that we make. Unlike linear designs, the linear patterns created by movement are through and through imaginatively constituted phenomena. Their spatial reality is such that they cannot be perceived. The patterns emerge in the form of imagined trajectories, *moving lines of force*, that a moving body draws in the process of moving, as when a dancer runs across stage, jumps in the air, and in landing, turns upstage and moves in a series of spirals downstage – or more simply, when we ourselves, in walking, turn a corner and proceed on our way down the different street.

Lines are clearly spatial entities, whether they are actually drawn and perceived as in paintings or perceived as linear designs of moving bodies as in dance and drama, or whether they are imaginatively constituted. When they are imaginatively traced or drawn and kinaesthetically or kinetically constituted, however – that is, when experienced as linear designs of our own moving bodies or as linear patterns created by movement, whether in art or in everyday life – they are not purely and solely spatial entities but spatio-temporal entities and in fact spatio-temporal-energic entities. We can appreciate this fact by way of the previous example of a dancer running across stage: the described movement pattern is a spatio-temporal phenomenon. We can appreciate the fact equally in our everyday lives when we zig-zag to avoid colliding with someone, for example, and experience that shifting movement as a linear pattern: again, the linear pattern is a spatio-temporal phenomenon. We can bring the inherent temporality of linear patterns to self-evidence in a focal and even striking way by moving apart from any task or activity. For example, when we draw a figure eight in the air, we experience the spatio-temporal nature of the imaginatively drawn line in terms of its rapidity, its pauses or rushes, and so on, and again, as indicated, in fact experience it as having a certain energic quality in terms of its fluidity, its strength, its softness, and so on.

While we kinaesthetically feel or have the capacity to experience on the basis of kinaesthesia the linear dynamics of our own moving bodies, these dynamics clearly enter into our perception of works of art. As noted earlier, we readily perceive the linear designs of moving bodies other than our own, and we readily constitute the linear patterns of others. Thus, in our perception of works of art, *depending upon the particular genre of art – whether music, dance, painting, theater, poetry, film, sculpture, architecture, or novel – and thus upon the particular kind of artist* – we can perceive and/or we can imaginatively constitute linear designs. Paintings, for example, obviously present us with lines, but they also propel us to follow the lines, thus to connect imaginatively the diagonal thrust of a straight line drawn at the lower left of a drawing with the diagonality of a straight line just above centre and continuing to the right beyond center. Distinctive lines that we perceive in paintings thus have the potential to become linear patterns. With respect to performing arts, while linear patterns are imaginatively experienced by audience and stage performer alike, the shifting linear designs that exist for the dancer and for the actor imaginatively are there perceptually for the audience. In sum, depending on the art work and the artist, linear dynamics can be both perceived lines and imaginative lines. In either instance, insofar as lines are in either case *drawn*, they are grounded in movement, hence in the kinaesthetic foundation of both linear designs and linear patterns.

A further line warrants specification in relation to the imaginative consciousness of movement. This line becomes evident in answer to the question, "What is there in the form that allows a composing artist to apprehend its dynamics and how does she or he do this?" I answered this question in terms of dance in a chapter titled "Dynamic Line" in *The Phenomenology of Dance*. My answer began as follows:

> Movement as a perpetual revelation of force creates a dynamic line. This is not an actual line, but "line" in the sense of an on-going projection of forces from a beginning point. Each dance creates its own dynamic line, a unique qualitative organization of forces from beginning to end.
>
> (Sheets-Johnstone 1966/2nd eds.1979/1980, p. 88)

I noted that this line is spatial as well as temporal, and this because "the spatiality created by any projection of force has to do not only with the *manner* in which space is created, but with the projected designs and patterns as well". I pointed out that "[i]t is precisely because each projection of force creates its own space as it creates its own time that the dynamic line of movement is spatially unified as it is temporally continuous" (ibid. p. 89).

Although described in terms of dance, the experientially-based concept of dynamic line is relevant equally to poetry, music, theatre, and film. A poem flows forth with a certain dynamic in virtue of its accentuations, metric pattern, repetitions, pauses, stopping points, and so on. As with dance, its dynamic line refers not to actual lines, but to the qualitative way in which the whole flows forth. Similarly, a Beethoven Sonata flows forth with a certain dynamic in virtue of its tempo, metric structure, repetitions, crescendos, fadings, rushes, ebbings, and so on. Were a poem read aloud, it too would have a filled out dynamics in which its intensities and amplitudes were audible. Dynamic line is in fact most simply exemplified in the classic idea of a play having a beginning, a climax, a dénouement, and an end, a classic idea that endures in novels, dramas, and films. It can be exemplified in more detailed ways by a child's recited verse: "Baa baa black sheep, have you any wool?" If the words are replaced by nonsense syllables – Ba ba Ba ba Babababa Ba – a certain qualitative dynamic is readily evident. Moreover that dynamic is mutable. We might, for example, intensify and extend the dynamic, and render it climatically as:

"Ba ba, Ba ba, BaBaaBaaBaa *BaaBaaBaaBaa* <u>*BaaBaaBaaBaa*</u> ***BAH!***"

Because the concern in the chapter on dynamic line was essentially compositional and a vocalization of dynamic line was considered an adjunctive tool through which the choreographer might enhance her grasp of a composition's dynamic flow more intimately, that is, kinaesthetically through its articulation and audibly in its sounding, a valid question arose that pertains to the challenge of artistic creation generally, namely: is there only one movement that correctly in an aesthetic sense follows a previous movement? – or, in terms of poetry, music, drama, novel, and film, only one word or sequence of words, for example, or one note or musical passage, or one scene or sequence of happenings, and so on, that correctly in an aesthetic sense follows the previous word or word sequence, note or musical passage, scene or sequence of happenings? The integrity of any work of art, after all, hangs on its formal relationships. Hence the significance of an artist's attunement to the dynamics inherent in the form he or she is creating. Hence too, then, the significance of dynamic line in the creation of an aesthetic form, even a painting or sculpture. In particular, what was said of dance in this context applies equally to creativity in all art forms:

> Tacit in the conception of dynamic line is the emphasis upon the movement itself, where it wants to go: the dance as an expressive art form must exist as a thing formally apart from the personal predilections of the dancer. The dancer, of course, controls her materials, but the control in the end is unseen or seen only as a function of the movement itself. Through the use of a vocalized dynamic line, the dancer becomes increasingly and more keenly aware of the dynamic flow of movement, the unity and continuity of each movement within the total form. Thus, the inclusion of extraneous movement is obviated, movement which one simply likes to do, movement which one includes because one does it well, etc. To develop the form is to create a dynamic line of sheer force which is logically [in an aesthetic sense] consistent with all that has gone before and all that will come to be. (Sheets-Johnstone 1966/ 2nd eds. 1979/1980, p. 93)

Susanne Langer, quoting Adolfo Best-Maugard in his book *A Method for Creative Design*, wrote, "Borders must move forward and grow as they move," and in turn asked, "What do the words 'move' and 'grow' mean in this context?" (Langer 1953, p. 63). She answers by showing how rhythm is a term "literally applicable to spatial as well as temporal forms", and concludes: "*All motion in art is growth* – not growth of something pictured, like a tree, but of lines and spaces" (ibid. p. 64). An artist in the process of drawing, a dancer in the process of choreographing, a playwright in the process of writing a play, a composer in the process of composing a concerto – all are involved in bringing something to life. If it is to live and live on its own, its creator must attend to its formal integrity, which means he or she must listen to its evolving dynamics and let those evolving dynamics lead the way.

4. The question of mirror neurons

The centrality of kinaesthesia to both our faculty to think in movement and our imaginative consciousness of movement clearly validates the notion of "bodily resonance" in the creation of art. That same bodily resonance and its linkage to our faculty to think in movement and our imaginative consciousness of movement have foundational significance to the appreciation of art as well. A sizeable hurdle, however, immediately confronts any effort to show this significance, a hurdle in the form of mirror neurons. Accordingly, we must first confront mirror neurons in greater detail and clear the hurdle they present.

The import of the discovery of mirror neurons and their relationship to multiple areas of research cannot be denied. Yet a fundamental question attaches to the discovery of mirror neurons, all the more so given the importance they have achieved in multiple areas of research. The fundamental question is a classic one in evolutionary biology. With respect to any particular aspect of a living creature, the question asks, "where does it come from?" or "how does it come to be?". While, as noted, there is no question of the signal significance of mirror neurons in present-day human brain research, there are grounds for question in the inductive use made of the research findings and in the way that inductive use snatches away and buries reference to anything other than *the brain*, thus bypassing the experienced, kinaesthetically-realised dynamics of real-life, real-time movement.

In mirror neuron texts, "embodied simulation" is invoked as the work of mirror neurons. Such "simulation" by mirror neurons is the source of "automatic empathetic responses" that enable "the direct experiential understanding" of a work of art". Art historian David Freedberg and brain neuroscientist Vittorio Gallese claim just this in their article titled "Motion, Emotion and Empathy in Esthetic Experience" (Freedberg & Gallese 2007, p. 202). Clearly, such reductionist explanations of experience push to the side – and in fact out of sight – real-life, real-time experienced dynamics as described above, all the more so when they are claimed to be the source of all kinds of "*direct*" human understandings. We should note that the claim has not gone unquestioned. Philosophers Roberto Casati and Alessandro Pignocchi, for example, title their article in *Trends in Cognitive Science* (2007), "Mirror and Canonical Neurons Are Not Constitutive of Aesthetic Responses".[6] Mark Johnson questions the claim more broadly and at greater length in his exposition of the "aesthetics of human understanding", specifically in his discussion of "embodied concepts". In this context, he characterises the claim made by Gallese and George Lakoff that "Understanding requires simulation" and their follow-up, more finely stated claim regarding concepts that "The understanding of concrete concepts – physical actions, physical objects, and so on – requires sensory-motor simulation" as a "bold claim" (Johnson 2007, p. 164). I would add,

6. In their article, Casati and Pignocchi write that Freedberg and Gallese's claim "is … open to the charge of irrelevance to the issues of aesthetic experience and of what constitutes artworks. Already the choice of artworks [that Freedberg and Gallese discuss in their article], such as Michelangelo, Goya, Caravaggio and Pollock … is open to objection: all the works are both famous, so as to suggest and emphasize the importance of this issue for art; and mostly gory, so as better to nail the empathic point" (Casati & Pignocchi 2007, p. 410).

and emphatically, that Gallese and Lakoff's claim is not only a "bold claim", but a claim that ignores a foundational fact; namely, that the body, from both an evolutionary and ontogenetic perspective, is a semantic template and that fundamental human concepts – "concrete concepts" of "physical actions, physical objects, and so on" – are nonlinguistic, corporeal concepts forged on the basis of that template (Sheets-Johnstone 1990). Indeed, fundamental human concepts inform paleoanthropological tool-making and paleolithic cave art, for example, just as they inform learning one's body and learning to move oneself. Concepts such as *in*, *far*, *sharp*, *open*, *strong*, *round*, and so on, are grounded in the tactile-kinaesthetic body, a body that clearly resonates throughout in the spatio-temporal-energic qualitative dynamics of its own movement, and that continues to resonate throughout life in just such qualitatively dynamic ways, ways that, it should be noted and in fact underscored, allow us to form habits that run off with a familiar dynamic, thus allowing us to be focally engaged elsewhere rather than claiming our central attention. *Understandings* of our surrounding world are rooted in just such bodily resonant tactile-kinaesthetic understandings that have allowed and continue to allow us to move about in the world effectively and efficiently. Edmund Husserl consistently observed and elucidated at length the way in which perceptions and cognitions in relation to a surrounding world are consistently informed by "the kinestheses", that is, by our moving bodies (Husserl 1970, 1980, 1989). In sum and in short, kinaesthesia is clearly of moment. Understood on its own, its import is heightened.

Its heightened import is pithily and straightforwardly captured in a statement by well-known neuroscientist Marc Jeannerod, a statement that bolsters the foundational significance of kinaesthesia recognised so prominently and consistently by Husserl. The statement occurs in the context of Jeannerod's discussion of what he terms "[the] longstanding controversy about the respective roles of the two main first-person cues in conscious knowledge of one's actions" and the anchorage of that controversy in the classic debate between Wilhelm Wundt and William James (Jeannerod 2006, p. 56): Wundt claimed that our knowledge "is based on a priori efferent information of a central origin", James that our knowledge is "based on a posteriori information from sensory organs" (ibid.). Jeannerod points out that the controversy is irresolvable experimentally, even by way of experimental research dealing with pathologically afflicted individuals, and this because kinaesthesia is an ongoing, insuppressible faculty. He states explicitly, "*There are no reliable methods for suppressing kinesthetic information arising during the execution of a movement*" (ibid.; italics added). We should take into serious account as well Jeannerod's answer to the question of "whether we consciously monitor our own actions and how we eventually become aware of them". His answer: "we remain unaware of most of our actions, unless an unpredicted event interrupts their course and brings them to consciousness" (ibid. pp. 58–59). Clearly, as observed elsewhere (Sheets-Johnstone 2011a), in light of *the insuppressibility of kinaesthesia*, we do not have to wait until something untoward occurs that awakens us into awareness and deters us from continuing on our way. On the contrary, precisely because movement is a dynamic happening and because the dynamics of our everyday movement are commonly habitual and thus within our everyday repertoire of our "I cans" (see, for example, Husserl 1980, pp. 106–12; Husserl 1989, pp. 13–15, 159–160, 228–31, 266–82, 340–43; Husserl 1970, pp. 106–108, 161, 217, 331–32; Husserl 1973, p. 97), we can consult them any time we wish in the course moving. In short, and as I have pointed out and emphasized many times over (Sheets-Johnstone 1999a/expanded 2nd ed. 2011), any time we care to pay attention to our own movement – our own so-called "action" – there it is. Not only this, but, as pointed out above, we all learned our bodies and learned to move ourselves as infants and young children. We did so by attending to our own movement and in the process forged an untold number of dynamic patterns that became habitual.

Given the above statements and discussion, it is surely evident that "embodied simulation" is a notion that totally bypasses the realities of kinaesthesia and our tactile-kinaesthetic bodies. In doing so, the basic evolutionary and logically pressing question of the provenience of mirror neurons is totally ignored: Where do they come from? How do mirror neurons come to be? We are clearly not born with them (for a vindication of these facts and a discussion of the seminal question of how mirror neurons come to be, see Sheets-Johnstone 2011c.). Moreover they are surely not within the tens of billions of neurons that sprout in foetal growth nor are they later prespecified genetically. Thus when Freedberg and Gallese claim that "a crucial element of esthetic response consists of the activation of embodied mechanisms encompassing the simulation of actions, emotions and corporeal sensation, and that these mechanisms are universal" (2007, p. 197), they are leading us to believe that mirror neurons – the "embodied mechanisms" of simulation – are not only at the heart of aesthetic appreciation but innate from the start. Indeed, *how we come by these "embodied mechanisms" is nowhere explained.*

Precisely in this context, it is notable that in their initial experimental research to determine whether mirror neurons exist in humans, Gallese, Giacomo Rizzolatti, and other major neuroscientists at the University of Parma did not utilise PET scan studies to determine neuronal activity in human brains; they utilised *neuromuscular* studies. They in fact pass quite breezily over this fact in their special 2006 neuroscience article titled "Mirrors in the Mind" in which they describe their first experiments with human subjects and give a background history and summary of their findings to date. They state with respect to those first experiments that their aim was to determine "whether a mirror neuron system also exists in humans". What they found is that,

> [a]s volunteers observed an experimenter grasping objects or performing meaningless arm gestures, for example, increased neural activation in their hand and arm muscles that would be involved in the same movements suggested a mirror neuron response in the motor areas of their brains.
> (Rizzolatti, Fogassi, Gallese 2006, p. 58)

They pass over the *kinaesthetically interesting neuromuscular finding* because of their desire to identify "the exact brain areas" that are activated when volunteers observe what they term "motor acts" (ibid.). Similarly, Freedberg and Gallese pass over this finding completely in their specification of embodied simulation in art appreciation, as when they state, "The discovery of mirror neurons illuminates the neural underpinnings of the frequent but hitherto unexplained feeling of physical reaction often in apparent imitation of the actions represented within a work of art or suggested by the implied movements involved in its making" (Freedberg & Gallese 2007, p. 197). Moreover they affirm that "mirror neurons also offer the possibility of a clearer understanding of the relationship between responses to the perception of movement within paintings, sculpture and architecture … and the emotions such works provoke" (ibid.). In the section that follows, we will take an alternative view of such "bodily resonance".

5. Experiential evidence

Even if we ourselves have never acted, danced, painted, or engaged in any other kind of artistic pursuit, we are – or can certainly be – moved by the artistic work of others.

When we are duly taken in by an aesthetic experience – when we are moved by a Bach Cantata, a Pina Bausch dance, a Shakespeare play, a Rodin sculpture – we are moved affectively within a certain dynamic peculiar to the affective character of the work as it unfolds itself to us. We are moved not to move in actuality as in everyday life, but moved in the sense of being caught up in affective feelings that spontaneously come forth in listening to or seeing the work, be it delight, sorrow, an entranced raptness, or a tense uneasiness. We are moved by the grandeur of a painting, for example, by the solemn speech of a lone figure on stage, and by the sonority and orchestral richness of the symphony. In being so moved, we are propelled to incipient movement responses, responses that consistently inform affective bodily experiences, as psychiatrist Nina Bull's studies so finely show (Bull 1951). Indeed, many years before the neuromuscular findings of the neuroscientists at Parma, body researchers discovered what they termed "tentative movements" (Washburn 1973 [1916]), "preparatory bodily attitudes" with respect to emotions (Bull 1951), "incipient motor responses" (Washburn 1914), and the like, by which they meant precisely the kind of neuromuscular findings that Rizzolatti, Fogassi, and Gallese found in their experimental study.[7]

What is of moment with respect to all of these findings is the fact that the nervous system is a whole body system, or in other words, that *the brain* exists and functions in relation to the whole of which it is a part. Laboratory and thought experiments to the contrary, it exists and functions neither in a vacuum nor a vat, but in whole living bodies. The brain is indeed what is *embodied*, and the fact that it is might in the hopefully not too distant future lead neuroscientists properly to study *the embodied brain*. Moreover the brain itself functions as a whole, meaning that all of its parts, as neuroscientists have identified and labelled them, are interrelated. Accordingly, if *connectivity* is the key to the brain's working and if *synapses* are key functional aspects of brains that are open to variation and can be newly created (Baars & Gage 2010), then surely we should realise that adhering to a reductionist notion of the brain which reduces human experience to particular neuron firings, that is, which stipulates that "embodied simulation" via mirror neurons is the source of "[a]utomatic empathetic responses" "enabl[ing] the direct experiential understanding" of a work of art (Freedberg & Gallese 2007, p. 202), is patently absurd. Clearly, the complexity of aesthetic experience is shortchanged by such reductionist "embodied" explanations as are the experiential learnings that necessarily precede any bona fide aesthetic experience, experiential learnings in the form of active artistic involvements: on the one hand, going to museums and seeing paintings, going to concerts and listening to music, going to the theatre and seeing dances and plays, and so on; on the other hand, playing an instrument, sculpting, acting in a play, and so on.

Through such experiences, we learn about the arts. On the one hand, we experience directly the dynamics of the work before us, and on the other, we experience directly the dynamics of the artistic effort in which we are engaged. In effect, not only do we first have to be effective and efficient movers in the world before the formation of mirror neurons and a mirror neuron system, i.e. kinaesthtically informed tactile-kinaesthetic bodies, but we need to experience the arts directly and learn more and more deeply from our experiences of them to develop aesthetic understandings.

A further point warrants attention and discussion. Margaret Washburn defines her coinage of the term "incipient motor responses" in reference to

7. Washburn's description of "tentative movements", for example, leaves no doubt about the correspondence: "These slight actual movements give rise to kinaesthetic excitations" (Washburn 1973, p. 48). It is furthermore notable that Washburn devotes a whole chapter to "Tentative Movements."

"the initiation of movements that are not fully carried out" (Washburn 1914, p. 376). While Washburn's aim in the paper is to show that "[t]here are grounds for thinking that "the association of movements is preliminary" to "that form of association which has traditionally been called the association of ideas" (ibid.), what is notable for us here is her definition of incipient motor responses. If incipient motor responses from a neurophysiological perspective are definable as "the initiation of movements that are not fully carried out", then experiential findings constitute the basis of the neurophysiological perspective. Moreover when we take the notion of "tentative movements", "preparatory bodily attitudes" with respect to emotions, and "incipient motor responses" into account in aesthetic appreciation, we are readily led toward a validation of the import not only of kinaesthesia, but of the relationship of kinaesthesia to affectivity, and further, to a straightforward recognition of the dynamic congruency of emotions and movement (Sheets-Johnstone 1999b).

Let us first recall that kinaesthesia attunes us in the most direct experiential sense to the inherent spatio-temporal-energic dynamics of movement. It provides us with a direct *felt* sense of the dynamics of any movement that we make – the way in which it flows: its surges, wanings, constrictedness, attenuations, and so on. We should add at this point that it provides us as well the possibility of *perceiving* the dynamics of our movement, perceiving those dynamics as taking place *in* time and *in* space. In other words, it provides us a direct perception of the exteriority of our own movement, its objective spatio-temporal-energic reality, its "timing" or temporal span and its "out-thereness" or three-dimensionality in relation to a surrounding world, as when we attend to just how our words resound when we are learning the lines of a scene in a play or film, or when we attend to the duration of an arm extension when we are learning a new movement sequence in a dance, or when we attend to just how we are brushing paint onto a canvas when we are attempting to fill out a background in a way that heightens the foreground. In doing so, it provides us a direct *experiential* foundation not only for appreciating the relationship between the spatio-temporal-energic dynamics of our own movement and the qualitative dynamics of what we are creating, but for appreciating the formal complexities and ultimate integrity of a work other than our own. Formal aspects of a work resonate on their own with a certain qualitative dynamic that is congruent with the formal dynamics of human feeling.

To demonstrate this congruency distinctly, consider first the words of Leo Tolstoy:

> *To evoke in oneself a feeling one has once experienced and having evoked it in oneself then by means of movements, lines, colors, sounds, or forms expressed in words, so to transmit that feeling that others experience the same feeling – this is the activity of art.* (Tolstoy 1959, p. 614; italics in original)

Consider next William Faulkner's implicit description of fear experienced by Temple in his novel *Sanctuary*:

> She surged and plunged, grinding the woman's hand against the door jamb until she was free. She sprang from the porch and ran towards the barn and into the hallway and climbed the ladder and scrambled through the trap and to her feet again, running towards the pile of rotting hay. Then suddenly she ran upside-down in a rushing interval; she could see her legs running in space, and she struck lightly and solidly on her back and lay still … (Faulkner 1953, pp. 75–76).

Faulkner's implicit description of fear illustrates how Temple's qualitative dynamics of movement are through and through congruent with the dynamics of fear: its felt urgency, clutchedness, stops and starts, desire for escape, sense of sudden impending disaster coming from everywhere and nowhere, and so on.

Now while we are moved to move in everyday life, propelled affectively toward a certain movement dynamic – flailing or curling up in grief, exultingly opening our arms and leaping about in uncontained joy, for example – and while these affective/kinetic dynamics are precisely what Faulkner describes, in our appreciation of art, we are not ourselves moved to move. We are not "surging" and "plunging" and "springing" and "running" and "climbing" and "scrambling", for example. On the contrary, we are stilled as it were by a work of art, but precisely in a resonant stillness, a stillness in which "tentative movements", "incipient movement responses", are present. Our tentative or incipient kinetic response is an aliveness to the affective/kinetic dynamics of the work before us. In effect, the dynamics of the work resonate kinetically and affectively, and we resonate in our rapt stillness before it. The research studies of Nina Bull referred to earlier corroborate this aesthetic reality. They demonstrate empirically how corporeal tonicities are congruent with specific emotions from their very beginning.

We should finally note with reference to the "bold claim", "Understanding requires simulation" ("The understanding of concrete concepts – physical action, physical objects, and so on – requires sensory-motor simulation") that our *understanding* of works of art, like our appreciation of works of art, rests precisely on our bodily felt resonance to dynamics, both affective and kinetic, and on the natural linkage of those experienced dynamics to our faculty of thinking in movement and our imaginative consciousness of movement. However distant we are from a reflective awareness, much less analytical investigation, of our faculty to think in movement and of our imaginative consciousness of movement, we are endowed *by nature* with these capacities. They are fundamental to the creation and appreciation of art and a testimonial to the dynamics that come to inform a work of art.

References

Arnheim, R. (1977). *The Dynamics of Architectural Form.* Berkeley, California: University of California Press.

Baars, B.J., & Gage, N.M. (2010). *Cognition, Brain, and Consciousness: Introduction to Cognitive Neuroscience* (2nd ed.). Amsterdam: Elsevier.

Bull, N. (1951). *The Attitude Theory of Emotion.* New York: Nervous and Mental Disease Monographs (Coolidge Foundation).

Casati, R., & Pignocchi, A. (2007). Mirror and Canonical Neurons Are Not Constitutive of Aesthetic Responses. *Trends in Cognitive Science, 11*(10), 410.

Faulkner, W. (1953). *Sanctuary.* Harmondsworth: Penguin Books.

Freedberg, D., & Gallese, V. (2007). Motion, Emotion and Empathy in Esthetic Experience. *Trends in Cognitive Science, 11*(5), 197–203.

Goethe, J.W. (1998), *Baukunst. Ästhetische Schriften 1771–1805* (Sämtliche Werke 18). Frankfurt/Main: Deutcher Klassiker Verlag.

Husserl, E. (1970). *The Crisis of European Sciences and Transcendental Phenomenology* (trans. by David Carr). Evanston, Illinois: Northwestern University Press.

Husserl, E. (1980). *Ideas Pertaining to a Pure Phenomenology and to a Phenomenological Philosophy, Book III* (trans. by T.E. Klein & W. E. Pohl). The Hague: Martinus Nijhoff.

Husserl, E. (1989). *Ideas Pertaining to a Pure Phenomenology and to a Phenomenological Philosophy, Book II* (trans. by R. Rojcewicz & A. Schuwer). Dordrecht: Kluwer Academic.

Jeannerod, M. (2006). *Motor Cognition: What Actions Tell The Self.* Oxford: Oxford University Press.

Johnson, M. (2007). *The Meaning of the Body: Aesthetics of Human Understanding.* Chicago: University of Chicago Press.

Langer, S.K. (1953). *Feeling and Form.* New York: Charles Scribner's Sons.

Rizzolatti, G., Fogassi, L., & Gallese, V. (2006). Mirrors in the Mind. *Scientific American, Nov.*, 54–61.

Rowlands, M. (2011). *The New Science of the Mind.* Cambridge, Massachusetts: Bradford Books/MIT Press.

Sheets-Johnstone, M. (1966). *The Phenomenology of Dance.* Madison, Wisconsin: University of Wisconsin Press (Second editions: 1979, London: Dance Books Ltd.; 1980, New York: Arno Press).

Sheets-Johnstone, M. (1990). *The Roots of Thinking.* Philadelphia: Temple University Press.

Sheets-Johnstone, M. (1999a/expanded 2nd edition 2011). *The Primacy of Movement.* Amsterdam/Philadelphia: John Benjamins Publishing.

Sheets-Johnstone, M. (1999b). Emotions and Movement: A Beginning Empirical-Phenomenological Analysis of Their Relationship. *Journal of Consciousness Studies,* 6(11), 259–277. This article also appears as Chapter VIII in Sheets-Johnstone, M. (2009). *The Corporeal Turn: An Interdisciplinary Reader.* Exeter, UK: Imprint Academic.

Sheets-Johnstone, M. (2010). Thinking in Movement: Further Analyses and Validations. In J. Stewart, O. Gapenne, & E. di Paolo (Eds.), *Enaction: Toward a New Paradigm for Cognitive Science* (pp. 165–182). Cambridge, Massachussetts: Bradford Book/MIT Press.

Sheets-Johnstone, M. (2011a). From Movement to Dance. *Phenomenology and the Cognitive Sciences, 11*(1), 39–57.

Sheets-Johnstone, M. (2011b). The Imaginative Consciousness of Movement: Linear Quality, Kinaesthesia, Language and Life. In T. Ingold (Ed.), *Redrawing Anthropology: Materials, Movements, Lines* (pp. 115–128). Surrey, England: Ashgate.

Sheets-Johnstone, M. (2011c). Movement and Mirror Neurons: A Challenge and Choice Conversation. *Phenomenology and the Cognitive Sciences, 11*(3), 385–401.

Sheets-Johnstone, M. (2012a). Steps Entailed in Foregrounding the Background: Taking the Challenge of Languaging Experience Seriously. In Z. Radman (Ed.), *Knowing Without Thinking* (pp. 187–205). London: Palgrave Macmillan.

Sheets-Johnstone, M. (2012b). Fundamental and Inherently Interrelated Aspects of Animation. In A. Foolen, U.M. Lüdtke, T.P. Racine, & J. Zlatev (Eds.), *Moving Ourselves, Moving Others* (pp. 29–55). Amsterdam/Philadelphia: John Benjamins Publishing.

Tolstoy, L. (1959). Emotionalism. In M. Weitz (Ed.), *Problems in Aesthetics* (pp. 612–621). New York: Macmillan Company.

von Uexküll, J. (1957 [1934]). A Stroll Through the Worlds of Animals and Men (trans. by Claire H. Schiller). In C.H. Schiller (Ed.), *Instinctive Behavior* (pp. 5–80). New York: International Universities Press.

Washburn, M.F. (1914). The Function of Incipient Motor Process. *Psychological Review, 21*, 376–390.

Washburn, M.F. (1973 [1916]). *Movement and Mental Imagery*. New York: Arno Press.

The moving body

Gestural recreation of the world in drama

Xavier Escribano
Universitat Internacional de Catalunya

1. Introduction

In his seminal work *Phénoménologie de la perception* (1945) and in many other writings from the same period, for instance those included in *Sens et Non-Sens* (1948), the French philosopher and phenomenologist Maurice Merleau-Ponty establishes a close parallel between the task of phenomenology and modern artistic creation, as in the works of figures such as Honoré de Balzac, Marcel Proust, Paul Valéry or Paul Cézanne. Indeed, both phenomenology and the various artistic disciplines, each with its own means of expression, bring into view and allow access to a layer or level of consciousness which has been forgotten or neglected, but which is however latent in all human and cultural endeavour: "the meaning of the world or of history as that meaning comes into being" (Merleau-Ponty 1945, p. xiv).

Here the author is referring to the level of sense experience and to the meaning of the world as perceived. Although the world of perception, that which our senses and everyday life reveal to us seems to be the most familiar of all, the fact is that to a great extent it remains hidden from us, while our attitude continues to be a practical or utilitarian one. The prestige which has accrued to scientific knowledge implies a devaluation of our lived experience of the world. Following the Cartesian tradition, it is generally considered that the progress of knowledge involves forgetting that which our senses convey to us in too simple a manner. The true world is the one which science describes and which is to be found behind such perceptible phenomena. In this way, perception is no more than a beginning, although a confused one, of science. Opposed to this, phenomenology and modern artistic creation, in the view of Maurice Merleau-Ponty, rehabilitate sense experience and revive for us the sense of the perceived world. This attempt at rehabilitation does not imply, however, a negation of the value of knowledge and scientific method; rather it combats the dogmatism of a science which sees itself as the be-all and end-all as regards knowledge. Art and modern thought have the merit of having stripped bare, of making us rediscover, the world in which we live, but which we are always tempted to forget (cf. Merleau-Ponty 2002, pp. 11–16).

There is no doubt that, of all art forms, it is painting which is foremost in the thought of Merleau-Ponty, not only because a reflection on pictorial art is present in all stages of his thought, but also because of the philosophical and metaphysical significance that the pictorial image has in his philosophy. Painting, by its very nature, places us in the presence of the lived world, presenting together things and the way they appear, and invites us to recognise the *logos* of the sensory world, that is, a sense which is not translatable or not replaceable by mere concepts. Merleau-Ponty even gives painting, especially in his last stage, as evidenced, for example, by his final work *L'Oeil et l'Esprit* (1961), an ontological function. He sees in it an ability to present the genesis of that which is visible, and its possibility of opening itself to Being without the strict limits imposed by conceptual logic (cf. Merleau-Ponty 1964, p. 43). Although one can certainly speak of Merleau-Ponty as a *philosopher of painting* (cf. for example, de Waelhens 1962; Taminiaux 1993) we could doubtlessly refer to him also as a *philosopher of pictorial gesture*, because the main subject of his reflection on painting and art in general is, rather than art itself, the perceptive, active and expressive body which gives rise to it.

The corporal subject able to perform artistically is not the objective body of naturalism, but the living and lived body, which synchronizes and recreates the forms of the perceptual world prior to any objectivisation. It is important to establish clearly the difference between the two perspectives of the body. The objective body means the body considered as a material reality, with physical properties (colour, texture, shape) similar to other objects. This objective body can be studied and analysed from outside, in the third person, with the view and perspective of the detached and the neutral knowledge of natural science, as in the case, for example, of anatomy, physiology or neurology. Unlike the former, the living and lived body refers to the body as it is experienced by the subject itself, as the centre of orientation around which the spatial dimensions of the world are organised, as the capacity of movement, and of action or of relationship with other beings, as an organ of the senses (capable of synchronizing with sensory qualities) and as a field of localization of sensations (cf. Husserl 1952, pp. 143–161). While the objective body occupies a position in space, together with other objects, with a spatiality which is geometrically determinable, the living and lived body inhabits space and maintains a vital relationship with it. That is, it is always directed toward certain tasks or polarised by certain objects. The fact of being directed towards the world is what Merleau-Ponty calls "motor intentionality".

In effect, Merleau-Ponty places "motility as basic intentionality" (Merleau-Ponty 1945, pp. 158–159, p. 450) at the core of perception and artistic expression which refers corporally and gesturally to the object, without the mediation of objectivising representations. Objective representation occurs at the conceptual level, is accomplished by the thinking subject and can be expressed in established language. In contrast, the corporal and gestural reference to an object occurs at the sensory level, is accomplished by the subject of the perception or the corporeal subject and cannot be replaced by any explanation or definition in established language. The first occurs therefore in terms of the conceptual *logos*, while the second is directed to the *logos* of the sensory world. For example, the pictorial work of Paul Cézanne constitutes for the author a clear illustration of the intrinsic interweaving between vision and movement, and between perception and expression: between the eye affected by the impact of what is seen and the hand which brings to completion the perceptive experience, without the need for conceptual mediation, since the artist "thinks in painting" (*pense en peinture*) as it was said by Paul Cézanne (Merleau-Ponty 1964, p. 60). Merleau-Ponty cites these words because, in his interpretation of the work of the artist from Aix-en-Provence, the painter does not try to translate a sensory experience into a conceptual language that would nullify and replace it, but attempts to show the *logos* of the sensory world, using its own means, in this case through what is visible.

Cézanne's quote is very pertinent, because it raises new possibilities in the relation between thought and art. Art conceived as the transferring of a previously developed thought to the exterior gives way to art which itself performs or completes the very process of thought, but in this second case utilising other means that are not conceptual. In terms that would probably be to the liking of Merleau-Ponty we could talk about the proposal of a *thinking art.*[1] Following precisely the same line of thought, Maxine Sheets-Johnstone uses the expression "thinking in movement", referring to dance and the possibility of developing thinking through body movement (cf. Sheets-Johnstone 1981). This possibility is evidenced, for example, in an improvisational dance, which is not the result of something planned and choreographed in advance, but rather expresses the dynamic and meaningful encounter between the subject and the world, here and now.

In improvising

> [...] I am exploring the world in movement; that is, at the same time that I am moving, I am taking into account the world as it exists for me here and now. As one might wonder about the world in words, I am wondering the world directly in movement; I am actively exploring its possibilities and what I perceive in the course of that wondering or exploration is enfolded in the very process of moving.
> (Sheets-Johnstone 1981, p. 403)

1. Our use of the expression *the thinking art* was inspired by the work of Paul Klee, *The Thinking Eye* (English translation: New York: George Wittenborn 1961). This is a work cited by Merleau-Ponty in *L'Oeil et l'Esprit* and, according to Galen A. Johnson, could have been the inspiration for Merleau-Ponty's choice of title (cf. Johnson 1996, p. 170).

I think what Maxine Sheets-Johnstone understands as "thinking in movement", i.e. "a way of being in the world, of wondering or exploring the world, of taking it up moment by moment, and living it in the flesh" (Sheets-Johnstone 1981, p. 406) expresses essentially the same idea, as we shall see in the authors that our study focuses on: the possibility possessed by human beings to take and recreate in their own flesh the forms and beings of the world, developing a kind of understanding of the world which in itself is corporal. "Thinking in movement is thus not a matter of a symbol-making body, but of an existentially declarative body" (Sheets-Johnstone 1981, p. 406).

But unlike the author above, Merleau-Ponty rarely uses the example of dance to illustrate the corporal *logos*. Sheets-Johnstone finds lacking a more serious treatment of dance in Merleau-Ponty, since it hardly appears in his writings and always takes second place: "Merleau-Ponty's aesthetic judgment of dance is surprisingly ill-informed and appears utterly lacking an experiential base" (Sheets-Johnstone 2009, p. 307). The absence of a careful reflection on dance as an art of body movement is even more surprising considering that, for Merleau-Ponty, the understanding of bodily existence is necessarily linked to the exercise itself, the practice of that bodily existence, and cannot be adequately provided by the theoretical consideration alone: "I cannot understand the function of the living body except by enacting it myself, and except in so far as I am a body which rises toward the world" (Merleau-Ponty 1945, p. 87). Despite this surprising forgetfulness, the poetics of body movement, present in drama and dance, in my view, allows one to see, even in the most illustrative way, the main theses of Merleau-Ponty's phenomenology of corporeality.

For this reason, the purpose of the following pages is to show that the disclosure of the perceived world through the motor intentionality of the corporeal subject, which Merleau-Ponty applies, among the arts, preferentially to pictorial art, can also be used with the dramatic arts and with arts of the moving body. By motor intentionality we mean the dynamic mode that the living body has enabling it to relate to the worldly objects that are around us and thus respond to their solicitation.[2]

Paradoxically Merleau-Ponty does not devote any explicit study to these, unlike the case of painting, literature or, even, cinema (cf. for example, Carbone 2011). In particular, I propose to show how the pedagogy of the dramatic expression of Jacques Lecoq, developed over more than forty years in the Paris

2. In other words, "the organic relationship between subject and world, the active transcendence of consciousness, the momentum which carries it into a thing and into a world by means of its organs and instruments." (Merleau-Ponty 1945, p. 176)

École Internationale de Théatre, constitutes another illustrative model of the theory of the corporal subject and artistic expression, essentially gestural, of Merleau-Ponty, an attempt that until now has not been made. Indeed, Jacques Lecoq speaks of this, using as his starting point distinctions attributable to Marcel Jousse, of whom we shall speak later. Jousse distinguished between *mimicry* (representation of the form) and *mimism* (a dynamic search for the sense). Lecoq makes a dramatic exploration of the cosmos through its elements and forms from the *resonance*, the *echo*, or the *reverberation* (Jousse) that the elements, forms and movements of nature produce in the artist. His purpose is to recognise this corporal manner of relating oneself to nature and the ability to incorporate it as material for artistic recreation. As we shall see below, the anthropology of gesture of Marcel Jousse allows one to link Merleau-Ponty's phenomenology of corporeality and the research on the poetics of body movement of Jacques Lecoq.

From the following analysis of the main concepts of both, the pedagogy of dramatic art of Jacques Lecoq and the anthropology of gesture of Marcel Jousse, a better understanding can be reached of the phenomenology of corporeality and, more particularly, of Merleau-Ponty's claim according to which the human body "uses its own parts as a general system of symbols for the world" (Merleau-Ponty 1945, p. 275), a pivotal statement for the understanding of the relation of body to world and to art. There is an obvious parallel, not noted so far, between the Merleau-Pontian proposal to reach an understanding of the body through the performance or exercising of bodily existence and the vital and pedagogical thesis that derives from the writings and practice of dramatic art of Lecoq. The latter consists of reaching an understanding of the world recreating it physically, thanks to the rediscovery of our intimate communication with it. In either case it is to achieve an understanding of reality through expressive action, in a relationship of identification and recreation, which is prior to and which underlies any posterior thematic or objectifying relationship to the world. The conception of the gestural, expressive and creative body, which Maurice Merleau-Ponty, Jacques Lecoq and Marcel Jousse all share, and which is able to symbolise all existing beings thanks to the identification and to the recreation of their gestural essence, seems an interesting key to understanding the motor and gestural dimension of our relation with art.

2. Lecoq and the poetry of motion in space

Jacques Lecoq began his career as an athlete and gymnast. Through sport he discovered the *geometry of body movement*, the type of abstract movements in space which gymnastic exercises require, and also developed his sensitivity to capture the *poetry of motion in space*, the germ of all his teaching:

> I adored running, but it was the pure poetry of athletics which attracted me the most: the contraction or elongation of the runners' shadows thrown by the sun slanting across the stadium when the rhythm of running sets in. This physical poetry had a powerful effect on me. (Lecoq 1997, p. 3)

We are not aware of any relationship or interaction between Lecoq and Merleau-Ponty during their lifetime. It is the remarkable coincidence of their theses, if *Phénoménologie de la perception* and *Le corps poétique* are read in parallel, which provides the conceptual links that are explained in this section. Both are concerned with the corporeal experience of reality, though initially they come from fields as diverse as philosophy and drama. Here we describe some fundamental aspects in Lecoq's pedagogy showing the points of convergence with Merleau-Ponty. There are remarkable similarities.

In 1956 Jacques Lecoq founded his own school in Paris, the École Internationale de Théatre. The teaching method developed has resulted in a two-year course which moves from silence towards the spoken word by means of the main training feature of the school: The Journey. In fact, the real educational journey begins with research into the dynamics of nature. That means that, before immersing the students in the different dramatic styles (which he called "territories") of tragedy, comedy or melodrama, Lecoq directs his attention for a period of one year – half the duration of the total learning programme – to the previous relationship (i.e. prior to any definite character or dramatic situation) between the actor's body and the elements, shapes and movements of nature. Lecoq and his students work on identification with the natural world. They seek the body formula that expresses or embodies the elements of nature, for example, water in the different forms of existence in which we may come across it: sea, rivers, lakes, drops of water. Then they go on to fire, air (wind, objects in motion), and earth. They also work on materials (wood, paper, cardboard, metal, liquids) and thus keep on expanding the repertoire of identities: colours, words, rhythms, spaces, etc. (cf. Lecoq 1997, pp. 43 and ff.) That level of corporeal relationship with reality is implicit in, and underlying, everyday situations of life or expressive drama situations. Only by making explicit that level of pre-personal relationship between the body and the world can one be aware of it and learn and explore its expressive possibilities. (Lecoq 1997, p. 48).

There is an interesting parallel between the two stages of the educational journey designed by Lecoq and the distinction between the pre-personal sphere and the personal dimension of our existence, as is sometimes used by Merleau-Ponty (cf. for example, Merleau-Ponty 1945, pp. 96–97). Indeed, the living body places us and binds us in a general and anonymous manner to a world in which there are colours, shapes, movements, dimensions which are not dependent on any previous decision by the subject. This pre-personal world is a base, a general pattern or, as Merleau-Ponty says, "a cleaving to the overall pre-personal form of the world" (Merleau-Ponty 1945, p. 97), from which we make personal decisions that shape our lives. Similarly, in parallel, the pedagogic journey of Jacques Lecoq begins by quietly exploring the territory to which perception and bodily movement give us access. Therefore, before taking on such and such a role or dramatic character, with his history, his decisions, his ambitions, etc. the actor goes over this (pre-personal) area that we share and experience together as incarnate subjects. In doing so, the actor enriches his ability to act: "Natural elements, materials, animals, colours, lights, sounds, and words are discovered through the miming body and then enrich character acting." (Lecoq 1997, p. 14).

The work done in the school of Lecoq is primarily a "school of observation" and students are invited above all to "go back to live observation" (Lecoq 1997, p. 31), to conduct an "analysis of movements in life" (Lecoq 1997, p. 27), in order to "bring[ing] the students into the closest possible contact with the world and its movements" (Lecoq 1997, p. 28), formulas that recall some characteristic expressions of Merleau-Ponty and his insistence on the need for "relearning to look at the world" (1945, p. xiii) or the importance of "return[ing] from the constructs to experience" (Merleau-Ponty 1960, p. 141). Certainly on many occasions, that which we know of things through objective or scientific knowledge makes us forget what is this contact or how this contact with things comes about. And this occurs with perception, which is buried or hidden under our ideal constructions, as if seeing, for example, were the act of a distant and disinterested spectator who has nothing to do with the object seen. The reality is that seeing, hearing and touching involve the ability of the corporeal subject to synchronise or adjust to the object. Perception, as we experience it, is not the presentation of an object to a subject, but "the assumption by the sentient subject of a form of existence to which the sensible points" (Merleau-Ponty 1945, p. 257). So, the true understanding of the forms or the movements of life cannot be obtained merely through an exterior observation, no matter how close or exhaustive it may be, but must necessarily involve an internal identification in the form of a corporeal recreation of that movement. For example, in the case of colours, it is necessary to discover bodily what the tempo of the colour is, the exact rhythm of each of them. If it is red, the general tendency is to confuse it with explosive movements, but true red is elsewhere: "True red exists only just before the explosion, in the powerful dynamic tension of the instant." (Lecoq 1997, p. 49).

Conforming closely to what has just been quoted, in the chapter in *Phénoménologie de la perception* devoted to sense experience, Merleau-Ponty opposes the conception of sensation as a mere state of consciousness. The sensory qualities – colours, sounds, etc. – are inserted in a certain form of behaviour. For example, each colour has a definite motor value: some colours favour adduction (the organism turns towards the stimulus and is attracted by the world) and other colours favour abduction (the organism turns away from the stimulus and withdraws towards its centre). Sensations have a motor accompaniment and "they impinge within me upon a certain general setting through which I come to terms with the world" (Merleau-Ponty 1945, p. 244).

Such synchronicity or that "motor grasping of a motor significance" (Merleau-Ponty 1945, p. 165) can only have one bodily exposure or explicitation, as in the case of "the powerful dynamic tension" of red, referred to by Lecoq, the bodily expression of which can be found only in the instant just before the recreation of the explosion. As we can see, Merleau-Ponty agrees philosophically and Lecoq artistically on a non-mentalist conception of colour, which is not a passive notation of an ineffable quality in a purely mental space, but a tension, a dynamism, a rhythm or intensity of existence to which our corporeal dimension can attune itself:

> the sensible has not only a motor and vital significance, but is nothing other than a certain way of being in the world suggested to us from some point in space, and seized and acted upon by our body, provided that it is capable of doing so, so that sensation is literally a form of communion. (Merleau-Ponty 1945, p. 246)

In his bodily exploration of the movements of nature, Lecoq begins with the elements: earth, water, air and fire. In phenomenological terms it would be to question and to describe how these elements appear in body experience: what is water for the body; what is for the body, for example, the first experience of the sea and how to incarnate or to express it. By doing this, Lecoq is developing a real *embodied phenomenology*, as his method not only asks how things appear to the body, but also involves body movement in the development of the research, in the line advocated by Maxine Sheets-Johnstone.

Although the body already knows it implicitly, it is necessary to rediscover it explicitly, bring it to light, in order to reappropriate and make it available as material for voluntary dramatic expression. The example put forward by Lecoq seems especially interesting to me – he carries out a phenomenological investigation on how the sea is experienced by the body:

> Water is a moving, resisting force, which can only be experienced by struggling with it. It is only from the pelvis that this overall sensation can be transmitted to the whole of the body. We emphasise the involvement of the pelvis so as to avoid arm- or hand-gestures which would tend to "signify" the sea without experiencing it. (Lecoq 1997, pp. 87–88)

This explanation of Lecoq corresponds to the original motor intentionality referred to by Merleau-Ponty, i.e. a way of relating to an object, which is not a representation, not determined by an objectifying relationship, but which is previous to this objectification. The type of research carried out here is the search for an essence, but not an ideal essence, capable of being represented, but a motor essence, which encapsulates and indicates to others the underlying dynamics of the situation. This motor essence can only be known by exercising it or putting it into practice, as for example, the motor essence of a natural phenomenon as the *hurricane* or the motor essence of a human situation such as the *farewell* (cf. Lecoq 1997, p. 41), in the sense of a structure that can be recognised by all and highlights the common denominator, recognisable by everyone, of every kind of farewell:

> This everyday theme is evoked with the people on the quayside, the mist and the ships' foghorns, but it could just as well be played out on the platform of a railway station, as a train is leaving, or anywhere else. It is not the incidental details of the exercise but the driving motor of the farewell which we are trying to bring out. In this way we can see how the farewell works, what are its dynamics. A genuine farewell is not just saying goodbye, it is an act of separation. […] This farewell is not an idea, it is a phenomenon which can be observed with almost scientific precision. Getting an actor to work on this theme is an excellent way of observing him, his presence, his sense of space, seeing if his movements and his body belong to everyone, if he can find the common denominator of a gesture, one which anyone could recognise: "The farewell of all farewells". (Lecoq 1997, p. 41)

In this section we found a close parallel between the phenomenology of corporeality of Merleau-Ponty and the pedagogy of dramatic art in Lecoq. Both are based on the assumption that the subject body is capable of an intimate communication (or even communion) with the world. Thus it is possible to reach an understanding of the world recreating it physically, through expressive action, in a relationship of identification and recreation. Now is the time to show that this teaching is inspired by the anthropology of gesture of Marcel Jousse. This new connection, besides establishing an interesting and little explored link between the three authors, offers a horizon of anthropological understanding of gestural recreation of the world, which is revealed, among other places, in drama and dance. From this viewpoint we can better evaluate the relevance of the phenomenon we are exploring.

3. Mimism and the dynamics of meaning

Lecoq refers to the gestural recreation of the world – following here the anthropologist of gesture Marcel Jousse – with the name of "mimism" (*mimage*). The corporeal recreation or *mimage* has an essential role in the pedagogy of movement and dramatic expression, but it has a wider application than that. To mime, that is to say, having the ability to play at being someone else and to summon illusory presences, besides being the foundation of dramatic creation is a fundamental action, a childhood action, through which children get to know the world and learn to live in it. Theatre takes this action and extends it in different ways (Lecoq 1997, p. 22). Natalie Depraz has quite rightly emphasised the importance of miming in childhood, precisely to the extent that it is not just an abstract and mere copying of the exterior appearance, but an "active, archaic and primordial involvement" (Depraz 2011, p. 78), which shows, especially in children, an infinite openness and receptivity, that breaks the boundaries, which are too rigidly defined, among all existing beings. This rediscovery, carried out by Jousse, of the virtue of internalised gestures, the ability to synchronise with the gestural significance and existential style of beings, an anterior and, in a way, a preparatory basis for any intellectual understanding (Depraz 2011, p. 78; cf. Jousse 1974, p. 43), is a key idea that also can be found in Merleau-Ponty, for example, in his theory of gestural significance of language, previous to the conceptual meaning:

> Before becoming the indication of a concept it [the word] is first of all an event which grips my body, and this grip circumscribes the area of significance to which it has reference [...] The word is then indistinguishable from the attitude which it induces, and it is only when its presence is prolonged that it appears in the guise of an external image, and its meaning as a thought. Words have a physiognomy because we adopt towards them, as towards each person, a certain form of behaviour which makes its complete appearance the moment each word is given. (Merleau-Ponty 1945, pp. 273–274)

To understand the interest of the proposal of Lecoq and its connection with the point of view of Merleau-Ponty, it is of utmost importance to distinguish the term "mimism" (*mimisme*), from the term "mimicry" (*mimétisme*). Mimicry is a "representation of the form", while mimism is the "search for the internal dynamics of meaning" (Lecoq 1997, p. 42; cf. Lecoq 1987, pp. 16–17). The concept of mimicry or imitation would correspond to the *mode* of an objectifying relationship with reality that uses representation, while mimism corresponds to the way of referring to an object not based upon objectification but on *co-existence*, *communion* or *familiarity*, as would be said by Merleau-Ponty, between the two realities. Mimism is based, therefore, on a direct and immediate relation that incorporates the corporeal, gestural quintessence of something and thus a better understanding of it is gained.

As has been suggested above, the *mimodramatique* of Lecoq, the key of his pedagogy in dramatic art, is inspired by the anthropological conception of

Marcel Jousse,[3] in particular the concepts of *mimème* and *mimisme*, which are explained in his *Anthropologie du geste* (1974). To Jousse, this singular anthropologist of gesture, the human being is essentially an *Anthropos mimeur*, who internalizes and recreates reality gesturally as a fundamental way of understanding and interacting with it: "The human being knows only what it incorporates into itself and recreates (*rejoue*)" (Jousse 1974, p. 55). The *Anthropos mimeur* understands reality, in the first instance, without objectifying, fixing or establishing a distance, but rather by recreating reality, identifying gesturally with it. The *mimeme* is "the reverberation of the transient or characteristic gesture of an object in the human ensemble" (Jousse 1974, p. 54), a kind of identification that is not, as has already been said, an imitation of the outward form, but a recreation of the "essential gesture" of the "essential action" (Jousse 1974, p. 52), of any being. Indeed, as highlighted by Jean-Louis Chrétien in his excellent book on the symbolism of the body, the extraordinary range of symbolic references to the human body is not so much due to the morphology of each of its parts – eyes, hands, feet, cheeks, belly, hair, etc. – but their way of acting or interacting. What is relevant for the symbolism is not how the body *appears*, but what the body *does* (cf. Chrétien 2005, p. 26).

In his particular dramatic exploration of the cosmos in its entirety, Lecoq can give us an example of the incorporation of other beings or forms of life into one's own bodily behaviour:

> Earth is any substance that can be shaped and moulded, but also the tree, which I consider to be its chief symbolic image, since it is planted in the earth. It is most important for an actor to work at the tree. He must be able to achieve a body that is in balance, positively planted in the ground. An actor preparing to play Nina in Chekov's *The Seagull* will be incapable of developing an aerial glide unless she has first acquired a basic rootedness. (Lecoq 1997, p. 44)

3. Marcel Jousse (1886–1961), ordained as a priest in 1912, joined the Society of Jesus in 1913. A student of Marcel Mauss, Pierre Janet, Georges Dumas and Jean Pierre Rousselot, he was professor of linguistic anthropology at the School of Anthropology in Paris (1932–1951) and visiting lecturer in the Turgot lecture hall in the Sorbonne (1931–1957). Interested in the oral transmission of the Bible, he was devoted to the anthropological study of the milieu where oral style was employed, especially the Palestinian. An initiator of the "anthropology of gesture", he studied the relationship between gesture, rhythm, memory and speech and its relevance to cognitive processes. Although his teaching was preferably oral, he produced a synthesis of his thought in *L'anthropologie du geste*, which was published posthumously in 1974 by his disciple Gabrielle Baron. We should also mention the various short scientific papers published by Jousse throughout his life, included in *La Manducation de la Parole*, Gallimard, Paris 1975 and *Le parlant, la parole et le Souffle*, Gallimard, Paris 1978. Recently, the anthropology journal *Nunc. Revue anthropologique 25*, Octobre 2011, has devoted one issue as a monograph to him.

To mime a tree, understanding it bodily, is not to imitate its external form (the trunk, the branches, the top), but to understand what it means to be *rooted*. It is not a matter of knowing what the tree is or what the tree is like, which implies an objective distance, but to answer the question what it is to be a tree; this understanding can only come about physically, through miming or mimodramatic identification, which involves the surprising ability to shift, even if only momentary, symbolically and virtually, from one's own body schema to the body schema of another being and to assume a "total awareness of [its] posture in the intersensory world" (Merleau-Ponty 1945, p. 114; cf. De Preester & Knockaert 2005).

It is, therefore, an understanding consisting of an incorporation, a search for the *echo* that a lived reality causes in the flesh, an account of the trace the world leaves in me, a kind of understanding that – as Jousse says – reminds one of *knowing* in the biblical sense, in the sense of two people becoming one flesh: "to become one sole living, acting, thinking and creating flesh with that person" (Jousse 1974, p. 79). Merleau-Ponty uses the same kinds of metaphors when he says that the body is "an object which is sensitive to all the rest, which reverberates to all sounds, vibrates to all colours" (Merleau-Ponty 1945, p. 275). With this we have a better understanding of Merlau-Ponty's claim according to which the human body is a general symbolic for the world:

> the body, in so far as it has *behaviour patterns*, is that strange object which uses its own parts as a general system of symbols for the world, and through which we can consequently *be at home in* that world, *understand* it and find significance in it. (Merleau-Ponty 1945, p. 275)

The bodily symbolism which the French philosopher is referring to is not based on an imitation of the form or outward appearance. The possibility of symbolising the world is based on the mimodramatic ability to identify oneself gesturally through an action, with the characteristic gesture of any existing thing. This symbolic corporeality manifests itself primordially as an "*I can*": "Consciousness" is in the first place not a matter of "I think that" but of "I can" (Merleau-Ponty 1945, p. 159), i.e. as a system open to behaviours and possibilities of action in the world, capable of synchronising or empathising with other rhythms of existence and in this way the amplitude of one's own reference to the world can be extended without limit. For this reason, Merleau-Ponty calls the symbolic body "natural symbolism" or even "undivided symbolism" (Merleau-Ponty 1995, p. 289), a kind of reference to things through existential identification, i.e. an understanding of things *being them*, different from the artificial or "conventional symbolism" of language, which understands them thematically, confining them in a characterisation or definition.

4. Conclusion

The pedagogy of movement and dramatic expression developed by Jacques Lecoq in his École Internationale de Théatre in Paris, between 1956 and 1999, the theoretical bases of which are set out in *Le corps poétique* (1997), is a highly instructive model of the originally bodily and pre-objective relationship of the human subject to the perceived world, as was also envisaged by the French philosopher Maurice Merleau-Ponty, for instance, in his main work *Phénoménologie de la perception* (1945). For this reason a close parallel can be established between the pedagogy of drama of Jacques Lecoq and the task that Merleau-Ponty attributed to art: to show the visible world *in statu nascendi*, i.e. to rediscover the world of perception in its pre-objective, pre-conceptual or pre-thematic stage. In either case it is to achieve an understanding of reality through expressive action, in a relationship of identification and recreation, which is prior to and which underlies any posterior thematic or objectifying relationship. After displaying the proximity between the philosophical and artistic approach of each one, through various examples, we can conclude that the arts based on bodily movement, such as drama, at a gestural level, or dance, to which Merleau-Ponty surprisingly gave little attention, provide the best possible illustration of a phenomenology of embodiment in which the expressive and symbolic relationship with the world occupies a prominent place.

Although some interesting attempts have been made (cf. for instance, Sheets-Johnstone 1966; Alarcón 2009), much remains to be done in using one to illuminate the other, the phenomenology of embodiment and the arts of the body in movement. The comparison between Merleau-Ponty and Lecoq shows an interesting way of reflecting on the two approaches. Precisely the rediscovery of Marcel Jousse and his conception of the *Anthropos mimeur*, which recreates the world gesturally identifying himself with it, i.e. with its essential action, allows us to understand more deeply the symbolic capacity of the human body, such as Merleau-Ponty does on various occasions and as Lecoq does by putting it into practice, drawing explicitly on the work of the French anthropologist.

References

Alarcón, M. (2009). *Die Ordnung des Leibes. Eine tanzphilosophische Betrachtung*. Würzburg: Königshausen and Newmann.

Carbone, M. (2011). *La chair des images: Merleau-Ponty entre peinture et cinema*. Paris: Vrin.

Chrétien, J.-L. (2005). *Symbolique du corps. La tradition chrétienne du Cantique des Cantiques*. Paris: PUF.

De Preester, H. & Knockaert, V. (Eds.). (2005). *Body Image and Body Schema: Interdisciplinary Perspectives on the Body*. Amsterdam/Philadelphia: John Benjamins Publishing Company.

De Waelhens, A. (1962). Merleau-Ponty philosophe de la peinture. *Revue de Métaphysique et de Morale, 67*, 401–409.

Depraz, N. (2011). Jousse et Merleau-Ponty: l'enfant en nous. Parole et mimisme. *Nunc. Revue Anthropologique, 25*, 75–80.

Husserl, E. (1952). *Ideen zu einer reinen Phänomenologie und phänomenologischen Philosophie – Zweites Buch* (herausgegeben von M. Biemel). Den Haag: Martinus Nijhoff.

Johnson, G.A. (1996). Thinking in Color: Merleau-Ponty and Paul Klee. In V. M. Foti (Ed.), *Merleau-Ponty: difference, materiality, painting* (pp. 169–176). New Jersey: Humanities Press.

Jousse, M. (1974). *L'anthropologie du geste*. Paris: Gallimard.

Lecoq, J. (1987). L'imitation: du mimétisme au mimisme. In *Le théâtre du geste: mimes et acteurs* (pp. 16–17). Paris: Bordas.

Lecoq, J. (2009 [1997]). *The Moving Body. Teaching Creative Theatre*. London: Methuen Drama.

Merleau-Ponty, M. (2002 [1945]). *Phenomenology of Perception* (transl. by Colin Smith). London: Routledge.

Merleau-Ponty, M. (1960). Le philosophe et la sociologie. In *Signes* (pp. 123–142). Paris: Gallimard.

Merleau-Ponty, M. (1964). *L'Oeil et l'Esprit*. Paris: Gallimard.

Merleau-Ponty, M. (1995). *La Nature. Notes cours du Collège de France*. Paris: Éditions du Seuil.

Merleau-Ponty, M. (2002). *Causeries.1948*. (Établies et annotées par S. Ménasé). Paris: Éditions du Seuil.

Sheets-Johnstone, M. (1966). *The Phenomenology of Dance*. Trowbridge and Esher: Dance Books Ltd.

Sheets-Johnstone, M. (1981). Thinking in Movement. *Journal of Aesthetics and Art criticism*, 39, 399–407.

Sheets-Johnstone, M. (2009). 'Man Has Always Danced' Forays into an Art Largely Forgotten by Philosophers. In *The Corporeal Turn* (pp. 306–327). Exeter: Imprint Academic.

Taminiaux, J. (1993). The Thinker and the Painter. In G. A. Johnson (Ed.). *The Merleau-Ponty Aesthetics Reader: Philosophy and Painting* (pp. 278–292). Evanston: Northwestern University Press.

Movement, gesture, and meaning

A sensorimotor model for audience engagement with dance

William P. Seeley
Department of Philosophy, Bates College

> Interpretation is often difficult in dance, since movements, unlike words, have few combinatory rules that guarantee a clear, unambiguous communication of ideas. Dance is unlike verbal language, for it usually credits meaning only vaguely. When it becomes more specific, it tends to move into the realm of pantomime, or sign language, or even to introduce verbal language.
>
> (Sally Banes 1995, p. 28)

The neuroscience of dance is a vibrant, fast growing field which embodies the promise of a genuine and productive interdisciplinary rapprochement between neuroscience and art. The strength of this field lies in the way it ties explanations of dance to an understanding of the sensorimotor processes that underwrite our ordinary perceptual engagement with the environment (see Bläsing, Calvo-Merino, Cross, Jola, Honisch & Stevens 2012; Cross & Ticini 2011). We use our own bodies to model observed behaviours in everyday contexts. Motor simulation and motor mimicry enhance our capacity to interpret the goals, motives, and emotions of others. These processes are critical to action understanding, empathy, and the social coordination of behaviour. A range of recent studies demonstrate that these same processes enable us to recognise abstract dance movements as intentional actions with emotionally expressive and semantic content constitutive of their artistic meaning. In what follows I examine this research with an eye to the potential contribution neuroscience can make to our understanding of choreographed movements as artworks, as dances opposed to ordinary everyday actions.

1. What is the neuroscience of art?

There is a natural methodological fit between cognitive science and art. Artworks are communicative devices. They are stimuli composed of abstract sets of marks, sounds, movements, etc. that are intentionally designed to trigger affective, perceptual, and cognitive responses in viewers constitutive of their expressive, aesthetic, and semantic content. This entails that questions about the understanding and appreciation of an artwork are, to a large extent, questions about the way consumers acquire, represent, manipulate, and use information carried in the formal structure of a work in order to recognise and evaluate its content (Carroll, Moore & Seeley 2012). Cognitive science, in its broadest sense, is the interdisciplinary study of the ways that organisms acquire, represent, manipulate, and use information in the production of behaviour. Theories and methods from cognitive neuroscience can therefore be used to model and explain the range of psychological processes that underwrite our engagement with artworks. Recent research in neuroaesthetics and neuroscience of art is dedicated to developing theories and methods to push this project forward (see Calvo-Merino, Jola, Glaser & Haggard 2008; Chatterjee 2012; Livingstone 2002; Seeley 2012; Zeki 1999).

A general model for neuroscience of art emerges from a standard story about artists' methods. The sensory inputs to perceptual systems are replete with information about the structure and dynamics of the local environment. However, only a small fraction of this information is salient to our current behaviour at any given time. Selectivity is, therefore, a critical feature of perception. Evidence suggests that we solve this problem by focussing attention on minimal sets of features *diagnostic for*, or sufficient to determine the identity, shape, location, and affordances of objects and events in the environment (see Schyns 1998). Perceptual systems can, in this regard, be conceptualized as evolved mechanisms for detecting the task salience of features of the local environment, or selecting information from the flux of sensory inputs sufficient for object recognition and action. Artists develop a suite of formal strategies for culling sets of *diagnostic features* from ordinary perceptual experience and rendering them in a range of media, e.g. colour studies and sketches in the visual arts. These productive strategies work as communicative strategies because they are directed at sets of diagnostic features sufficient to trigger the ordinary operations of perceptual systems. This, in turn, entails a tight coupling between artists' productive strategies and the operations of perceptual systems.

A significant amount of research in the neuroscience of art is devoted to teasing out the productive relationship between artists' formal and compositional strategies and the neurophysiological operations of perceptual systems. However, correlations between these productive strategies and the operations of perceptual systems do not alone suffice to explain the artistic salience of the formal and compositional elements of an artwork. What one needs is a story that links explanations of how artworks work as perceptual stimuli to explanations of how we recognise and understand the artistic salience of their formal, expressive, and semantic features. This kind of an explanation is forthcoming in a standard story about artists' methods (Gombrich 1960). Consider the case of realistic depiction in landscape painting. Productive practices in this context include colour studies, formal studies, preliminary drawing studies, and a range of other strategies that are designed to recover sets of environmental features sufficient for adequate depiction. However, there is no ideal formal solution to the problem of depiction. Any of a range of formal/compositional strategies will suffice to render these environmental features. This entails that artists must choose how to execute their subject matter from a broad range of potential strategies. What are the constraints that guide these choices – the perceptual, expressive, aesthetic, and semantic effects, the artistically salient experiences and interpretations, that artists intend to induce in consumers. In this regard artworks can be conceptualised as *attentional engines*, or stimuli intentionally designed to direct attention to their artistically salient diagnostic features. Neuroscience is a tool that can be used to explore, model, and explain the psychological processes that underwrite the success of artworks as attentional devices. Therefore, neuroscience can contribute to our understanding of the artistic salience of the formal and compositional features of artworks.

2. What is the neuroscience of dance?

A set of core critical questions frame the application of this model for neuroscience of art to any particular artform. First, what are the general formal/compositional strategies constitutive of productive practices in that artform? Second, how are they used to carry and communicate diagnostic information? Third, what accounts for the artistic salience of these features and strategies? In framing these questions I do not mean to suggest that artforms are taxonomised by, or restricted to, particular media. Nor do I mean to imply that they are constrained by rigidly defined productive strategies. My claim is simply that these are questions that must be addressed in order to distinguish artworks from other classes of perceptual stimuli. Categories of art are flexibly defined by the range of productive practices associated with them at a time. These productive practices determine a common formal/compositional framework for artworks in that category and the nature of consumer engagement with them.

The building blocks of dance are expressive movements. We express any of a range of mental states, e.g. goals, intentions, or emotions, when we publically display them in our movements and postures. We orient our bodies towards the objects of our actions in everyday behaviour. Our bodies thereby display the explicit goals of our actions. Likewise, the character of our postures and movements carries information about the tenor of our actions, e.g. we are curious, cautious, or eager to achieve a goal, which also indicates our emotional disposition towards the object of our actions, e.g. we are fascinated, frightened, or overjoyed respectively. Further, the expressive capacities of our bodies are not limited to explicitly goal directed actions. We often recognise the behaviours of others as more generally furtive, anxious, or cheerful. Therefore, postures and movements also carry information about the abstract inner dispositions and mental states of agents. Together these bodily expressions display where the current behavioural strategies of an agent sit on the continuum between approach and withdrawal, and signal to others how to engage with them in the social context of collective behaviour. The diagnostic features that enable us to recognise the expressive character of movements are *biological motion cues*, stereotyped and patterned relationships among joints that enable us to recognise and track animate movements. Dance, therefore, depends on a general gestural semantics built from biological motion cues.

Point-light displays can be used to illustrate the expressive power of biological motion cues. Point-light displays are constructed by attaching lights to a target agent (directly, digitally in post production, or in the production phase in animations) and adjusting the brightness and contrast in the resulting video so that these points of light are the only thing that remains visible (Johansson 1973). Viewers easily recognise the movements depicted in the display if the point-lights are attached to the joints of a human actor. This is also true for the movements of animals. However, it is not the case for the animated movements of abstract geometric figures. Nor is it the case if the point-lights are attached between joints on the limbs of biological actors. This demonstrates that the relative positions of, and dynamics among, the joints of biological actors are configural cues that carry information about the stereotyped patterns of biological movement that support ordinary behaviour.

Biological motion cues also carry information about the goals, intentions, and emotions of actors. Viewers are able to recognise the actions depicted in point-light displays, e.g. ball throwing or interpersonal dialog (Ahlstrom, Blake & Ahlstrom 1997).[1] Viewers easily recognise gender, personality traits, and current emotional states in point-lights displays of a range of human gaits (Troje 2008).[2] Viewers are able to recognise both who is speaking and the emotions expressed by speakers and listeners in point-light displays of interpersonal dialogue (Clarke, Bradshaw,

1. See retrieved April 1, 2004: http://www.psy.vanderbilt.edu/faculty/blake/BM/BioMot.html

2. See retrieved April 1, 2004: http://www.biomotionlab.ca/Demos/BMLwalker.html. Claire Roether and her colleagues used a sample of 25 walkers to isolate a set of affective postural and biological movement cues which enabled them to generate computer animated artificial walkers with recognisably expressive gaits (Roether, Omplor, Christiansen & Giese 2009).

Field, Hampson & Rose 2005; Rose & Clarke 2009). Similarly, and more to the point of the current discussion, viewers are able to recognise the range of basic emotions expressed by choreographed dance movements in point-light displays, i.e. anger, fear, grief, joy, love, and disgust (Dittrich, Troscianko, Lea & Morgan 1996; Krumhansl & Schenk 1997). Point-light displays carry information about the dynamics of biological motion in the absence of any perceptual information about the appearance of the actors or the more general context, e.g. facial expressions, scene, setting, or sound. Although it is certainly the case that this broad range of perceptual information contributes to, and likely enhances, our capacity to recognise and understand expressive movements, these studies demonstrate that biological motion cues are alone diagnostic for, or sufficient to express, the goals, intentions, and emotions of an agent.

It has been argued that stereotyped expressive movements are decoupled from their natural contexts and used symbolically in a language of dance (Beardsley 1982; Langer 1953). However, the appeal to a language of dance is, at best, metaphorical. Natural languages are composed of abstract symbols stitched together into meaningful sequences by formal systems of strict syntactic rules. The meaningfulness of symbols employed in natural languages is, therefore, an artefact of the way they are used, of the way they can be combined and related given these grammatical rules. No such rules exist for an expressive language of dance, nor are any needed.[3] Rather, we recognise the expressive qualities of dance movements because they are tuned to our natural capacity for *kinaesthetic empathy*, our capacity to recognise the goals, intentions, and emotions of other agents in the interplay of tension and relaxation in their ordinary, everyday movements. Further, violations of syntactic rules in natural language produce nonsense sentences. Not so for dance. The stylistic conventions that define different genres of dance, e.g. classical ballet, modern ballet, modern dance, etc. are rules of thumb, not strict syntactic rules. Violations of these rules do not make a work incomprehensible. Rather, they call on us to make sense of them, to fit them to the more general critical context of dance history. Violations of stylistic rules are, as result, a fertile source of expressiveness in dance.

Some knowledge of salient conventions is necessary to understand how recognisably expressive movements are being used in dance. These movements are, after all, abstracted from the context of everyday behaviour in all but the most literally narrative dance contexts. However, the way consumers learn the stylistic conventions that define categories of dance is nothing like the way we generally learn second languages. Second language learning is a long an arduous process that

3. See Carroll and Seeley (in press) for a similar argument against semiotic theories of film.

requires us to learn to forget the rules governing our primary language in order to become immersed in the rules governing another. Learning the conventions of dance, on the other hand, requires nothing more than our natural capacity to recognise and contextualise expressive movements. We may need help identifying the relevant art critical diagnostic cues at first. But, with some modicum of familiarity with these parameters, we can easily bootstrap our way into novel categories of dance.

The central claim of the neuroscience of dance is that our understanding of the expressive qualities of choreographed movements emerges from the role motor simulation, motor mimicry, and affective mimicry play in ordinary perceptual contexts. A range of studies demonstrate that these processes underwrite a more general capacity to use our own bodies to model the actions and mental states of others in everyday perceptual contexts (for a review see Decety & Grèzes 2006). Topologically organised areas in premotor cortex that code for the orientation and movement of muscles and limbs in ordinary actions are recruited in passive perceptual contexts where viewers merely observe the actions of another agent. Activation of these premotor areas is associated with increased electromyographical activity in the muscles that would be recruited to perform the perceived action. Further, stereotyped actions are associated with stereotyped emotional responses in ordinary contexts, e.g. smiles are associated with positively valenced emotional responses, frowns with negatively valenced emotional responses (Niedenthal 2007; Niedenthal, Barsalou, Winkielman, Krauth-Gruber & Ric 2005). These responses become paired to one another over time. The net result is that adopting an expressive posture triggers the activation of the same neural processes that would be activated with the associated gut reaction and emotional response. Finally, motor simulation and mimicry are used to generate forward models of perceptual changes associated with the predicted behaviours of others in ordinary contexts. These processes enable us to recognise, understand, and track the behaviours of other agents, and interpret their emotional states. These same processes are used in the more abstract context of dance to motivate an embodied understanding of character, and where appropriate story, constitutive of the expressive content of a work, e.g. the approach and withdrawal behaviour exhibited in the first and second pas de deux in Sergei Prokoviev's *Romeo and Juliet* (expressing the hopefulness of new love and the unhappy desperation of their circumstances respectively), the pas de deux in George Balanchine's *Diamonds*, and the duets in Kate Weare's *Bridge of Sighs*.[4]

4. See for instance, Kate Weare, *Bridge of Sighs*, retrieved April 1, 2012: http://www.kateweare.com/work/bridge_of_sighs#; http://www.youtube.com/watch?v=p6y315Mys0o&list=UUaAZvX9Di5Yfq04U9nhY8fw&index=9&feature=plcp

3. Art, aesthetics, and the neuroscience of dance

The grounding assumption of the neuroscience of art is that, through trial and error, artists develop formal strategies and vocabularies that are fine-tuned to the neurophysiological processes that underwrite our cognitive capacities as normal perceivers in ordinary contexts. In the case of dance, the claim is that the productive practices of choreographers and performers are fine-tuned to our capacities to recognise and understand the expressive qualities of biological movements. This claim is supported by a range of behavioural studies which demonstrate that premotor and limbic system processes underwrite our capacity to recognise the expressive content of a dance in the movements of dancers. These studies shed light on the way stereotyped choreographic strategies are used to communicate the expressive content of their works. In this section I turn to the third core critical question: what accounts for the artistic salience of expressive movements in the context of a dance?

There is a general assumption within neuroscience of art that the close coupling of formal/compositional strategies with perceptual capacities yields a focused, or enhanced perceptual experience in consumers, a heightened perceptual awareness constitutive of aesthetic experience (see for instance Zeki & Lamb 1994, p. 607). This assumption reflects a bias towards aesthetic theories of art. Aesthetic theories of art define artworks as artefacts intentionally designed to trigger aesthetic experiences in consumers (Davies 1991). A lot of philosophical ink has been spilled over the question of just what exactly an aesthetic experience is. I would like to bracket that issue here. I assume that the artistic salience of some works does lie in their capacity to induce aesthetic experiences in consumers. However, in this section I would like to rehearse a range of objections which demonstrate that neuroscience of dance doesn't succeed as an aesthetic theory of art (even granting that in some cases the intuition is sound).

The first difficulty is a familiar problem from the philosophy of art. Whatever else we want to say about the generality of a theory of art, it ought to suffice to discriminate artworks and aesthetic experiences from non-art artefacts and ordinary experiences. Theories of art are, after all, theories about the nature of art and associated behaviours. Consider the claim that the artistic salience of artworks somehow lies in their capacity to focus our perceptual awareness on key structural features of experience. This has been a central claim of formalist theories of aesthetics, e.g. Immanuel Kant (1790); Clive Bell (1914); Jerome Stolnitz (1960); and Monroe Beardsley (1981). Sometimes this feature of aesthetic experience is referred to as *disinterestedness*, or attention focused on structural features of experience independent of either their representational content or their utility for the perceiver. The thought is that, through trial and error, artists develop formal strategies coupled to the neurophysiological structure of perceptual systems that focus, and thereby enhance, a consumer's awareness of some phenomenal aspects of perceptual experience. In the case of dance these productive practices are thought to yield a heightened awareness of the expressive qualities of movement dynamics. The trouble is that laboratory stimuli and demonstrations are also explicitly fine-tuned for the focused perception of target features. For instance, point-light displays are an efficient means to achieve a focused, heightened awareness of the expressive qualities of movement dynamics. Therefore, on this account, point-light displays should be experienced as artworks because they should suffice to induce an aesthetic experience in experimental contexts. But they aren't because they don't. This problem illustrates a general difficulty for any attempt to explain the nature of art and aesthetic experience in terms of ordinary perceptual or cognitive processes: what, if anything, would then differentiate them from non-art artefacts and ordinary experiences?

Neuroscience of dance has emerged as a stand alone field in the context of research on the role of motor expertise in perception. The well developed motor expertise of expert dancers is coupled to well defined categories of perceptual stimuli. Consequently, measuring the perceptual sensitivity of expert dancers to a range of dance styles and genres has been used as a means to test the generality of motor expertise effects in perception. The canonical work in this regard is Beatriz Calvo-Merino's fMRI study of perceptual differences between ballet and capoeira dancers (Calvo-Merino et al. 2005). Capoeira is a contemporary Brazilian dance form that is compositionally similar to, but formally distinct from, ballet – the leaps, spins, and duets of the former are choreographed from a unique set of formal movements derived from martial arts. Calvo-Merino and her colleagues measured the relative cortical activation among three groups of participants: dancers from the Royal Ballet of London, expert capoeira dancers, and non-dancers, while they watched clips of choreographed ballet and capoeira solos and duets. The results showed significant differences between all three groups. Ballet dancers showed heightened activation in premotor areas and parietal areas associated with action observation and kinaesthetic empathy for videos of ballet movements compared to capoeira dancers. Capoeira dancers showed heightened relative activation in premotor areas and parietal areas associated with action observation and kinaesthetic empathy for videos of capoeira movements compared to ballet dancers. The relative activation in target premotor and parietal areas was significantly lower among non-dancers than either ballet or capoeira dancers, and, more importantly, there was no significant difference between the two conditions for this group.

Calvo-Merino's study is interesting and important. It suggests a neuroscientific method for studying the influence of particular stylistic conventions in our engagement with dance. However, the promise of the study comes with a caveat. The controls, naïve viewers who lacked salient motor expertise, were not sensitive to perceptual differences necessary to discriminate ballet and capoeira from one another as categories of dance. Of course, the goal of the study was to explore motor expertise effects in perception, not the aesthetic responses of naïve viewers to dance. Naïve viewers do exhibit aesthetic responses to some types of abstract movement features (Calvo-Merino et al. 2008). However, and this is the critical point, non-dancers in the study were not perceptually sensitive to the biological motion cues diagnostic for the appropriate categories of art. This entails that non-dancers were not perceptually sensitive to those aspects of the choreographed movements hypothesised to be diagnostic for the artistic salience of particular works of dance. Therefore, it is not clear that kinaesthetic empathy is sufficient to provide viewers access to the range of artistic conventions necessary to recognise and understand choreographed movements as works of dance.

The problems identified here present a general challenge for the methodology of neuroscience of art. The identification of a close coupling between the formal/compositional structure of an artwork and the structure of perceptual systems is not alone sufficient to explain the artistic salience of the features of particular artworks. Although this may be a sound strategy for explaining how artworks perceptually communicate their content, it does not suffice to explain how consumers recognise the artistic salience of that content. Analogous difficulties arise when we turn to the dance side of neuroscience of dance. Consider Yvonne Rainer's solo in *Trio A* and the duet in Merce Cunningham's *Septet* (Atlas 2001).[5] The female lead in *Septet* plays the role of an inanimate partner, expressively inert, manipulated like a marionette, wholly dependent on the support of the danseur. The focus of the dance is, as a result, the detached form, the kinaesthetics and dynamics, of her movements. Likewise, the generation that followed Merce Cunningham in New York embraced pure movement. The anti-expressionist flavour of the works performed in the early 1960s at the Judson Dance Theatre, like *Trio A*, embraced the often invisible, expressively neutral, repetitive, stereotyped movements of everyday activities. Of course the extreme expressive neutrality of the movements in these pieces is striking, and strikingly expressive in its own right. But, whatever their artistic salience, it is not identical to, nor adequately captured by focused attention on the perceptual experience of, their explicit expressive quality, *neutrality*. It lies somewhere else.

Sometimes conceptually difficult artworks like *Septet* and *Trio A* are singled out and set aside as aesthetic outliers. This is a common strategy used to handle counterexamples to aesthetic theories of art. Seen against the context of the broad range of aesthetic objects we favour in our everyday lives. e.g. design items and

5. See Yvonne Rainer, *Trio A: The Mind is a Muscle, Part I* (1966), retrieved April 2, 2012: http://video.google.com/videoplay?docid=7807527461347231697

architectural spaces, this strategy may have some merit. But it is out of place within the context of the category "art." The self-reflective conceptual play these works exhibit is a canonical artistic practice that has transparently defined our engagement with artworks since at least the advent of modernism in the mid-Nineteenth century, and arguably has covertly always defined art (Danto 1983).

4. Art, meaning, and perception

The crux of the problem for neuroscience of dance is that the expressive properties of choreographed movements are not generally ends in themselves, they aren't alone the point of the work. Rather, they are a means for the expression of a range of ideas. Arthur Danto makes a distinction between *what is seen* and *what is shown* in our engagement with artworks that can be used to elucidate this point (Danto 2003a). What is seen in a work of visual art is what is explicitly visible in its surface, its formal properties and the depictive content that emerges from their compositional relationships. What is seen is transparently visible to any organism with perceptual capacities like ours, e.g. pigeons in Danto's assessment (Danto 2003b). What is shown, in contrast, emerges from a relationship between what is seen and what Danto calls *an atmosphere of theory*, or the contextual background of artistic practices against which the work was constructed and within which it is engaged (Danto 1983). What is seen is a tool used by artists to communicate what is shown, the meaning, or perhaps better the content of the work. The diagnosticity of the formal features of a work, their artistic salience, is thereby a function of what is shown, not what is seen.

Danto's classic example is a hypothetical exhibition of red canvases that he describes at the beginning of *Transfiguration of the Commonplace* (Danto 1983, p. 1). The first work in the show is a fictional painting of the Israelites crossing the Red Sea mentioned by Søren Kierkegaard in the aphorisms at the beginning of *Either/Or* (1843/1987, p. 28). Kierkegaard described the painting as a representation of the spiritual turmoil that haunted his life (apparently associated with the panic, fear, and claustrophobia of a displaced people being chased down the narrow corridor of a dried sea bed, closely pursued by the world's most powerful army, towering walls of water threatening to collapse and drown them). This painting is followed by an anonymously painted abstract portrait called *Kierkegaard's Mood*, a Suprematist composition by Kazimir Malevich called *Red Square*, a painting called *Nirvana*, a still life by an embittered disciple of Henri Matisse called *The Red Table Cloth*, a canvas grounded in red lead that Giorgione had intended to use for an unpainted masterpiece, and a rag from a garage workshop stained with red lead paint from a weekend project. These works are, at first glance, perceptually indiscriminable red canvases. However, they are quite distinct artefacts. *Israelites Crossing the Red Sea,* I take it, isn't much of an artwork, but it would be a philosophical curiosity of some value if it existed, an interesting intellectual artefact. The portrait of Kierkegaard, on the other hand, would be seen as a canonical example of early modernist expressionism. *Nirvana* would be of interest as a contemporary postmodernist painting that comments on attitudes towards religion (Danto tells us that "red dust" is a term used by detractors to refer to the Samsaric order that leads to Nirvana). The still life after Matisse is stylised and derivative. But perhaps it would be of art historical interest as an example of the value of originality in art (or its limits). Giorgione's canvas is not an artwork. It would nonetheless be an interesting artistic artefact, a physical trace of his presence. The rag bears no relation to art at all. Of course, it is important to note that the works aren't really perceptually indiscriminable. We could easily tell them apart. But, and this is Danto's point in the end, whatever perceptual differences we would use to physically sort them one from another would not, in and of themselves, suffice to distinguish them from one another as the particular artworks that they are, or even mark them as belonging to one category of art or another.

Where do Danto's distinctions leave us? An artist uses what is seen, or better perceived, to communicate ideas, to show consumers the content of her work. The content of a work need not be an explicit propositional meaning. It may be that the artist intends for the consumer to apperceptively reflect on some aspect of experience, or simply to enjoy the perceptible features of the work. Nonetheless, in each of these cases a consumer would have to tease out the relationship between what is seen and what is shown, the communicative intent of the work, in order to understand its artistic salience, in order to recognise it as the artwork it is, and even to understand how to engage with it in the first place. Let's return to *Septet* again. Carolyn Brown describes the experience of dancing the piece as a feminist nightmare (Atlas 2001). The following interpretation of the piece emerges from Brown's comment and a reading of Ann Daly's, "The Balanchine Woman: Of Hummingbirds and Channel Swimmers" (Daly 1987). The romantic ballerina was a celebrity and the focus of attention in part because she was presented as enticing, alluring, and elusive. Analogously, the ballerina is the focus of attention in Balanchine's modern ballets. But here her strength and independence is signalled by the athleticism of her postures and movements. The role of the danseur in this context is to display the ballerina's strength. Her movements are framed and aided by his muscular control. He supports her poses and provides the extra energy necessary to facilitate her acrobatic movements…and herein lies both the art critical problem and the artistic salience of the work. The ballerina's postures and movements are constrained, controlled, contorted, and coerced by the will of her masculine partner, some of which she could not accomplish without him.

This entails that she is not actually treated as a strong, independent character. Rather, she is passively displayed, presented as an object of manipulation and voyeuristic regard by a male choreographer. Against this art critical backdrop, the numbed neutrality of Carolyn Brown's modernist performance in *Septet* is deeply expressive – it portrays the emotional retreat of a powerless participant in a coerced activity. A similar kind of story can be told about *Trio A*. Interpreted against the overwrought metaphysical and psychological weight of abstract expressionism and modern dance, the pedestrian playfulness of Yvonne Rainer's movement in the piece is expressive of the mischievous reflective irreverence that defined early conceptual art. Seen against the conceptual backdrop of Balanchine's modern ballet this irreverence can, in turn, be interpreted as an expressive act that wrests the strong individuality of the dancer away (or maybe better back) from the danseur.

These examples illustrate a *functionalist account of artistic form* (Carroll 1999; Carroll & Banes 1982). How do we delineate artistically salient features from the range of formal features and compositional relations present in a work? We ask ourselves why the work was made the way it was, what its purpose is, or how the formal choices made by the artist contribute to its content. In difficult cases we may have to engage in explicit interpretive activities in order to tease this out of the work. But in the vast majority of cases a tacit understanding of the general practices that define common categories of art, the stylistic conventions and productive practices that define schools of art, artistic movements, or the body of work of an individual artist, will suffice.

5. A sensorimotor model for audience engagement with dance

The presence of a heightened focused awareness of the expressive qualities of movement in our engagement with dance does not suffice to explain the artistic salience of the choreographed movements from which they are constructed. What matters is the semantic salience of these features, or how they contribute to the more general content of the work. The semantic salience of an artwork, in turn, is not an intrinsic property of any of its features. Rather it emerges from the context of our engagement with the work, from the range of artistic conventions that define artistic practices and consequently constrain artistic production. The challenge for neuroscience of dance is, therefore, to understand how choreographers and dancers use kinaesthetic empathy in the context of artistic conventions to express the content of the work. In what follows I will sketch out a sensorimotor model for audience engagement with dance derived from a diagnostic recognition framework for object recognition and a biased competition model for selective attention. This model can serve as a framework for understanding how dance can communicate the artistic salience of its formal and compositional features.

The sensory inputs to perceptual systems are, as discussed above, replete with information about the local environment. Cognition is, in contrast, a limited capacity resource. Selectivity is, as a result, a critical feature of perceptual processing. This raises a question. How do we assign salience to local environmental features? One way is simple *perceptual salience*. Some features stand out because they are distinct from their surround, e.g. high colour contrast or sharp differences in the relative motion of a target and its surround. However, it is not always the case that the features salient to our current behavioural context are also the most perceptually salient. This entails that perceptual systems need an independent mechanism to bias perception to the behaviourally salient features of an organism's local environment. Biased competition models for selective attention demonstrate that cortico-thalamic attentional networks bias perception by priming sensory systems to the expectation of features diagnostic for the identities, shapes, and affordances of task salient objects and their parts at particular locations, enhancing the perceptual encoding of expected targets and inhibiting the encoding of local distractors. Selective attention is, therefore, a mechanism through which we flexibly bias basic sensory processes to our current behavioural context on the fly relative to our changing needs in a dynamic environment.

Diagnostic features are defined as sets of sensory features sufficient to enable an organism to perceptually recognise the identity, shape, and affordances of objects and events in the local environment (Schyns 1998). Diagnosticity is a task specific notion (Palmer 1999). Altering our behaviour, changing a target task, changes the way we categorise objects and events. Changing the way we categorise objects and events alters the way we assign salience to its parts and features. Given the framework of a biased competition model for selective attention, this entails that changing the way we categorise an object or event quite literally influences the way we perceive it.

How do biased competition models propose that task salience is integrated into sensory information in goal directed behaviour? Feedback projections from prefrontal areas associated with spatial working memory and object recognition, e.g. dorsolateral prefrontal cortex (dlPFC), and premotor areas associated with the implementation of motor programs for motor preparation and planning, e.g. supplemental premotor (SMA) and premotor areas (PM), to areas throughout the visual system enhance the firing rates of populations of neurons that would encode for target objects and features at expected locations and inhibit the firing rates of populations of neurons that would encode for task irrelevant distractors (Kastner 2004; Schubotz & Von Cramon 2003). These processes include top down projections to subcortical areas like the lateral geniculate nucleus (LGN) and pulvinar (PUL) in the thalamus and the superior colliculus (SC). LGN is the primary relay station for sensory information between the retina and the visual system. Pulvinar is reciprocally connected to SC and all areas of the visual system (Pessoa & Adolphs 2010). SC is a multisensory area involved in directing eye movements and the crossmodal integration of visual, auditory, and somatosensory information (Beck & Kastner 2009). Analogous stories can be told about the architecture of attention in auditory and somatosensory processing (MacLauchlan & Wilson 2010; Stein, Stanford, Wallace, Vaughan & Jiang 2004; Winer 2006). Affective processing influences perceptual processing via a similar cortico-amygdala network that includes reciprocal connectivity between areas associated with assessments of the predictive value and behavioural significance of objects and events, i.e. orbitofrontal cortex (OFC), visceromotor control and gut reactions, i.e. ventromedial prefrontal cortex (vmPFC) and anterior cingulate cortex (ACC), and the amygdala (Duncan & Barrett 2007). Amygdala is reciprocally connected with the visual, auditory, and somatosensory systems. These cortico-thalamic and cortico-amygdala attentional networks are mechanisms through which cognitive assessments of object identity and behavioural context influence sensory processes at their very earliest stages. The result is an integrated, crossmodal biased competition model for perception that is a means to direct attention, encode the semantic, task, and emotional salience of objects and events, and facilitate embodied responses to affective and sensorimotor contingencies in the local environment.

What is the take home message for neuroscience of dance in this laundry list of neurophysiological processes? Artworks are attentional engines (Carroll, Moore & Seeley 2012; Carroll & Seeley in press; Rollins 2004). Object recognition is a goal directed task in which perceptual systems parse sensory inputs into salient cues and group them together into objects relative to available perceptual categories. Artworks are communicative devices that are designed to focus attention on minimal sets of perceptual cues diagnostic for their content. How might this work in practice? The conventions governing consumer engagement with artworks within a medium or genre are strong constraints on artists' productive practices. Cues diagnostic for the categorical intentions of an artist, for the category of art an artist intends a work to belong to, e.g. modern dance, modern ballet, or capoeira, shape the attentional strategies adopted by consumers in their engagement with dance – instruct consumers what to look for and where to look for it. These diagnostic cues include sensorimotor cues which trigger the activation of motor programs that encode the kinaesthetics and dynamics of perceived choreographed movements in a genre. These processes, in turn, facilitate tracking expressive cues embedded in the postures and movements of the dancers, perceptual cues that trigger affective embodied appraisals of the expressive content of the work in consumers.

The artistic salience of these cues is determined by, and so only emerges in the context of, the role they play in communicating the content of the work, e.g. the expressive qualities of Carolyn Brown's movements in *Septet*.

6. The neuroscience of dance redux

The sensorimotor model that I have proposed is not offered as a definition of dance. It is rather offered as a model for how the neuroscience of dance can contribute to our understanding of a range of artistic practices associated with the medium. The model resolves questions about how consumers discriminate artworks from non-artworks in dance contexts. The artistic salience of a dance does not lie in the expressive qualities of choreographed movements per se, but rather in the way these expressive qualities are used as communicative devices to convey the content of the work. e.g. the expressive neutrality of the woman's part in the duet from *Septet* can be interpreted as a reflection on the relationship between the compositional structure of Balanchine's modern ballets and our conception of gender roles in traditional dance genres, an interpretation suggested by the dancer herself (Atlas 2001).

What about questions raised by the observation of expertise effects in our sensorimotor engagement with dance? These are concerns that emerge from the observation that familiarity with the motor skills required to perform an action may be needed to recognise the sensorimotor contingencies constitutive of an embodied response to it. The integrated biased competition model for selective attention sketched above suggests an alternative possibility. Perhaps the pairing of generic motor programs that encode the kinaesthetics and dynamics of everyday actions with knowledge of the formal and compositional conventions governing different types of dance would suffice to bias perception to biological motion cues diagnostic for the expressive content of a particular dance – just as the conjunction of generic motor programs and general world knowledge do when we use sensorimotor process to track and predict the movements, actions, moods, and emotions of others in everyday contexts (see Calvo-Merino et al. 2008). If so a general knowledge of artistic conventions might suffice to bootstrap embodied responses to artistically salient expressive features of choreographed movements.[6] Dance is a hard medium to understand in part because it is abstract, or, as Sally Banes argues, constraints on

6. But see Calvo-Merino, Grèzes, Glaser, Passingham and Haggard (2006) and Calvo-Merino, Ehrenberg, Leung and Haggard (2010) for a discussion of the relative influences of visual and sensorimotor familiarity in viewers embodied responses to capoeira and ballet stimuli.

production within the medium limit the clarity with which it can convey ideas. But this is only part of the story. Dance history, the story of the conventions that define categories of dance, is not transparently part of our everyday engagement with public media in the same way that the history of painting is. This raises the possibility that non-dancers may simply have lacked sufficient contextual information to tease out what was shown in what was seen, to recognise the experimental stimuli as exemplars of different categories of dance. Or, it may be the case that the dance stimuli used lacked the compositional depth necessary to carry categorical artistic salience for naïve viewers. One means to evaluate these possibilities would be to include a control group of dance critics who were familiar with capoeira and ballet, but were not themselves dancers, in an experiment with the same design. However, independent of the validity of this alternative explanation of the performance of non-dancers in Calvo-Merino's study, the take home message in the proposed model is that methodological objections to the neuroscience of dance, and neuroscience of art more generally, can be overcome by paying closer attention to the full range of variables that contribute to our understanding of artistic salience in ordinary contexts.

References

Ahlstrom, V., Blake, R., & Ahlstrom, U. (1997). Perception of biological motion. *Perception, 26*(12), 1539–1548.

Atlas, C. (2001). *Merce Cunningham: A lifetime in dance*, American Masters Series [Television Program]. United States: PBS.

Banes, S. (1995). On your fingertips: Writing dance criticism. Reprinted in *Writing dancing in the age of postmodernism* (pp. 24–43). Middletown, Connecticut: Wesleyan University Press.

Beardsley, M. (1982). What is going on in dance? *Dance Research Journal, 15*(1), 31–36.

Beardsley, M. (1981). *Aesthetics*. Indianapolis: Hackett Publishers.

Beck, D.M. & Kastner, S. (2009). Top-down and bottom-up mechanisms in biasing competition in the human brain. *Vision Research, 49*(10), 1154–1165.

Bell, C. (1914/1981). *Art*. New York: Pedigree Books.

Bläsing, B., Calvo-Merino, B., Cross, E.S., Jola, C., Honisch, J. & Stevens, C.J. (2012). Neurocognitive control in dance perception and performance. *Acta Psychologica, 139*, 300–308.

Calvo-Merino, B., Ehrenberg, S., Leung, D. & Haggard, P. (2010). Experts see it all: Configural effects in action observation. *Psychological Research, 74*(4), 400–406.

Calvo-Merino, B., Glaser, D.E., Grèzes, J., Passingham, R.E. & Haggard, P. (2005). Action observation and acquired motor skills: An fMRI study with expert dancers. *Cerebral Cortex, 15*(8), 1243–1249.

Calvo-Merino, B., Grèzes, J., Glaser, D.E., Passingham, R.E. & Haggard, P. (2006). Seeing or doing? Influence of visual and motor familiarity in action observation. *Current Biology, 16*(19), 1905–1910.

Calvo-Merino, B., Jola, C., Glaser, D.E., & Haggard, P. (2008). Towards a sensiromotor aesthetics of performing art. *Consciousness and Cognition, 17*, 911–922.

Carroll, N. (1999). *The philosophy of art*. New York: Routlege.

Carroll, N. & Banes, S. (1982). Working and dancing: A response to Monroe Beardsley's, "What is going on in a dance?" *Dance Research Journal, 15*(1), 37–41.

Carroll, N., & Seeley, W.P. (in press). Cognitivism, psychology, and neuroscience: Movies as attentional engines. In A. Shimamura (Ed.), *Psychocinematics: Exploring Cognition at the Movies*. New York: Oxford.

Carroll, N., Moore, M., & Seeley, W.P. (2012). The philosophy of art and aesthetics, psychology, and neuroscience: Studies in literature, music, and visual arts. In A. Shimamura & S. Palmer (Eds.), *Aesthetic Science* (pp. 31–62). New York: Oxford University Press.

Chatterjee, A. (2012). Neuroaesthetics: Growing pains of a new discipline. In A. Shimamura & S. Palmer (Eds.), *Aesthetic Science* (pp. 299–317). New York: Oxford University Press.

Clarke, T.J., Bradshaw, M.F., Field, D.T., Hampson, S.E. & Rose, D. (2005). The perception of emotion from body movement in point-light displays of interpersonal dialogue. *Perception, 34*, 1171–1180.

Cross, E.S. & Ticini, L.F. (2011). Neuroaesthetics and beyond: New horizons in applying the science of the brain to the art of dance. *Phenomenology and the Cognitive Sciences, 11*(1), 5–16.

Daly, A. (1987). The Balanchine woman: Of hummingbirds and channel swimmers. *The Drama Review, 31*(1), 8–21.

Danto, A. (2003a). Seeing and showing. *Journal of Aesthetics and Art Criticism, 59*(1), 1–9.

Danto, A. (2003b). The pigeon within us all: A reply to three critics. *Journal of Aesthetics and Art Criticism, 59*(1), 39–44.

Danto, A. (1983). *The transfiguration of the commonplace*. Cambridge, Massachusetts: Harvard University Press.

Davies, S. (1991). *Definitions of art*. Ithaca, New York: Cornell University Press.

Decetey, J. & Grèzes, J. (2006). The power of simulation: Imagining one's own and other's behaviour. *Brain Research 1079*, 4–14.

Dittrich, W., Troscianko, T., Lea, S.E.G. & Morgan, D. (1996). Perception of emotion from dynamic point light displays represented in dance. *Perception, 25*(6), 727–738.

Duncan, S. & Barrett, L.F. (2007). Affect is a form of cognition: A neurobiological analysis. *Cognition and Emotion, 21*(6), 1184–1211.

Gombrich, E.H. (1960). *Art and illusion*. Princeton, New Jersey: Princeton University Press.

Johansson, G. (1973). Visual perception of biological motion and a model for its analysis. *Perception & Psychophysics, 14*, 201–211.

Kant, I. (1790/1989). *A critique of judgment* (Translated by J. Creed Meredith). New York: Oxford University Press.

Kastner, S. (2004). Attentional response modulation in the human visual system. In M. Posner (Ed.), *Cognitive neuroscience of attention* (pp. 144–156). New York: Guilford Press.

Kierkegaard, S. (1843/1987). *Either/Or, volume 1* (Tranlated by E. V. Hong & E. H. Hong). Princeton, New Jersey: Princeton University Press.

Krumhansl, C.L. & Schenk, D.L. (1997). Can dance reflect the structural and expressive qualities of music: A perceptual experiment on Balanchine's choreography of Mozart's Divertimento No. 15. *Musicæ Scientiæ, 1*, 63–85.

Langer, S. (1953). *Feeling and form*. New York: Prentice Hall.

Livingstone, M. (2002). *Vision and art: The biology of seeing*. New York: Harry N. Abrahams.

McLachlan, N. & Wilson, S. (2010). A central role of recognition in auditory perception: A neurobiological model. *Psychological Review, 117*(1), 175–196.
Niedenthal, P.M. (2007). Embodying emotion. *Science, 31*, 1002–1005.
Niedenthal, P.M., Barsalou, L.W., Winkielman, P. Krauth-Gruber, S. & Ric, R. (2005). Embodiment in attitudes, social perception, and emotion. *Personality and Social Psychology Review*, 9(3), 184–211.
Palmer, S.E. (1999). *Vision Science: Photons to Phenomenology.* Cambridge, MA: MIT Press.
Pessoa, L. & Adolphs, R. (2010). Emotion processing and the amygdala: From a "low road" to "many roads" of evaluating biological significance. *Nature Reviews Neuroscience, 11*(1), 773–783.
Roether, C.L. Omlor, L., Christiansen, A., & Giese, M.A. (2009). Critical features for the perception of emotion from gait. *Journal of Vision*, 9(6), 1–32.
Rollins, M. (2004). What Monet meant: Intention and attention in understanding art. *The Journal of Aesthetics and Art Criticism, 62*(2), 175–188.
Rose, D. & Clarke, T.J. (2009). Look who's talking: Visual detection of speech from whole-body biological motion cues. *Perception, 38*(1), 153–156.
Schubotz, R.I. & von Cramon, D.Y. (2003). Functional-anatomical concepts of human premotor cortex: Evidence from fMRI and PET. *NeuroImage, 20*, S120–S131.
Schyns, P. (1998). Diagnostic recognition: Task constraints, object information, and their interactions. *Cognitio, 67*, 147–179.
Seeley, W.P. (2012). Hearing how smooth it looks: Selective attention and cross-modal perception in the arts. *Essays in Philosophy: Aesthetics and the Senses, 13*(2), 498–517.
Stein, B.E, Stanford, T.R., Wallace, M.T., Vaughan, J.W., & Jiang, W. (2004). Crossmodal spatial interactions in subcortical and cortical circuits. In C. Spence & J. Driver (Eds.), *Crossmodal space and crossmodal attention* (pp. 25–50). New York: Oxford University Press.
Stolnitz, J. (1960). *Aesthetics and the philosophy of art criticism.* New York: Houghton-Mifflin.
Troje, N.F. (2008). Retrieving information from human movement patterns. In T. F. Shipley and J. M. Zacks (Eds.), *Understanding events: How humans see, represent, and act on events* (pp. 308–334). New York: Oxford University Press.
Winer, J.A. (2006). Decoding auditory corticofugal systems. *Hearing Research, 207*, 1–9.
Zeki, S. & Lamb, M. (1994). The neurology of kinetic art. *Brain, 117*(3), 607–636.
Zeki, S. (1999). *Inner vision.* New York: Oxford University Press.

Achieved spontaneity and spectator's performative experience – The motor dimension of the actor-spectator relationship

Gabriele Sofia
Dipartimento di Storia dell'Arte e Spettacolo, Sapienza Università di Roma

1. Introduction

The work of the actor is first of all a work on the action. For the actor, the action is not just the motor dimension of his own creative and imaginative processes but it is rather the matter as well as the dimension of his creativity. The work of the actor does not entail any dichotomy between imagination and motion, since both belong to the same circular process of constructing *another* reality, different to everyday reality. This reality is constructed in order to be shared with another human being, the spectator, who cooperates in its construction and takes part in it with his whole body-mind system.

The motor dimension of the actor's imagination is the mine of his art. For the actor the action is exactly what marble or wood is for the sculptor. The actor is at once instrument, music and musician able to echo "within the biographic caves of every single spectator" (Barba 2010, p. 33).

Analysing the motor processes on which the actor's creation lies, we can start a new approach to investigate the actor's creativity and its effect on the spectator's experience.

2. Entailed hypotheses and methodologies

By the expression "spectator's performative experience" we want to indicate that peculiar kind of experience that concerns every human being, while this latter is involved in an intersubjective relation with an actor – a dancer, a mime, etc. – during a performance.

Such experience is characterised by several particular personal events that make it different from other kinds of experience in which a human being is involved every day. My hypothesis is that such a difference – from which the spectator's associative and imaginative activities arise – is due to neuromotor processes different from those operating in everyday imaginative activities. I suppose that these differences can be assumed and analysed taking into account the subjective value that the spectator attributes to his own experiences. In this sense, the present chapter follows Francisco Varela's considerations, according to which experience can be thought of as the convergence of phenomenology and neurosciences, given that "Experience is clearly a personal event, but that does not mean it is private" (Varela 1996, p. 340). The phenomenological and neuroscientific perspectives will be used here as complementary to two other disciplines dealing with the performative activity and its reception, i.e. Theatre Anthropology (Barba 1995; Barba, Savarese 2005), and Ethnoscenology, (Pradier 1990, 1996, 2001). These two latter disciplines recently have been increasingly concerned in neuroscientists' and phenomenologists' studies.[1] Furthermore, these epistemological bases of work have constantly been flanked and informed by the direct experience of the author of this paper as actor, director and of course also as theatre spectator.

3. Determination of the matter of the research

Within the Euro-American culture the word "theatre" is employed to signify a great deal of events that are not always similar nor conform one to the other. It is therefore necessary to specify that in this chapter we refer to the definition of "theatre" provided by the Polish director Jerzy Grotowski in his work *Towards a Poor Theatre*:

> Can the theatre exist without costumes and sets? Yes, it can. Can it exist without music to accompany the plot? Yes. Can it exist without lighting effects? Of course. And without a text? Yes; the history of the theatre confirms this. […] But can the theatre exist without actors? I know of no example of this. […] Can the theatre exist without an audience? At least one spectator is needed to make it a performance. So we are left with the actor and the spectator. We can thus define the theatre as what takes place between spectator and actor. All the other things are supplementary. (Grotowski in Richards 1993, p. 32)

1. Vittorio Gallese, one of the neuroscientists who discovered the mirror neurons' mechanisms, highlighted that the Theatre Anthropology and its way of considering the human body according to levels of organisation is a perfect link to the neurosciences: "The Theatre Anthropology, breaking down the actor's behaviour, traces his whole dimension of expressions back to many levels of organization of the body's motor practices. This represents a perfect link to the cognitive neurosciences that inquire the role of the body-brain system within the social cognition." (Gallese 2010, p. 251)

Dealing with theatre is an inquiry into a peculiar *intersubjective relation*. Unlike most other arts, the object produced by the theatre lasts and exists as long as the relation exists; when this relation fades the object disappears. We can generally state that analysing the theatre event means analysing the direct *experience* of this event. Mentioning Varela, we can say that whoever analyses theatre cannot have any idea apart from his own experience of it.[2] Whoever analyses theatre is part of the object of his analysis and must therefore overcome the traditional distinction between subject and object. In this sense, in the history of theatre studies it is possible to identify a change of paradigm similar to the revolutionary effects of the theory of relativity and the discoveries of the sub-nuclear physics within the scientific world.[3] The theatre relation may then be described as a system arising from the interaction actor-spectator: a system that cannot be understood by analysing either the actor or the spectator outside of their mutual relation.[4]

Such inter-dependence between the actor and the spectator is to be highlighted, especially if we consider the way in which contemporary neuroscientific researches use the performers (for a review: Bläsing et al. 2012). Although we do not intend to reduce the important role of these researches within the studies of the theatre event, it is probably useful to consider that most of them have so far disregarded not only the influence of the spectator on the performer but also the fact that the performer's psychophysical organisation is not the same when he relates with a human being rather than with a camera. In this perspective watching *footages* of the actions performed by an actor or a dancer may lead to some misleading generalisations, which do not take into account the basic element of the performative event: the co-presence of an actor and a spectator at the same time.[5]

I dilate on this aspect in order to highlight that gathering scientific data essential for analysing the spectator's experience is not enough, but a *disciplined* analysis

2. In 1996, Francisco Varela remarked that "Science of cognition and mind must, sooner or later, come to grips with the basic condition that we have no idea what the mental or the cognitive could possibly be apart from our own experience of it." (Varela 1996, p. 331)

3. This change of paradigm has been remarked by the scholar Marco De Marinis who considered it as the distinguishing mark of a "new theatrology" (De Marinis 1988 and 2011).

4. I draw on the definition of emergent system proposed by Edgar Morin in the first volume of *La Méthode*: "We can call "emergence" the features or the properties of a system which present a characteristic of novelty with respect to the features or properties of the components taken into account in isolation." (Morin 1977, p. 106, my translation).

5. A notable exception is the work of Corinne Jola showed during the Fourth International Conference "Dialogues between theatre and neuroscience" (Rome, April 2012). Jola presented some first experiments with spectators and dancers in co-presence (Jola et al. 2012).

of the direct experience as spectator of a theatre event is also required, as proposed by Varela.[6]

Theatre Anthropology and Ethnoscenology, sometimes defined as "schools of the gaze", have led to a number of particular methodologies teaching people to organise their own experience as spectators and, by doing that, to focus their analyses not only on contemporary performative practices but also on several forms of theatre through history. This is the direction recently followed by the so-called *Embodied theatrology*, proposed by Marco De Marinis: "an embodied theatrology, in which the researcher's body as well, and his subjectivity too, are somehow involved" (De Marinis 2012, p. 82).

4. The actor's creative processes and their motor dimension

Considering how theatre people and neuroscientists have been holding a "dialogue" for over four years,[7] we can notice that one of the greatest difficulties lies in the neuroscientists' prejudices about the actor that are still widespread in the Euro-American culture. One of the toughest prejudices considers the actor as someone who is very good at *imitating* reality. The actor is thought of as someone who "walks in the character's shoes" so that he lives somehow through the situations experienced by the character he has to play. Neuroscientists are rarely aware that what they watch results from the creation of different dynamics that may sometimes be opposed to those ruling everyday life. In other words, neuroscientists remain bound to a sort of "spectator ethnocentrism" (Barba 1995, p. 42), which leads them to consider an actor appearing perfectly natural on the stage as someone who is perfectly "repeating" reality. They ignore that such a naturalness is just an *effect* made possible by the actor's technique. This "spectator ethnocentrism" (which is the dangerous side of the mentioned perspective arising from direct experience) disregards an element that may be supposed to have precise physiological consequences: stage acting is not merely acting on a stage, but a kind of acting that is supposed to constantly keep, feed and rule the attention of

6. I follow here Varela's considerations: "The novelty of my proposal is that *disciplined first-person* accounts should be an integral element of the validation of a neurobiological proposal, and not merely coincidental or heuristic information. This is why I choose to describe the situation by the hypothesis that both accounts be mutual *constraints* on each other" (Varela 1996, p. 344).

7. Such a dialogue resulted in an International convention of four meetings titled "Dialogues between theatre and neuroscience" (Sofia 2009; Falletti, Sofia 2011 and 2012).

the spectator. A practical example may make this concept clearer: if an actor has to drink from a glass on the stage, every motor act he is going to activate ("grabbing the glass", "bringing the glass to his mouth", "swallowing the water", "putting the glass again on the table") will be aimed at performing the act of "drinking a glass of water", but, though the action is factually the same and follows *the same series of motor acts*, it will be different, since the actor is here supposed to stimulate the spectator's attention. The actor's action is not only directed to an on-stage aim (drinking the glass of water) but also to the audience (stimulating the spectators' attention). In the same time the same action has two different aims. This gives rise to a "double intention" of the actor or better to a *dilated intention* that broadens from the performed action out to the audience. We can reasonably suppose that such a "broadening" of the intention concerns a peculiar neuromotor dimension.

Beside the "dilated intention", we have to mention another theatrical constraint that affects the actor's organisation: unlike everyday life where every action gets reorganised according to the particular situation and unexpected events, on stage the actor knows the complete sequence of the events that will take place during the performance, so that any possible contingency is minimised. However the actor must be able to not anticipate the actions that follow and to render all the dynamics and ways of restructuring and reacting to unexpected events as they occur in everyday behaviour. Although he knows exactly what is going to happen, the actor must recreate on the stage such an *effect* that makes the spectator "believe" that what is going on is "really" unexpected and incidental, as it "naturally" occurs in the everyday life.

These two examples show the difference between the everyday and the on-stage action and allow us to remark that, considered in neurophysiological terms, this difference is probably quite relevant, since it may concern the processes of action planning, postural control, decision making, body schema, etc.

It is then necessary to understand how the actor factually reorganises his actions in order to reach what Jacques Coupeau used to define as *achieved spontaneity* (Copeau 1955). This will probably allow us to get partially rid of the spectator ethnocentrism that still affects theatre studies as well as neuroscientific studies on the performative arts.

5. Motor dynamics of believable action

It's now important to underline that the efficacy of an action on the spectator's perception is not directly linked to the similarity of this action to everyday actions. Our experience as spectators tells us that an action of a modern dancer or of an

Indian Odissi performer should be really believable and effective also if their motor patterns are very different from everyday life. On the other side, the actions of a poor-trained "naturalistic" actor should be perceived as really false also if they are similar to everyday forms. The process of "believing" to the performer's actions deals with the entire psychophysical process of the actor. In order to *achieve an effect of spontaneity* for the spectator, the actor's actions must above all be *believable*, which does not entail that they have necessarily to be *similar to everyday action*. It is well-known that Constantin Stanislavski, father of the contemporary theatre, used to rebuke the actors by saying: "I don't believe it!" (Stanislavski 1956). His way of determining whether the actor was good at acting did not depend on an "objective" or "objectivisable" method but on the direct experience of the first spectator par excellence: the director.

Of course, the recent studies on the mirror neurons mechanism provide information about the neurobiological processes determining the believability of the action. Without going into detail (for a review in this regard, cf. Rizzolatti & Sinigaglia 2008), it is still necessary to consider some aspects that are particularly important in analysing the believable action.

The first and probably best known aspect is given by the peculiar mechanism of mirror neurons, which, connecting immediately the sensory information with the motor mechanisms, shows that, on the stage as well as in everyday life, understanding the others' actions does not depend on a cognitive effort but on an actual "resonance" of the executer's motor acts through the observer's motor areas. But what is the difference between this 'resonance' as occurring in everyday life and as occurring at the theatre? The answer to this question requires an analysis of the mirror neurons mechanism. A relationship between the intentional character of the action and its ability to resonate through the observer has often been proposed. For instance, in 2001 Maria Alessandra Umiltà carried out an experiment showing that the macaque's mirror system activated only when the actions were 'real' and not imitated. (Umiltà et al. 2001). However the interesting point is that in this experiment the subject charged to "mime" or "realise" the action was a neuroscientist, that is someone not trained to make his mimed action *believable*. Another similar experiment, carried out on human beings by using as stimulus the actions performed by actors, showed that the "mimed" actions, too, resonated through the observer's mirror system (Buccino et al. 2001). A further experiment, carried out in 2008 in collaboration with Rizzolatti, highlighted that among three kinds of *non-object-related* actions – mimed, symbolic and meaningless – only the mimed actions seemed to let the observer's mirror system resonate (Lui et al. 2008). Apparently actions implying an actual interaction involve the observer into a resonance of mirror mechanism much more than those actions that require an explicit cognitive effort, such as symbolic actions. We could state that the "actuality" of the action's objective is an essential issue even when such an "actuality" is only *imagined* by the performer. Of course, there are many ways of "imagining". Mere "imagination" is not enough, a good training is also required, in order for the motor dimension of this process to be effective. Other recent studies on the mirror system seem to suggest that the resonance of the actions is due less to the form of the observed action than to the motor purpose of the action (Umiltà et al. 2008). This consideration is not surprising for theatre experts, given that all the greatest theatre protagonists of the 20th century have stressed the importance of working on the actor's intention. In *The Work of the Actor on Himself*, Stanislavski defines a believable action as: "The well-founded action that corresponds to a purpose" (Stanislavski 1956, p. 44) whereas Meyerhold set the intention as basis of any on-stage action: "Every element of the acting process is made of three fundamental moments: (1) Intention, (2) Realization (or Execution), (3) Reaction." (Meyerhold 2009b, p. 138). Similarly, Jerzy Grotowski employed the concept of intention to describe the psycho-muscular unity of the action[8] whereas the Odin Teatret actress Roberta Carreri defined theatre as "the dance of intentions" (Carreri 2007, p. 81).

It is always worth quoting Peter Brook's well-known sentence (which Giacomo Rizzolatti wanted on the first page of his book on mirror neurons) according to which, by discovering the mirror neurons, "neurosciences had finally started to understand what has been long common knowledge in theatre." (Rizzolatti & Sinigaglia 2008, p. ix).

Now we should focus on a peculiar aspect shown by the research on the mirror mechanism: any motor act is aimed not only at reaching the objective but also at preparing and anticipating the actions that follow. Such anticipation of the motor acts that follow immediately resonates in the observer's body-mind, who – as suggested by some experiments (Umiltà et al. 2001; Fogassi et al. 2005) – can foresee and implicitly anticipate the outcomes and the consequences of the observed action.

If applied to the theatre, these complex processes of anticipating another's action suggest that the spectator always tends to make some implicit motor forecast of the actor's actions. For the actor this is a double-edged weapon, since it can be a help as well as a hindrance to his performance.

8. "In/tension-intention. There is no intention if there is not a proper muscular mobilization. This is also part of the intention. The intention exists even at a muscular level in the body, and is linked to some objective outside you […]. Usually, when the actor thinks of intentions, he thinks that it means to pump an emotional state. It is not this. Intentions are related to physical memories, to associations, to wishes, to contact with the others, but also to muscular in/tensions." (Grotowski 1986, p. 96).

6. Surprising and suspending. The actor's advantage over the spectator

One of the actor's "advantages" consists in his power of playing with the spectator, by leading him to have precise expectations and then surprising him by a sudden change of intention. As Roberta Carreri, actress of the Odin Teatret, explains:

> If during a scene I must stoop to pick up a notebook from the floor, my eyes would not immediately stare at the object, but I would, for example, look left and right before stooping down. My aim is to avoid anticipating the action, but I must also be able to justify what I'm going to do by providing it with a logical reason: I look about me to make sure that no one can see me, or maybe I wonder why no one else picks it up, or perhaps just in order to verify whether there are some other objects on the floor I might pick up. Only at the last minute I fix my eyes on the notebook and I stoop down. At this point I will be able to use my "*in-tension*"[9] to pick it up as if it was a feather. In order to pick the notebook up, I will grasp its cover with two fingers. It is essential to me that I do not execute the action in a mechanical way, following the shortest path I would follow in everyday life, but that I succeed, by its phrasing, in evoking images able to change my *in-tensions* and to let associations arise in the spectator's mind, offering him several levels of interpretation. (Carreri 2007, p. 88)

Similarly the actor can suspend the action, in order that the spectator, who has probably already formulated some hypothesis, is left waiting in a condition of suspense. In the Odin Teatret this moment is denoted by the Norwegian term *sats*:

> In the action of sitting, for example, we can single out the moment when, as we bend, we are no longer able to control our weight and the body descends. If we stop just before that moment we are in a *sats*: we can return to a standing position or decide to sit. To find the life of the sats, the performer must play with the spectators' kinaesthetic sense and prevent them from foreseeing what is about to happen. The action must surprise the spectators. (Barba 1995, p. 56)

7. Foreseeing and anticipating: The spectator's advantage over the actor

The negative aspect of the spectator's tendency to anticipate the action lies – as we have already seen – in the difficulty for the actor to render an effect of unforeseeability. For example, if in the stage pretence somebody is supposed to

9. (Translator's note) By translating *in-tension* we try to render the pun implied by the original Italian expression *in-tensione*, which is a word crossing the similar word *intenzione* (intention) and the expression "*in tensione*" (under tension, which refers to the muscular tension of the actor while he executes actions provided with a real intention).

suddenly knock at the door, the actor must be able to reproduce his own reaction so that this event can appear as "unforeseen", although this same event has been repeated several times by the actor during rehearsals. This moment is very difficult because, unless the actor controls precisely his whole body, some parts of it – such as the legs that are not directly involved in the action – may unconsciously move in advance towards the door, in order to make easier the action following the unforeseen event, but in this case the "surprising" event will be revealed as merely pretended. These anticipating mechanisms then are not only related to the action but involve the whole body of the actor, who is usually completely exposed on stage. A better comprehension of this stage problem requires further consideration of the notion of *body schema*.

Shaun Gallagher, one of the scholars most committed to analysing this mechanism, defined the body schema as

> A non-conscious system of processes that constantly regulate posture and movement – a system of motor-sensory capacities that function below the threshold of awareness, and without the necessity of perceptual monitoring. (Gallagher 2005, p. 234)

The studies concerning the notion of *body schema* teach us that our body-mind system is a widespread mechanism that cannot be reduced to a "pure central mechanism" supposed to combine the information concerning the outer ambient with the information concerning the position of our body in space, our posture and our possibility of interacting. Furthermore the *body schema* also regulates the pre-reflective organisation of the whole body towards a precise goal. It is then absolutely related to the intentional dimension of the action. According to Dorothée Legrand, "To have an intention is not only to have a reason to act, but also to have a body oriented toward a goal" (Legrand 2010, p. 166). In everyday life the whole body reorganises itself according to each intentional event. For the actor the important point is that such an organisation or combination of egocentric and allocentric information, is not a conscious process:

> If the behavior monitored through the body schema does not necessitate conscious control, it is not reducible to a mere reflex either. Such behavior can indeed be precisely modulated according to the conscious intentions entertained by the agent rationally and consciously. For instance, if a subject holds out his or her hand to reach a glass of water to drink, the subject's hand forms a grip adapted in size to this goal automatically and in an anticipated way. (Legrand 2010, p. 167)

The body schema operates so that several body mechanisms cooperate at a pre-conscious level in preparing the concatenation of action. This means that, in a stage condition where the actor already knows the concatenation of actions, his body schema may naturally anticipate the following actions even if they are supposed to be a reaction to an incidental event. This is why the actor needs to control his body schema at a higher level than usual, and to this end he elaborates special psychophysical strategies that are the exercises the actor does during his training.

8. Fragmentation and reconstruction: The artificial body schema

As we have already seen, the pre-reflective status of the body schema's activation prevents the actor from willingly inhibiting it, so that he has to construct a rather *artificial body schema* in order to attend a higher pre-reflexive control, different from our daily pre-reflexive experience of it. The processes of constructing such an *artificial body schema* take different forms depending on the performative tradition. Most of them are founded on two basic moments, i.e. the fragmentation of the everyday neuromotor routines and the reconstruction of other routines at a different level of control. An actor is required not only to reproduce the suitable intention but also to have an unusual control of his *whole body* during the performance. For instance, Meyerhold considered this aspect as the basis of the whole system of biomechanics: "The whole biomechanics is based on this fact: if the nose works, the whole body works as well." (Meyerhold 2009a, p. 100).

In the 20th century the pedagogy of acting provides several examples of "fragmentation" of everyday routines: Stanislavski's decomposition into "tasks" – "a turkey can be eaten in pieces!" (Stanislavksij 1956, p. 123), the dialectics of *otkaz-posil-stoika* of the theatre biomechanics, Decroux's contemporary mime's *grammaire*, footage of which is available on the DVD *Enfin, voir Decroux Bouger* (2006). Furthermore, the same dialectics can be detected in Eastern performative practices, such as the *yo-ha-kyu* of the Japanese Kabuki theatre.

The conscious awareness provided by fragmenting the action is necessary to the actor not only to inhibit the unwished anticipating movements but also to reconstruct the fluency the action requires in order to appear effectively spontaneous.

The conscious control of a motor act is not enough. The actor must reach a new *pre-reflective* control, which, unlike the everyday pre-reflective control, has to allow his intention to broaden out to the spectator, so that the actor can play with him, surprise him, listen to his breath, feel his level of attention. By doing so, he can make every performance a unique experience, an authentic complex relationship instead of a mere automatic repetition of a series of acts. This is the aim of constructing an *artificial body schema*. Precisely as the everyday body schema is continuously modified and cannot be reached by a conscious effort, so the artificial body schema can be constructed only *through experience*, i.e. only by unceasingly and physically experiencing a lot of non-daily situations that develop several thought-action dynamics through the actor's body-mind:

> Exercises are small labyrinths that the actors' body-minds can trace and retrace in order to incorporate a paradoxical way of thinking, thereby distancing themselves from their own daily behaviour and entering the domain of the stage's extra-daily behaviour.
>
> Exercises are like amulets, which the actor carries around, not to show them off, but to draw from them certain qualities of energy out of which a second nervous system slowly develops. An exercise is made up of memory, body-memory. An exercise becomes memory, which acts through the entire body. (Barba 1997, p. 128)

In my opinion, when Barba says "An exercise becomes memory, which acts through the entire body", he is tracing an alternative way of describing the process of embodying the artificial body schema, which operates *as* body and body memory.

In this sense, the work of a "naturalistic" actor is not very different from the work of an actor or a dancer who comes from a high-codified performative tradition (i.e. classical ballet, Indian Odissi dance or Decroux's corporal mime, etc.). We can thus come back now to the discourse on the *believable action* that we started in the fourth paragraph of this chapter. Either the "naturalistic" actor or the "codified" one provides for himself an *artificial body schema* able to assure that the whole body *coherently* moves towards a goal. We notice again that the effectiveness of an action on the spectator does not depend on its level of *similarity to everyday life* but on how *coherently the body organises itself in aiming at a goal.* An action is felt as intentional and therefore believable, if the actor takes care of the details of the action as well as of the coherence of the collateral movements.[10] For instance, Indian performative practices develop ways of acting on stage that are far distant to the usual acting and they nevertheless keep the "naturalness" of the action, as if it was a quite natural way of interacting with space. Considering how long and complex an Indian actor's training is, we realise that such an effect of naturalness results from a long and careful work of fragmentation, new composition and organisation of the performer's body.

Similarly, in order to be effective, even the most "naturalistic" theatre practices do not require the actor just to evoke a precise intention or to identify with a particular condition. They rather require him to demolish and to work, to dig, to

10. In this regard the philosopher Pierre Livet has remarked in a recent contribution that the collateral movements are essential for identifying the intention: "Adjustments like collateral movements, or like updatings of the position of the body and its limbs relative to the environment, are required both from the observer's and the agent's perspective in order to feel the movements as intentional." (Livet 2010, p. 189).

split and to reconstruct the deep motor mechanisms ruling any action. Here we return to our starting point, according to which the work of the actor on his own motion is not a "dimension" of his creativity but *is* his actual creative work.

We would like to consider how such *achieved spontaneity* can affect the spectator's way of experiencing the actor and the stage set.

9. The spectator's performative experience

The spectator's performative experience, like any other human experience, can be considered as resulting from the interaction between many different mechanisms, which we could not list here, unless approximately. We shall focus on what, in my opinion, makes this experience different from any other.

In neuroscientific terms, the mechanisms operating between actor and spectator, as they are both present, are still unexplored. It is nevertheless possible to propose some hypotheses in this regard. For this purpose we can start by some considerations arising from the interdisciplinary cooperation between neuroscientists and phenomenologists in analysing a human being's intersubjective processes.

In a paper written with Marco Iacoboni, a neuroscientist at the University of Los Angeles, Dorothée Legrand shows that any intersubjective relation is primarily founded on the sharing of a same space, which comes to be the common *goal* for the intentions of the interacting individuals:

> A primary intersubjective relation is made possible through the sharing of a common world, by virtue of the execution and observation of goal-directed actions: the goal of one's action becomes represented as something that can be shared in the sense that the object is not only one's own intentional object but also the intentional object of others. (Legrand & Iacoboni 2010, p. 238–239)

Another interdisciplinary project, carried out by the neuroscientists Marcello Costantini and Giorgia Committeri in collaboration with the philosopher Corrado Sinigaglia, resulted in some experiments (Costantini et al. 2010; Costantini et al. 2011) that suggest that each of us experiences through motion the world as *goal* of the others' potential actions:

> Overall, our findings indicate that the visual features of an object may suggest or even demand a motor behaviour to the observer not only when the object is located within her own reaching space, but also when it falls within the reaching space of another individual. Our proposal is that such an effect is likely to be due to a mapping of one's own and others' arm reaching space. (Costantini et al. 2011, p. 4)

In fact phenomenology had already stated something similar, i.e. Husserl's notion of *Mitkonstitution* that has recently been drawn on by Jean-Luc Petit and Alain Berthoz (2008), who proposed the translation *co-constitution of the world*. The notion of co-constitution belongs to the phenomenological perspective according to which there is no "pre-determined" world, because the world itself is constituted, modified and perceived by the subject through a circular process of perception-action (Varela, Thompson, Rosch 1992), so that the world is not separated from the subject, but rather composes the latter, it is part of him. In this perspective two interacting subjects do not "share" the same pre-determined world but actively co-constitute it. The world perceived as "already constituted" is an effect due to the fact that the subject has always been experiencing a context shared with other subjects, who interact with the world through the same motor dynamics of the subject.

> If I am ever to able to think of the world as already constituted, it is only because it has already been constituted by another subject who co-constitutes it along with me. It is constituted, let us add, by an other who is, initially precisely not one among other constituted objects (constituted by a solitary subject) in the world but an other altogether, another man or woman, completely different from myself but already equipped with the afferent transcendental prerogatives belonging to a co-constituting subject. (Berthoz & Petit 2008, p. 256)

This is how we can realise that my way of perceiving the world depends on the way in which the other subjects interact with me, co-constituting the world.

However if, as we have said above, the actor adopts different techniques in order to interact with his stage world, the way of perceiving by the spectator (who is co-constituting the world along with the actor) will also be modified somehow. In other words, the mechanisms of the actor's interaction with the world, according to different and unusual rules, *do modify the world itself*, allowing the spectator to experience the co-constituted world differently from the usual way of experiencing it. This concept may be explained by quoting a well-known work by Adolphe Appia, who describes the process by which the stage set, interacting with the actor, comes to life in the spectator's perception:

> Let's consider a vertical pillar, squared with sharply defined angles. This pillar rests, without basement, on horizontal slabs. It gives the impression of stability and strength. A body comes close. The contrast between its movement and the stillness of a quiet pillar already provokes a feeling of expressive life, as the body without pillar and the pillar without this moving body would not achieve.
> (Appia 1921, p. 372)

Appia already understands here that the interaction of the actor's body with space is precisely what produces such an expressive effect. The Swiss director goes even further in his considerations:

> Here the actor's body touches the pillar; now the opposition is stronger. Then the body leans against the pillar whose stillness offers it a solid point to lean against: the pillar holds out. It acts! The opposition has created the life of an inanimate form. The space has become a living space! (Appia 1921, p. 373)

The space described by Appia is now "living". But living with respect to whom? With respect to the spectator's performative experience.

The space comes to life precisely because the spectator tends to "remap" it according to the actor's actions and potentiality of acting. The *artificial body schema* used by the actor, while he interacts on stage, *modifies* not only the perception of the stage world but also the mechanisms of co-constituting the world on which the intersubjective relation of actor and spectator is based. The spectator *experiences in a different way the world co-constituted* along with the actor. In my opinion, this different way of experiencing the world characterises the spectator's performative experience.

As we have already seen, the spectator's attention is based on mechanisms of hypothesis, anticipation and concatenation of motor acts; they are choices that the spectator continuously makes in a more or less explicit, automatic or pre-reflective way. The actor can play with these automatisms, if he reaches a psychophysical control different from the "usual" control belonging to the spectator. The actor plays on the physically unbalanced nature of the spectator's attention, and he opens alternative ways, he surprises, he proposes unexpected associations of ideas that lead the spectator to actively recall his imagination.

The theatre spectator's imagination does not arise from a straightforward process of constitution, the spectator is not taken by the hand towards his own imaginative processes. On the contrary the actor lets the spectator fall into the action's distances, lacks of balance, surprises, unusual associations, uncommon perception of the world. This is exactly why the spectator *turns* to his imagination, clings to it in order to fill in these gaps, he uses his imagination as bridge between these unexpected experiences, among different *performative experiences*. Not accidentally Alain Berthoz identified the imagination as a resource of the attention:

> For me the attention is not only a mechanism connected with perception, as a commander in chief who would decide where and what to watch; perception is an anticipation mechanism that prepares for action, a mechanism that sets the world for our actions and intentions whose traces we find the at every level of our nervous system, from the elementary to the higher cognitive levels. Attention is not only the conscious perception of real stimuli and small perceptions, attention can use imagination. (Berthoz 2009, p. 57, our translation)

Without knowing it, the spectator creatively operates in the performance. His function is not a passive observation, but a reconstruction, a steady psychophysical interaction with what is going on the stage. It is a long time since the theatre studies started dealing specifically with the *dramaturgy of the spectator* (De Marinis 1987).

The spectator's performative experience is not only the result of the actor's resonating actions, but it is also and especially a process of reacting to them, reorganizing the stimuli, making links to his own personal experiences, co-constituting a reality different from the usual one. It is an ineluctably creative experience: "The theatre's raw material is not the actor, nor the space, nor the text, but the attention, the seeing, the hearing, the mind of the spectator. Theatre is the art of the spectator." (Barba 1995, p. 37)

10. Conclusions

We have proposed some hypotheses on how the work intended to get an *achieved spontaneity* could change the motor organisation of the actor. My opinion is that this change is not only a "propaedeutic" training for the actor but it is the fundamental key to study the motor dimension of the imaginative processes that rend the actor-spectator relationship an artistic experience. Future researches both theoretical and empirical on human intersubjective dynamics could offer some new epistemological tools. Anyway, we can set a real interdisciplinary dialogue only if the discussion takes into account the creative process of the actor and the creative dynamics of the spectator's performative experience. We should thus try to develop a collaboration focused more on the *processes* than the *results*. A collaboration where the actor is not considered only a "test case" but the owner of a refined extra-daily embodied knowledge. Theatre doesn't need the answers of science but its questions.

Translation by Gennaro Lauro

References

Appia, A. (1988 [1921]). *L'Œuvre d'Art Vivant*. In *Œuvres Complètes*, Vol. III. Lausanne: L'Âge d'Homme.

Barba, E. (1995). *The Paper Canoe. A Guide to Theatre Anthropology*. London: Routledge. [Original version: *La canoa di carta. Trattato di Antropologia teatrale*. Bologna: Il Mulino. 1993].

Barba, E. (1997). An Amulet Made of Memory. The Significance of Exercises in the Actor's Dramaturgy. *The Drama Review, 156*: 127–132. [Original version: Un amuleto fatto di memoria. Il significato degli esercizi nella drammaturgia dell'attore. In M. De Marinis (Ed.), *Drammaturgia dell'attore* (pp. 11–18). Bologna: I quaderni del Battello Ebbro. 1997].

Barba, E. (2010). *On Directing And Dramaturgy. Burning The House*. New York & London, Routledge. [Original version: *Bruciare la casa. Origini di un regista*. Milano: Ubulibri. 2009].
Barba, E. & Savarese, N. (2005). *The Secret Art of the Performer*. London/ New York: Routledge. [Original version: *Anatomia del teatro*. Firenze: La Casa Usher. 1983].
Berthoz, A. (2009). *La simplixité*. Paris: Odile Jacob. [English version: *Simplexity. Simplifying Principles for a Complex World*. New Haven/London: Yale University Press. 2012].
Berthoz, A. & Petit, J.-L. (2008). *The physiology and phenomenology of action*. Oxford: Oxford University Press. [Original version: *Phénoménologie et physiologie de l'action*. Paris: Odile Jacob. 2006].
Bläsing, B., Calvo-Merino, B., Cross, E.S., Jola, C., Honisch, J. & Stevens, C.J. (2012). Neurocognitive control in dance perception and performance, *Acta Psychologica, 139*, 300–308.
Buccino, G., Binkofski, F., Fink, G.R., Fadiga, L., Fogassi, L., Gallese, V., Seitz, R.J., Zilles, K., Rizzolatti, G. & Freund, H.J. (2001). Action observation activates premotor and parietal areas in a somatotopic manner: an fMRI study. *European Journal of Neuroscience, 13*, 400–404.
Carreri, R. (2007). *Tracce. Training e storia di un'attrice dell'Odin Teatret*. Milano: Il Principe Costante Edizioni.
Copeau, J. (1955). Réflexion sur le "Paradoxe" de Diderot (1929). In Copeau, J., *Notes sur le métier du comédien* (Ed. by Dasté, M.-H.) (pp. 15–33). Paris: Michel Brient Éditeur.
Costantini, M., Ambrosini, E., Tieri, G., Sinigaglia, C. & Committeri, G. (2010). Where does an object trigger an action? An investigation about affordances in space. *Experimental Brain Research, 207*, 95–103.
Costantini, M., Committeri, G. & Sinigaglia, C. (2011). Ready Both to Your and to My Hands: Mapping the Action Space of Others. *PLoS ONE, 6*(4), e17923.
De Marinis, M. (1987). Dramaturgy of the Spectator. *The Drama Review, 31*(2), 100–114.
De Marinis, M. (1988). *Capire il teatro. Lineamenti di una nuova teatrologia*. Firenze: La Casa Usher.
De Marinis, M. (Ed.) (1997). *Drammaturgia dell'attore*. Bologna: I Quaderni del Battello Ebbro.
De Marinis, M. (2011). New Theatrology and Performance Studies: Starting Points Towards a Dialogue. *The Drama Review, 55*(4), 64–74.
De Marinis, M. (2012). Corpo e corporeità a teatro: dalla semiotica alle neuroscienze. Piccolo glossario multidisciplinare. In C. Falletti & G. Sofia (Eds.), *Prospettive su teatro e neuroscienze. Dialoghi e sperimentazioni* (pp. 68–82). Roma: Bulzoni.
Falletti, C. & Sofia, G. (Eds.) (2011). *Nuovi dialoghi tra teatro e neuroscienze*. Roma: Editoria & Spettacolo.
Falletti, C. & Sofia, G. (Eds.) (2012). *Prospettive su teatro e neuroscienze. Dialoghi e sperimentazioni*. Roma: Bulzoni.
Fogassi, L., Ferrari, P.F., Gesierich, B., Rozzi, S., Chersi, F. & Rizzolatti, G. (2005). Parietal lobe: from action organization to intention understanding. *Science, 308*, 662–667.
Gallese, V. (2010). Corpo e azione nell'esperienza estetica. Una prospettiva neuroscientifica. In U. Morelli (Ed.), *Mente e bellezza. Arte, creatività, innovazione* (pp. 245–262). Torino: Umberto Allemandi & C.
Gallagher, S. (2005). Dynamic Models of Body Schematic Processes. In De Preester, H. & Knockaert V. (Eds.), *Body Image and Body Schema: Interdisciplinary perspectives on the body* (pp. 233–250). Amsterdam/Philadelphia: John Benjamins Publishing Company.
Grotowski, J. (1968). *Towards a Poor Theatre*. Holstebro: Odin Teatrets Forlag.

Jola, C., Abedian-Amiri, A., Kuppuswamy, A., Pollick, F.E. & Grosbras, M.H. (2012). Motor Simulation without Motor Expertise: Enhanced Corticospinal Excitability in Visually Experienced Dance Spectators. *PLoS ONE, 7*(3), e33343.

Legrand, D. (2010). Body Intention and the Unreasonable Intentional Agent. In F. Grammont, D. Legrand, & P. Livet (Eds.), *Naturalizing Intention in Action* (pp. 161–180). Cambridge, Massachussets: MIT Press.

Legrand, D. & Iacoboni, M. (2010). Intersubjective intentional actions. In F. Grammont, D. Legrand, & P. Livet (Eds.), *Naturalizing Intention in Action* (pp. 227–246). Cambridge, Massachussets: MIT Press.

Livet, P. (2010). Recursivity, Control, and Revision in Intention in Action. In F. Grammont, D. Legrand, & P. Livet (Eds.), *Naturalizing Intention in Action* (pp. 181–198). Cambridge, Massachussets: MIT Press.

Lui, F., Buccino, G., Duzzi, D., Benuzzi, F,. Crisi, G., Baraldi, P., Nichelli, P., Porro, C.A. & Rizzolatti, G. (2008). Neural substrates for observing and imagining non-object-directed actions, *Social Neurosciences, 3*, 261–275.

Meyerhold, V. (2009a). Principes de Biomécanique (1921–22). In *Écrits sur le théâtre. Tome II, 1917–1929. Nouvelle édition revue et augmentée* (pp. 100–103). La Cité-L'Age d'Homme: Lausanne.

Meyerhold, V. (2009b). L'emploi de l'acteur (1922). In *Écrits sur le théâtre. Tome II, 1917–1929. Nouvelle édition revue et augmentée* (pp. 138–147). La Cité-L'Age d'Homme: Lausanne.

Morin, E. (1977). *La Méthode, 1. La nature de la nature*. Paris: Éditions du Seuil.

Pradier, J.-M. (1990). Towards a Biological Theory of the Body in Performance. *New Theatre Quarterly, 6*, 86–98.

Pradier, J.-M. (1996). Ethnoscénologie: la profondeur des emergences. *Internationale de l'Imaginaire, 5*, 13–41.

Pradier, J.-M. (2001). Ethnoscenology: the Flesh is Spirit. In G. Berghaus, (Ed.), *New Approaches to Theatre Studies and Performance Analysis* (pp. 61–81). Tübingen: Max Niemeyer Verlag.

Richards, Th. (1993). Conference at Liège, Cirque Divers, 2 January 1986. Unpublished transcription of a tape recording of Jerzy Grotowski (1986). *At work with Grotowski on physical actions*. London and New York: Routledge. [Original version: *Al lavoro con Grotowski sulle azioni fisiche*. Milano: Ubulibri. 1993]

Rizzolatti, G. & Sinigaglia, C. (2008). *Mirrors in the brain. How our minds share action and emotions*. Oxford: Oxford University Press. [Original version: *So quel che fai. Il cervello che agisce e i neuroni specchio*. Milano: Raffaello Cortina. 2006].

Sofia, G. (Ed.). (2009). *Dialoghi tra teatro e neuroscienze*. Roma: Edizioni Alegre.

Stanislavski, C. (1956). *Il lavoro dell'attore su se stesso*. Roma-Bari: Editori Laterza. [Original version: *Rabota aktera nad soboj. Dnevnik učenica*, Moskva, 1938].

Umiltà, M.A., Kohler, E., Gallese, V., Fogassi, L., Fadiga, L., Keysers, C. & Rizzolatti, G. (2001). I know what you are doing: a neurophysiological study. *Neuron, 32*, 91–101.

Umiltà, M.A., Escola, L., Intskirveli, I., Grammont, F., Rochat, M., Caruana, F., Jezzini, A., Gallese, V. & Rizzolatti, G. (2008). When pliers become fingers in the monkey. *Proceedings of the National Academy of Sciences, 105*(6), 2209–2213.

Varela, F. (1996). Neurophenomenology: a methodological remedy to the hard problem. *Journal of Consciousness Studies, 3*(4), 330–350.

Varela, F., Thompson, E. & Rosch, E. (1992). *The Embodied Mind. Cognitive Science and Human Experience*. Cambridge, Massachussets: MIT Press.

The digital body in contemporary American cinema

Marco Luceri
Università di Firenze

1. A transformation of American cinema

Contemporary American cinema is undergoing a period of rapid and profound transformation due to the increasing use of digital technology. *Motion capture* and *facial performance replacement* are two of the most significant and recent innovations. Both allow creating a virtual image of the actor's body. Motion capture has first been used by Robert Zemeckis in *Polar Express* (2004) and was then further developed in his two subsequent films, *Beowulf* (2007) and *A Christmas Carol* (2009). Facial performance replacement has been pioneered by James Cameron in *Avatar* (2010).

Motion capture allows electronic sensors, which are placed on the body, to track and record the movements of the actor. This animation data is mapped to a 3D model so that the model performs the same actions as the actor. The results are rather realistic movements. The spectators are able to recognise in the characters of Zemickis' films the features of the famous Hollywood stars (like Tom Hanks, Angelina Jolie, Jim Carrey and many others) who interpret them. There is however a significant difference between *Polar Express* and *A Christmas Carol*: in the first movie all the facial expressions, gestures and, to a certain extent, Tom Hanks' entire way of acting are still rather uncertain and not quite fluid, whereas in the second film a technological improvement has allowed the image of Jim Carrey to appear in a more structured and realistic way. Still, the limit of motion capture is that it only *partially* succeeds in supplying a virtual mirror image of the real actor, and this is verifiable even in the most recent films which have been made with this technology, such as *The Adventures of Tin Tin – The Secret of the Unicorn* (2011) of Steven Spielberg.

Facial replacement performance, developed by Cameron's collaborators for the film *Avatar*, largely overcomes the difficulty presented by motion capture. Actors wear a helmet equipped with a sophisticated micro-camera in HD positioned about 20 cm from the face. In this way, it is possible to record all movements of the facial muscles, capturing facial expressions with a precision that has never been reached before. The use of this technology enables a kind of "pure" interpretation: not having to focus on their physical appearance, actors can concentrate on the character itself. "Real" actors give life to their virtual *alter ego*, increasing thereby the spectators' sense of participation and emotion during the movie. In *Avatar* facial performance replacement allows a veritable *mise en abyme* of the narrative discourse of the double: if on the diegetic level (that what belongs to the story and to the world created by the cinematographic fiction) humans give life to their avatar, then on the extradiegetic level (that what does not belong to the world created by the cinematographic fiction) real actors are creating their own virtual image. This phenomenon, which is undoubtedly one of the most interesting aspects of *Avatar*, gives the entire film a meta-linguistic character (*Avatar* is a film that continually enacts the practices of cinema itself). Moreover, insofar many sequences show how the "human" characters transform themselves in virtual beings or avatars, one could even argue that *Avatar* is a kind of *mise-en-scène* of the technological nature of the film itself.

Motion capture and facial performance replacement have given rise to the notion of digital performance and are part of a broader transformation of the role of the actor (and of the representation of the body in general) in American cinema over the last fifteen years. In addition to motion capture and facial performance replacement there are other technological innovations which influence the way of acting and the use of the body of the actor. Due to lack of space, we will only list some of the most important ones here. The Chroma Key, also referred to as colour keying or colour-separation overlay, is a technique characterised by the actor standing in front of a large blue or green screen and acting out the scene by himself. The background is then replaced with footage either taken from another location or created digitally by a computer. Chroma key was used for the first time in 1982 for the film *Tron* of Steven Lisberger. Mocap Toon, a technique deployed in animation films, uses the movements of the body of the actor as dynamic structures for characters. In the technique of retargeting, the body of the actor provides algorithms to the machine, defined by the movement of points in space fixed on the body of the actor, which then put into relation the dynamic and physical structure of the actor with the skeleton of the modelled creature (Spanu 2011, pp. 168–169). Bullet Time, used in films like *The Matrix*, *300* and *Avatar*, is a spatial and visual effect that refers to a digitally enhanced simulation of variable-speed photography. It is characterised both by its extreme formation of time (slow enough to show normally imperceptible and un-filmable events, such as flying bullets) and space (by way of the ability of the camera angle to move around the scene at a normal speed while events are slowed). This is almost impossible with conventional slow-motion as the physical camera would have to move impossibly fast. Digital Matte painting is a painted representation of a landscape, set or distant location that allows filmmakers to create the illusion of an environment that would otherwise be too expensive or impossible to build or visit. Historically matte painters and film technicians have used various techniques to combine a matte painting image with live-action footage. Dragon Effect consists in the manipulation of the images through the increased contrast and sharpness and the alteration of the colour of the body of the actor (Terzo 2011, pp. 78–80).

It may be clear from the above that the use of digital technology has taken many forms. Some famous film directors have used digital technology to make their actors perform movements which would have been almost impossible to obtain in analogue: one just has to think of the bloodthirsty dances of Keanu Reeves in *The Matrix* (1999) or those of Uma Thurman in *Kill Bill* (2004) or of the entirely artificial landscapes in which the numerous stars (like Bruce Willis, Micky Rourke, Benicio Del Toro, Jessica Alba etc.) move themselves in an intermediate (between cinema and comics) film as *Sin City* (2009). Moreover, under the impetus of animated film – and in particular under influence of John Lasseter's Pixar – the idea that a movie can be made entirely in computer graphics, that is, by creating "abstract" images without a real referent (as the actor) – has caught on rapidly. The Japanese-American movie *Final Fantasy* (2001) was the first long-feature film in the history of cinema entirely made in three-dimensional computer graphics: everything that the spectator sees, including actors and spaces, are digital models. One could speak therefore of a kind of "digital object that asks the public to make an ambitious perceptual "jump": to believe in the images one sees as if one was looking to an "ordinary" film" (Amaducci 2011: 31, our translation).[1] *Final Fantasy* is a digital film based on a video game with the same name. It is a typical cross-media product: the persons who designed and produced the film are also those who produced the video game.

What are the consequences – ontologically and historically speaking – of the frequent use of techniques (which, and let's not forget, are continuously evolving) as motion capture and facial performance replacement in this vast landscape in which the language of cinema defiles with that of other media (like television, comics, video games, etc.), giving rise to an increasingly widespread hybridisation?

2. Second lives

From an *ontological* point of view the use of digital technologies in the film industry seems to have strengthened the broader tendency, typical of today's society and

1. "[…] oggetto digitale che chiede al pubblico un salto percettivo ambizioso: credere alle immagini che vede come se fosse un film "normale"." (Amaducci 2011, p. 31)

culture, to leave behind the limitations of corporeality. This trend started in the 1980s with the wider diffusion of information technology. In William Gibson's cyberpunk novel *Neuromancer* (1984), for example, the subjectivities which operate in cyberspace are described as de-contextualized, quantifiable entities, so-called *patterns*, with no physical *presence*. Their bodies are disparaged as dead meat which exists primarily to sustain their consciousness until the next time they will enter cyberspace. If the body is only "data incarnate", that is, a mere accidental accessory to a more essential thinking mind, then it is only a small step to erase our bodies and to leave the precariousness of our physical existence behind. Hans Moravec's book *Mind Children: The Future of Robot and Human Intelligence* (1988) is, to a certain extent, the culmination of this way of thinking about our bodies. In this work Moravec makes a shocking announcement: "soon, he says, it will be possible to download human consciousness into a computer" (Moravec 1988, pp. 109–110). At the end of the process, the person in question will find himself inhabiting the metallic body of the computer in which his consciousness is located, without any loss of meaning or form. It may be clear that in both cases the writer's imagination outstrips the hitherto existing technologies in which our access to cyberspace still depends in complex and highly specific ways on our embodiment (Hayles 1999).

The attempt to liberate humanity from its bodily burden is not confined to the cyberpunk movement of the 1980s, but has swept through the cultural mindset of the, so-called, "flesh-eating" 1990s and is still a feature of today's cultural perception, as is evidenced by the many internet sites which promise their users a safer and a more pleasant life by abolishing the physical body, prone to violence and unknown gazes, in exchange for a self-created pattern or avatar (De Clercq 2009, pp. 201–202). The (in)famous internet site "Second Life" is exemplary here: "Second Life"[2] (from now: SL) is an online three-dimensional virtual world, imagined and created by its residents. To begin your SL, you first have to create an avatar, an electronic representation of yourself – faithful or invented – in three dimensions. Simple basic controls allow you to change your hair colour, the size of your breasts, hips, nose and so on. As an inhabitant of SL you can never truly die, which means you can fly or fight without fear of harm. If you are worried about what will happen to your avatar in the event of unfortunate circumstances in your "first life" you can always indicate in your will the name of the person who you want to inherit your SL account. Basically, life in SL is really whatever you make of it. Hence, the slogan "your world, your way". This was also the dream of Linden Lab, the founder of SL: to create a world where people could live without

2. For this presentation of Second Life see *What is Second Life?*, retrieved March 2012 from www.secondlife.com.

any social, cultural or religious boundaries; a place where people could really be themselves. What does this brief outline tell us about the conception of the human body in SL? The "body" in SL is not a physical presence but a three-dimensional pattern, an avatar, which cannot die. Human enhancement technologies that try to overcome the physical limitations of the "normal" human body through medicine or technology share a similar desire to obtain the ultimate privilege of immortality. Although some forms of human enhancement are not yet available and may appear to belong to the realm of science fiction, others are already widely used: cosmetic surgery, the use of mood altering substances, drugs to improve physical strength and so on. The presupposition behind these techniques is that human perfectibility is infinite and that human faculties can and will constantly improve through science and reason. They give people the possibility to become who they always wanted or felt to be, be it through physical, personality or cognitive enhancement.

3. Body, space, movement, image, acting: From theatre to cinema

From a *historical* point of view technology seems to have realised, more than a century later, that what the European symbolists of the late 19th and early 20th century dreamed about: a spectacle in which the physical presence of the actor has vanished in favour of a pure image. Symbolism was an attempt to elevate art over science in the name of a higher knowledge than that of the contingent empirical world; a knowledge of a spiritual reality made of pure forms. This kind of knowledge is difficult to realise in theatre by virtue of the fact that the actor due to his physical presence inevitable refers to the empirical world. This explains why all symbolists, from Stéphane Mallarmé to Albert Mockel and even Maurice Maeterlinck, when writing about theatre, have argued against the presence of the actor on stage. As such, symbolist theatre comes very close to the expressive characteristics of the figurative arts of this period. The function of the actor was so drastically reduced to the role of a mere executor of the project of the director-demiurge that Maeterlinck came to foresee a theatre where the presence of man was no longer indispensable:

> One should perhaps eliminate the living being from the stage [...]. Will the human being be replaced by a shadow? A reflection? [...] a projection of symbolic forms, or a being who would appear to live without being alive? I do not know; but the absence of man seems essential to me.
>
> (Maeterlinck (1890), quoted in Dorra 1994, p. 145).

For Charles Baudelaire and Stéphane Mallarmé dance, with its ability to be "pure" sign, was the form of expression closest to symbolist poetry. Symbolist theories have had a strong influence on the activities of two Parisian theatres, the *Théâtre d'art* founded in 1891 by Paul Fort and *L'Oeuvre* founded in 1893 by

Aurelien Lugné-Poe. The *mise-en-scène* of *La Gardienne* of Henri de Ragnier, staged at the theatre *L'Oeuvre* in 1894 is exemplary here: "the sole intention of the staging was to deprive the actors of their bodily weight, reducing them to fantastic shadows, making them play behind a veil while speaking in an ecstatic and mellifluous tone" (Molinari 1996, pp. 251–252, our translation).[3]

Gordon Craig is one of the most important "heirs" of this symbolist utopia of the first half of the 20th century. Craig dreamed about a kinetic-visual spectacle without interpreters in flesh and blood. His notion of theatre as *Total Art* was in strong contrast with the naturalist tendency which had diffused itself in Europe during the second half of the 19th century and which tried to restore the authenticity of the "real". The influence of symbolism on Craig's scenographic theory and practice is evidenced by his idea that theatre should open new horizons of imagination, starting from a new understanding of the actor. As an important exponent of the avant-garde theatre that promoted the craft of the director, Craig put into question the mimetic style of acting because he deemed it inadequate to the "theatre of the future". Influenced by his relationship with the famous American dancer Isadora Duncan, who made him discover the value of a suggestive, abstract interplay of form, light, music and movement, Craig turned motion into the most important vehicle of theatrical expression (Attolini 1996, p. 61). In fact, from this moment on dynamism will become a crucial element in his project to revolutionize theatre. He asserted further that the director was the true artist of the theatre and he suggested viewing actors as mere marionettes, clearly with the aim of totally removing their presence on scene. In fact, in one of his most famous texts, the *Actor and the Über-marionette* (1911), Craig seems to want to do away with the living actor, replacing him with a larger-than-life puppet. Still, it remained an idea on paper only and it was probably intended as a provocation to draw the actor's attention on the inadequacy of naturalistic acting, impelling them to revise their own role in relation to the totality of the theatrical show (Attolini 1996, p. 62). Craig tried to overcome the physical presence of the actor on scene with the use of neutral and mobile screens, an idea that he developed in Florence in 1907: rectangular screens of a neutral colour were composed and recomposed according to taste and their kinetic and expressive force was enhanced by a skilful play of light and shade. Drawing on the interpenetration of sight and movement, Craig managed to create a dynamic vision of the scenographic space in which every aspect was a matter of free poetic creation; a vision devoid of any reference

3. Our translation of "in cui è chiara l'intenzione di togliere agli attori il loro peso corporeo, riducendoli a ombre fantastiche, facendoli recitare dietro un velo con un tono estatico e cantilenante." (Molinari 1996, pp. 251–252)

to physical reality, realising, in his own way, the idea of the Über-marionette: the screens became a kind of artificial actor thanks to which (as the symbolists hoped for) the spiritual was freed from the physical, an essential requirement in order "to reach the true essence of the theatrical spectacle, namely, movement" (Artioli 1972, p. 252, our translation).[4]

Although Craig's ideas have had a strong influence on the theatre of the early 20th century, they did not undermine the tendency, typical of that period, of what historians have named the "retheatralization of the theatre", a movement based upon a new "dramaturgy of space" (De Marinis 2000) and a redefinition of the role of the actor as the main creative subject. Still, the actor's position was no longer that of the 19th century either because it was reduced to its "basic dimension, to a moving body in space" (De Marinis 2000, p. 38, our translation),[5] yet it was also different from Craig's Über-marionette because the movement absolutely required a body or a physical presence. This is why the theatrical research of the first decades of the 20th century shows important connections with modern dance and mime (Isadora Duncan, Rudolf Laban, Jacques Dalcroze & Étienne Decroux); two performing arts which faced similar changes during the same period and often intermingled in a hybrid form known as "theater-dance" (Casini Ropa 1990, p. 137). In the 1920s, therefore, prior to Decroux, the analysis of the relation between the human figure in motion and space was at the center of the research conducted by Oscar Schlemmer at the Bauhaus on "abstract" dance and theatre, as he called them. In a text of 1925, which is his best known essay, *Man and Artistic Figure*, Schlemmer argues that the dynamic relations between the human body and space are regulated by two fundamental, but very different, types of laws, that of three-dimensional space and that of the organic man. According to Schlemmer, who was in search of a theatre-dance that is not natural and not illustrative, but that at the same time does not lose contact with biological organicity, none of these two types of law must prevail in an exclusive manner: the actor-dancer must follow both the law of the body and that of space, trying thus to reach a higher level of organic authenticity, which is not realistic and not mimetic (De Marinis 2000, p. 40–41).

Thus, despite the attempts of Craig and the symbolists to eliminate the actor, the actor's physicality and kinetic force not only did not disappear, but became an essential condition of the retheatralisation hoped for at the beginning of the 20th century. The question then becomes why? The main reason for this can

4. Our translation of "per giungere all'essenza del fatto scenico, ovvero il Movimento." (Artioli 1972, p. 252).

5. Our translation of "dimensione basica, ovvero un corpo in movimento in uno spazio" (De Marinis 2000, p. 38).

be found in the strong attack during this period on "the word" and "the text" as the main means of expression. For centuries one had been witnessing a total enslavement of theatre to literature and psychology and this in turn had led to a distortion of theatre's original physicality (De Marinis 2000 p. 129). But if word and text are put on the sideline, then what remains is precisely the body of the actor with its gestures and movements. This explains why, despite their differences, the most important drama theories of the 20th century all share the idea that one cannot do away with the actor's physicality. The most eminent figures who have carried forward this idea, both in their theories and on stage, are Georg Fuchs, Jacques Copeau, Antonin Artaud and Vsevolod Mejerchold. The latter invented Biomechanics, a theatrical vision completely founded on the art of the actor as plastic art; an art in which the physical presence of the actor is at the basis of the spectacle and in which the human body becomes totally independent from the word.

In the same years, a new art, cinema arrived which ended up prevailing in collective imagination. What consequences did this have? Throughout the entire 20th century cinema renegotiated the relationship between reality and its representation, turning the physical presence of the actor in an image (as predicted by the symbolists), but always in a direct (photographic) relationship with reality (through the representation of movement). Cinema, in substance, found a certain "equilibrium" between the ideals of the symbolists and the idea of retheatralisation (a discussion which emerged in theatre between the end of the 19th and the beginning of the 20th century) because on the one hand it safeguarded the original function and physicality of the actor, but on the other hand it offered the viewer a *realistic image* in motion, preserving thus the emphatic relationship between actor and spectator that the avant-garde theatre had been unable to preserve. Still, the use of technologies as motion capture and facial performance replacement seems to have awakened again the "problem" of the actor due to the attempt to overcome the actor's physicality by replacing it by an abstract digital image. The question then becomes whether contemporary American cinema has been able to (finally) realise the dream of the symbolists. Before dealing with this problem more thoroughly, it is important to highlight the difference, from an expressive point of view, between film actors and actors in theatre.

In film history the actor interprets and represents a character that adheres to the actor himself, setting off all those mechanisms of empathy between the spectator and the actor which are at the basis of a phenomenon like stardom. This phenomenon does not occur in theatre: there may be countless interpreters of Hamlet, while in cinema that peculiar actor is forever "fixed" in that specific character of that precise film (James Dean is the one and only interpreter of *Rebel Without a Cause*, as Audrey Hepburn is the one and only interpreter of *Roman Holiday*, etc.). Things are different, however, in the case of films that use motion capture or facial performance replacement because here we are dealing with a pure interpretation: actors act *without* representing (because the representation is almost entirely in the hands of the film director and of technology). In this way, the definition of a precise physiognomy, which hitherto has been a fundamental principle of acting, becomes less important. When actors wear tights full of sensors that are connected to the computer or when they play in front of a small HD camera, they no longer need make-up and costumes to define their character expressively (technology takes care of this aspect). This change might represent an important "loss" because make-up and costumes are important tools of support in the construction of a character. However, the absence of these external instruments can also prompt the actor to focus more intensively on the internal characteristics of the character. American actors are in a certain sense more suited for this kind of "interiorisation" of the character because unlike their European counterparts, they generally rely on the technique of identification rather than on that of imitation. The technique of identification allows the actor to interpret the characters as real, unique individuals, reproducing not only general emotions, but also more nuanced and subtle mood swings. These procedures have been introduced by some great theatre actors of the mid-19th century, particularly then by Tommaso Salvini, the great tragic actor of that time. They have been reinterpreted by Constantin Stanislavski and after the Second World War they have circulated in America, with significant variations, thanks to the work of Stella Adler and Lee Strasberg at the Actor's Studio in New York.

At this point, and in light of the above considerations, it is time to answer the question raised above regarding contemporary American cinema and its aim to transform and even substitute the body of the actor by virtue of the new technological advances like motion capture and facial performance replacement. The question at issue here is: does contemporary American cinema has been able to realise this ambitious project?

4. To be or not to be: The actor, the spectator and the representation of movement

Let us start our discussion by returning to the first film entirely made in computer graphics: *Final Fantasy*. The spectator's reaction to the virtual humanoids of *Final Fantasy* has been mixed and on the whole rather negative because although the film does not represent a major linguistic break nor a significant change in narrative, the spectator is thrown in a totally incomprehensible hyperrealistic dream world. Perhaps the surrealists, the futurists and Gordon Craig could have liked *Final Fantasy*, but most people, even those more familiar with digital images, were rather disappointed by it, as is testified by the fact that the film did very bad at the box office. Some people contend that this failure has something to do with a phenomenon which is known by the name of "Uncanny Valley" (Plantec 2007). According to the uncanny valley hypothesis robots and virtual characters that approach human-likeness cause a negative response among human observers precisely because they look and act almost, but not perfectly, like human beings. The term was coined by the Japanese professor of robotics Masahiro Mori in 1970. The hypothesis is linked to Sigmund Freud's concept of the uncanny, indicating the uncomfortable feeling when something is familiar and unfamiliar at the same time. The valley refers to a dip in a proposed graph of the positivity of human reaction as a function of human-likeness (Mori 1970: pp. 33–35). One could argue that the same mechanism is at work when people watch a film like *Final Fantasy*. The animated characters of *Final Fantasy* look very much like actual people, but there is something about them that does not fit quite with what we usually understand by the human, this provokes cognitive dissonance and this in turn triggers the feeling of uncanniness. This is a possible reading, but in what follows we will try to show that the "failure" of a film like *Final Fantasy* has rather something to do with a shortcircuit in the ontology of the cinematographic image.

There is a close relationship between the cinematic representation (photography) and its object. According to André Bazin photography (and cinema) distinguishes itself (affirming in this way its originality) from painting thanks to its essential objectivity (Bazin [1958] 1973, p. 7). In virtue of this close relationship with the corporeal, photography and cinema are iconic arts (according to Charles Pierce (Luisi 2009) the icon is a sign in which the relation with the referent is based upon a relation of similarity, i.e. it physically resembles what it stands for). Thanks to elements of visual similarity, offered by photographic and cinematographic reproduction, the spectator is not only able to recognise anthropomorphic simulacra, but also capable of attributing a certain degree of existence to them. This is why the presence of human referents has become one of the main criteria in the making of a film: the technical reproduction of what is human and its function to create the illusion of reality determine the form and the limits which the film characters can take. This explains why even today, despite the enormous appeal and power of technology, it is very difficult to conceive of fiction films without the presence of human simulacra. A film as *Final Fantasy* offers the viewers nothing more than pale ghosts which they will easily forget because of the lack of a human referent. Without this link with reality (with an object, in this case the body of the actor) the spectators are unable to recognise these characters as truly "cinematographic" and this triggers feelings of alienation and dullness, rather than of uncanniness. This is why *Final Fantasy* works as a videogame, but not as a film: in the first case the adventure has to be constructed subjectively, whereas in the second case it is presumed to be objectively given.

Still, not all films made by computer graphics have the same limits as *Final Fantasy*. Think for example of the many success movies produced by John Lasseter's Pixar. These animation movies (like the ones in the past) are built upon the process of identification between the actor and the spectator thanks to an anthropomorphisation of the characters. In *WALL-E* (2009), for example, a film based upon a classical narrative structure and language, the two protagonists Wall-E and Eve – two robots – seem more human than the humans themselves because they are gifted by those feelings and moral sentiments that the human beings seem to have lost. Although the actors, like in *Final Fantasy*, do not "create" the images, in *WALL-E* the absence of a true human referent is considered to be "normal"; it is seen as an essential part of any animation movie. This is why the spectator is more prone to identify himself with an anthropomorphised machine than with an anonymous humanoid.

In films as *Polar Express*, *Beowulf* and *Avatar* the motion capture technology enables the spectators to identify themselves with their favourite actor in the character on screen and thanks to the technique of facial performance replacement they are able to recognise that corporeal dimension which technology is unable to eliminate. This demonstrates that all the technologies that aim to make the invisible (emotions, feelings etc.) visible, not only fail to diminish the importance of corporeality, but make the body's presence even more necessary. The film *Avatar* fits perfectly within this context. The protagonist of the story, Jake Sully, is an invalid ex-marine. As an avatar he is able to move freely and this is why he, at the end of the story, decides to abandon his human body forever, transforming himself into his avatar. In a certain sense, the film foresees the possible realisation of the Platonic dream to liberate humankind from the carnal prison of the body. The question, however, is whether this dream is still a *human* one. In *Avatar* the technique of facial performance replacement is not an end, but rather a means to concretise this utopia from a visual point of view. Yet, the nature of this medium shows us that we cannot do without the body. We are clearly facing a contradiction here: in order to create a pure image the facial performance replacement technique definitely needs the body of the actor to give origin to the image. Although playing a crucial role in all phases of a film, technology seems so far unable to eliminate the body. In fact, despite all technological advances, the corporeal dimension continues to determine the relationship between cinematographic representation and sensible reality. The attempt to create pure forms or images entirely made by computer graphics which are able to preserve the empathy between viewer and actor or star has (at least until now) failed.[6] Given the impossibility to ignore the physical body of the actor, one could speak in a certain sense of a kind of "ultra-body" (Uva 2011, p. 104), that is, of a physicality that can move beyond old limits and explore new horizons. Of course, this is possible because this process does not only affect the perception of the image and the emphatic relation between actor and spectator, but regards the ontology of the filmic image itself. Digital technology has been unable to reformulate the relationship between actor and character (given that the actor continues to be a physical subject on whose performance the "life" of the characters in the movie, be it in analogue or digital, depends) because the character, like all other elements of the film is always already the product of a *mise-en-scène*, always already part of a representation and therefore already an image; "the product of a process of artificialisation and simulation" (Bertetto 2007, p. 23, our translation).[7] If the filmic image, from its very beginnings, is distinguished by its ability to capture and make visible the bodily movements in space and time (Gunning 2007), then digital techniques as motion capture and digital performance replacement capture the image of this movement, or, if one wishes, the movement of a movement. Hence, one could argue that despite the technological evolution, nothing has really changed compared to the times in which the pioneers of cinema, Étienne-Jules Marey and Eadweard James Muybridge, tried to capture locomotion in a sequence of so-called "freeze-frames". All of this gives evidence of the fact that not everything is representable by technological means and that the body can never be completely erased. Not only the function of the actor, but also the nature of the cinematographic image prevent us from doing so.

5. Conclusion

The advent of the modern world (in the second half of the 19th century), characterised by the rise of mass communication, the technological acceleration of the means of transport, the triumph of the capitalist system and the establishment of an industrial visual culture, has profoundly altered the representation of the human in the visual arts. The body has always been an important source of information for this type of art by virtue of its visual essence, and this is especially the case with cinematic representation. The birth of cinema, at the end of the 19th century, not

6. In addition, one must not forget that *Avatar* is a film made for stereoscopic 3D, with the result that very little use has been made of rhetorical figures, such as close-up, which are very important to an actor.

7. Our translation of "il prodotto di un processo di artificializzazione e simulazione". (Bertetto 2007, p. 23).

only offered a new way to perceive and think about images, but it also gave these images the capacity to represent something real. The cinematographic actor continues to be perceived on the basis of a representation destined to provide a corporeal simulacrum body to an audience ready to believe in his moving image. This is exactly what Jacques Aumont intends with "the quality of the effects of reality" (Aumont 1991, pp. 12–13).

References

Amaducci, A. (2011). Un cinema senza film. In M. Gerosa (Ed.), *Cinema e tecnologia* (pp. 30–41). Genova: Le Mani.

Artioli, U. (1972). *Teorie della scena dal naturalismo al simbolismo, Vol. 1: Dai Meininger a Craig.* Firenze: Sansoni.

Attolini, G. (1996). *Gordon Craig.* Roma-Bari: Laterza.

Aumont, J. (1989). *L'Œil interminable. Cinéma et peinture.* Paris: Lignes (Italian tranlation (1991). *L'occhio interminabile. Cinema e pittura.* Venezia: Marsilio).

Bazin, A. (1958). *Qu'est ce-que le cinéma?* Paris: Cerf (Italian translation (1973). *Che cos'è il cinema?* Milano: Garzanti).

Bertetto, P. (2007). *Lo specchio e il simulacro. Il cinema nel mondo diventato favola.* Milano: Bulzoni.

Casini Ropa, E. (Ed.) (1990). *Alle origini della danza moderna.* Bologna: Il Mulino.

Craig, E.G. (1911). The Actor and the Über-Marionette. In *The Art of the Theatre* (pp. 80–94). London: Heinemann.

De Clercq, E. (2009). The Seduction of the Female Body and the Ambiguity of Love. *Theoria, Metamorphoses of Love, 29*(2), 198–206.

De Marinis, M. (2000). *In cerca dell'attore. Un bilancio del Novecento teatrale.* Roma: Bulzoni.

Dorra, H. (Ed.) (1994). *Symbolist Art Theories: A Critical Anthology.* Berkeley: University of California Press.

Gunning, T. (1995). Tracing the Individual Body: Photography, Detectives and Early Cinema. In L. Charney & W.R. Schwartz (Eds.), *Cinema and Invention of Modern Life* (pp. 15–45). Berkeley/Los Angeles/London: University of California Press.

Hayles, K. (1999). *How We Became Posthuman: Virtual Bodies in Cybernetic, Literature and Informatics.* Chicago/London: University of Chicago Press.

Luisi, M. (Ed.). (2009). *Esperienza e percezione: percorsi nella fenomenologia.* Pisa: ETS.

Molinari, C. (1996). *Storia del teatro.* Roma-Bari: Laterza.

Moravec, H. (1988). *Mind Children: The Future of Robot and Human Intelligence.* Cambridge Mass.: Harvard University Press.

Mori, M. (1970). The Uncanny Valley. *Energy, 7*(4), 33–35.

Plantec, P. (2007). Crossing the Great Uncanny Valley. *VFX World Magazine.* Retrieved from www.awn.com/articles/production/crossing-great-uncanny-valley/page/1%2C1, May 2012.

Spanu, M. (2011). Al cinema con gli occhiali. Regia, spazio, attore al tempo di Avatar. In M. Gerosa (Ed.), *Cinema e tecnologia* (pp. 164–177). Genova: Le Mani.

Terzo, M. (2011). Ambienti digitali. In M. Gerosa (Ed.), *Cinema e tecnologia* (pp. 73–81). Genova: Le Mani.

Uva, C. (2011). L'attore e la digital performance nel cinema sintetico. In M. Gerosa (Ed.), *Cinema e tecnologia* (pp. 93–106). Genova: Le Mani.

Embodiment

Technologies and musics

Don Ihde
Department of Philosophy, Stony Brook University

1. Introduction

The history of humans producing and experiencing music is probably at least as ancient as *homo sapiens sapiens* and Neanderthals or older, and just as diverse as every culture known to anyone. In this chapter I want to take both a long and broad look at music production and experience, but also focus particularly upon "musical technologies" or instrumentation. The perspective I take here is triply "phenomenological". First, it is descriptive: I take it the phenomenon of music is a highly varied one – I shall use the term "musics" in the plural to emphasise this point. I shall also avoid any ideological preference which favours one style, culture, or type of music and retain a musically relativist stance (which can, however, emphasise virtuoso results over novice ones). Second, I shall use variations in the form of concrete illustrations to exhibit this musical richness which the phenomenon displays. And third, I shall take note of the different forms of embodiment which the different music productions take.

2. Where we are

If we begin from the here and now, and primarily in the context of late modern, global culture, I suspect the single largest set of produced "musics" is that which is usually called recorded or re-produced music, i.e. the many varieties of records, CDs, iPods, tapes, broadcast recordings (both aural and audio-visual) and the rest. The electronic and digital explosion of music dissemination is so pervasive that it is simply taken-for-granted and therefore it is easy to miss its implications for a deeper understanding of the human experience of music. The above should be obvious to anyone. In the context here, I shall refer to such musics as *constructed musics* which are complex and entail both performances, constructing technologies ("studios") and production technologies.

When we turn to the very special world of musicians and musicologists, we might find a different take on this dominant technological embodiment of music. Musicians, of course, do have a unique perspective upon music insofar as they are the humans who *produce* the original musical performances which their audiences or listeners experience. Musicologists (and I include composers here) are more the theoreticians and critics of music production and, from their perspective again, have a unique take upon musical performance and production. Stop! This is already taking too much for granted since it already presupposes a contemporary set of socially embedded practices which must take place within a much larger and more complicated scene. So, I shall open this analysis anecdotally: I was once a Dean of Humanities and Fine Arts in my university. In this setting the Music Department was clearly the premier arts department and its dominant and large graduate program emphasized performance – but it also had a core of *avant-garde* composers and musicologists. In the context of a highly charged tenure case, I had to learn something about the "sociology" of this group to be informed about the case at hand. What I learned was that the perspective which the majority of our musicologist-composers took upon music was focused upon a very specialised experiential technique: to "experience" music and judge it; one *read and analysed the score,* a form of "text" as it were. But, specialised training also allows such "readers" to imaginatively *hear* the music through this reading. I understood this phenomenologically – but it also seemed strange since this type of music was clearly *technologically disembodied* and not fully a perceptual listening. Then, I learned something more – associated with this specialised visual score-imagined music experience, there was also a more selective musical ideology. Now while I would argue, phenomenologically, that any kind of music should be able to be so specially experienced by the trained score reader-imaginer, in this case the preferred style of music was that of a kind of pure atonality, a highly abstract, and "mathematised" music. This should not actually come as a surprise since the phenomenological practice of this kind of "reading-imagining" pretty neatly fits into something similar to a mathematical experiential practice. Unfortunately and precisely because such expert experience takes this shape, it also leaves out of account many, many other varieties of possible experience and styles of music.

Second anecdote: A decade later, after completing my learning experience in deaning, I became interested in so-called "synthesised" music. My son, Mark, at that time was taking pre-college composition classes using digital computational devices, and simultaneously I was communicating with and learning from Trevor Pinch about the history and sociology of analog synthesizers. The three of us did a panel on synthesised music in Vienna (2001), and I returned to Vienna again the following year and gave a paper to an interdisciplinary group at the university, using some examples from electronically produced music. During the discussion, a couple of musicians, performers, chided me for allowing such a drift away from "pure music". In this case, unlike the previous example, "pure music" turned out to be music performed and played only with the instruments appropriate to the periods in which the music was composed, i.e. early music called for early instruments. In this case the narrowing of the "pure" was a performer's sense of "authenticity" determined by a peculiar historical sense. Apart from possible historiological problems to be found here – how can one know the precise instrumentation and arrangements from four centuries ago? – my interest was again more phenomenological. What is the range of musical possibility and its variations?

3. Where does music come from?

To open up the questions I have raised, I will first turn to some anthropological-archaeological speculation concerning human music origins. To this I will add observations related to the history of technologies. To find actual origins is probably a hopeless task – yet perhaps the simplest and most "bodily" origin of human produced music must include *singing*. I, myself, suspect that singing and some of its variants may precede or accompany the rise of language itself. Language itself is, after all, musical in some sense too. There is cadence, tone, pitch and the like, although usually highly conventionalised. Singing can be at the least a sort of exaggeration of the sound patterns which are more limited in ordinary language. Nor would I want to exclude other bodily expressed musical or proto-musical sounds: whistling, yodelling, throat singing, individual and social musical expressions, clearly must go back as far as early humanity. But – so far – we have no way of recovering such sounds.[1]

What about *instrumentally* produced music? Again, the task of finding the first uses of extra-body instruments is equally hopeless. Using a stick or other object to "drum" could be as old as humans, maybe even some animals. Woodpeckers with hard beaks are springtime drummers. In 1997 a cave bear bone flute, carbon dated back to 43,000+ BP was found and thought to be associated with Neanderthal sites and when analysed with respect to its tuning style, it turned out that distances between the holes yield an acoustical result which produces a diatonic tone scale

1. There have been some attempts to find proxy sounds, for example in materials which harden rapidly, such as some paints which may "record" sound vibrations during the hardening process, but to date there is very limited success with such techniques.

not too dissimilar to that of much later Greek tuning systems 40 millennia later![2] And how far back do stringed instruments go? These would not be easily preserved since sinew and wood are unlikely to survive the millennia of their origins. My own suspicion is that since the technology of archery – string under tension in a bow arrangement – can have a musical variation by plucking or rubbing, and since any archer can hear the bow string make its "musical" sound when fired, some form of stringed instrument could be at least as old as archery which can be dated back at least to 20,000+ BP. Finally, in my anthropological-archaeological-historical speculation I will surmise that just as archery was invented by almost all pre-historical cultures, so, likely were simple stringed musical instruments – I will add that I suspect the antique musical instrument kit included wind (Kudu horns in Africa; rams horns or shofars in the Middle East), percussion (drums are everywhere) and the previously mentioned string variants (in addition to the bodily expressive musics noted previously).

4. A phenomenology of instrumentation

In the previous illustrations and speculations, I have differentiated between two types of human musical production. In one set of examples, under "singing" and its variants, one may note that this type of musical production is directly *bodily expressive.* I have not even come close to exhausting such direct bodily musical expressivity. Singing, whistling, varieties of bodily sound production should also be expanded to variations upon whole body movement such as dance, even self-percussion such as slapping oneself or other objects.

In the second set of examples, I began to suggest varieties of musical *technologies,* or instruments, at first directly incorporated into bodily practices. Flutes, simple stringed instruments, percussion instruments such as those suggested, arise many millennia ago and all fall under a distinctive human-technology use which I have earlier called *embodiment relations.*[3] By this I mean that the human or humans producing the music, do so *through* material artifacts or instruments. The simple examples cited are all "played" by bodily using these artifacts to produce musical sounds. Going into this practice, of course, there can be a learning, the development of special techniques, higher and higher skills of sound and music making, the development of styles, schools of musical traditions

2. One cave bear flute with four holes has been dated to 43000+ BP and associated with Neanderthal tools. See *The AAAS Science News Service,* April 3, 1997.

3. My phenomenology of human-technology relations may be found in *Technics and Praxis* (1979) and in more detailed form in *Technology and the Lifeworld* (1990).

and instrumental developments. All this is presupposed by our instant ability to differentiate between the novice and the virtuoso performers in musical performances. Early instruments tended to be fairly simple even if widely varied, and I want to say, such simpler instruments also tended to demand highly skilled bodily movement. To produce overtones with simple string instruments or with wind instruments, very fine skills and much practice are needed.

The bone flute mentioned clearly called for fine fingering and exquisite breath techniques for any musical nuance; early stringed instruments usually utilised a small number of strings, but over time often became more and more complex with larger numbers of strings. These were plucked – with or without plucks, often with specially trimmed fingernail shapes – bowed, and later mechanically played. I have often been fascinated with instrument museums, particularly in Europe, which display the history of experimentation upon stringed instruments. In this Eurocentric case it is interesting to note in passing that from a small number of strings (one to six) in early instruments, there was a period when the numbers increased (from six to twelve and more) but then returned to the now "classical" (from four to six) set on violins through guitar string numbers for concert uses, that is with instruments which call for primarily hand play (the exceptions are harps and zither-like instruments with many more strings, see below).

These are "technological" innovations, but remain within the range of clear bodily hand and finger capacities. By "classical" times, however, harps, zithers, and multi-string instruments also appeared which were still finger or finger plus pluck played. In all these cases musical nuance was again attained through skilled hand/finger motion. A second step occurs once the playing was "mechanised" by using keys with mechanical plucks (claviers, harpsichords) or valves (brass and woodwinds). Here something quite interesting happened in music history. Arguments broke out concerning the alienation of "pure" hand playing as it "degraded" into "mechanical" playing. This happened in the transition from the harp to the keyboard instruments, and again from the simplest plucking devices to the more complex ones of the piano-forte (Pinch & Bijsterveld 2000, pp. 3–5). And it happened with winds and the introduction of valves over fingers in both woodwind and brass instruments. Objections regarding the loss of expressivity, the loss of nuance, the "mechanisation" of music, and the loss of "romanticism" occurred (ibid., pp. 6–7). This was a "Heidegger"-like response to modern technology now concerning musical technologies.[4]

4. Martin Heidegger disliked any writing technologies other than the pen – even the typewriter detracted from the preferred, primordial practice of penmanship. See Michael Heim, *Electronic Language: A Philosophical Study of Word Processing* (1987, pp. 210 ff).

One set of resistances is understandable: musicians had to learn new skills; such skills take time and discipline; and one does not immediately produce virtuoso performances – yet, once attained, who can doubt the expressivity of any master piano player over a novice, or take appreciative note of the new capacities of the human-instrument result. One can imagine, too, that with each style of production, it is possible for one to reify some kind of "purity". Did our ancestors who sang claim that only singing was "pure" music? There have been moments in our histories in which only singing, and within song, only sacred tones are worthy, and there were times when polyphony was eschewed. And there have been religions which allow only a capella hymns with no organs or other instruments allowed (except a tuning device!).[5] But then, once a new human-instrument relation is attained, there can again emerge a sort of tradition-of-the-instrument which stabilises and allows the sorting out of the virtuosi on the concert circuit. In short, I am suggesting that modern musical experience is contexted in a history-of-technologies setting in which instrumental innovation plays a major role.[6]

5. Instrumental trajectories

I am now ready, finally, to turn to *late* modern music and its embeddedness in late modern musical technologies, which introduce new complexities and possibilities for musics. For a brief moment I shall leap over the earliest, still mechanical technologies which allowed *recording,* and continue the ever more complex trajectory of human-instrument music transformations by taking initial note of *electric and electronic* technologies. These technologies might be added onto historically extant acoustic instruments, or they might also become part of the sound production itself. To make things simple, I shall first focus upon *amplification.* Today, even acoustically good auditoria often also use amplification – as in most opera houses. Here the attempt is to make the amplification as inobtrusive and "transparent" as possible, to have technologies which make it seem as if the singer were *not* technologically assisted. At the

5. Strictly a cappella singing was the tradition amongst many of the Germanic religious groups familiar to me as a boy in Kansas; my own equally Anabaptist group did allow a piano.

6. It is interesting to note in passing that instrumental history in science differs with that of instrumental history in music. In science it is presumed that many and newer instruments are better; one does not go back to "historical" instruments to perform science. But in music, historical instruments continue to be played and have value, and may even be thought of as having higher value.

other extreme, amplification can take on its own unique preferred sound quality and becomes identified with the style of music itself – Rock music is an example. In the first case, the musical tradition wants the *prima donna* to sing as if not amplified; in the second case the mike-amplified voice *is* the preferred voice of the rock singer. We do not want to hear the non-amplified voice of the rock singer.[7] Amplification "magnifies" sound, but unavoidably it also transforms it. All technologies are non-neutrally transformational, including musical ones. In the two examples noted, amplification ranges from a minimalist and transparent capacity to an enhancement of the amplificational transformation from the technology's own unique transformational capacities. Thus while the performer remains "bodily" active in producing the song, the singer+instrument can vary away from direct, body-only activity.

But this has always been so. If I take the Xhosa Uhadi as an example, this African single stringed instrument is constructed very much like an archery bow, with a curved wooden tensioner, to which is attached an open ended gourd resonator. The string is played with a second bow and its music utilises basically two tones, but the virtuoso player can produce overtones within a minimalist style of playing which is then highly expressive and appreciated by the trained listener. The resonator both "magnifies" the sounds, but also transforms them. And, there is an obvious art to producing excellence even with simple resonating acoustical amplification – thus the sought after Guarneri and Stradivari violin phenomenon. I am claiming that electronic amplification lies on the same trajectory as resonation amplification, but its electronic possibilities are much more "active" than those of classical echo or resonance amplification. Electronic amplification carries the possibility of moving to a much more active sound transformation and even to sound production itself, as in electronic synthesizers, a possibility to be explored below.

I am, of course suggesting that not only do instruments – musical technologies – play an essential role in music production, but the history of instruments parallels that of technological history itself. The move is from simpler to more complex and compound technologies, and although this has been a background feature of this analysis, also this history evidences a move from direct bodily expressive musics to more instrumentally mediated musics, and in late modernity, on to musics which are or can be more *indirectly* related to first-person practices. The "same" musical piece can be repeatedly played both temporally and spatially. This is to say that the when and where the human player takes in musical production can also vary.

---

7. My "Bach to Rock", in *Technics and Praxis,* (1979) analyses this difference in detail.

6. Digital postmodernism

In simplest terms, I now have several styles of human-technology music production: direct bodily production (singing-dancing variants), body-instrument variants, and then the "constructed" add-ons to simple instruments which include amplification and digitally produced technologies and on to studio settings. I have suggested in all the "histories" with each new musical technology, there is a time of experimentation and performance "tuning" which is entered. To listen to constructed music however, may entail a certain blindness to this process. Constructed music entails a studio which is a complex location with new processes involved. Acoustical space is constructed; takes, re-takes, and increasing musical editing goes into the development of constructed music such that a simple live-performance recording becomes but one possibility out of many. Active "construction" is the norm. The editing process "picks and chooses" the best takes (the analog with cinema editing is obvious) to produce the "best" result. Time forward and we enter the age of the "remix".

It is here that we also reach *postmodernity*. One of the themes concerning postmodernity, sometimes nostalgically decried, is the "death of the author" or the "subject". And, there is the blurring of the boundaries between different "texts", those of the author of the novel, for example, and the critic who increasingly claims equal rights as writer. My point takes its departure by my focus upon the materiality of the technologies with which our writers, authors, subjects – now composers, performers, listeners interact. The musics which are studio and recording produced are no longer merely materialised performances; they are "constructed" pieces of repeatable musics. And a new set of possibilities begins to shape a new trajectory here as well. Note that this is a historical trajectory which entails much more than first-person to bodily-instrumental mediation. It is also a movement to variations upon "corporate" or social complexity. The remixer, the DJ, is a new actor in constructed musics.

Related, in constructed music, is the process of machine produced sound such as occurs with digital and analog synthesised sound. Trevor Pinch and Frank Trocco (2000) have noted this in *Analog Days: The Invention and Impact of the Moog Synthesizer.* Electronic music was experimental in several forms by the mid-20th century. Strange instruments like the theremin were played by hand motion within an oscillator generated electric field and produced weird "whining" sounds – these sounds were picked up by movie producers for sound effects. The theremin turned out to be a very hard to play instrument since the player simply had to make hand motions within the electric field and had no felt resistance such as frets or keys to feel. In more classical acoustic instruments, a material feed-back provided a different "feel" through which the player could learn.

A single machine which could produce whole sets of electronically produced sounds was invented only in the '60's by Robert Moog and, separately, by Don Buchla. Electronic oscillators, feed-back circuits, filters and dampeners were combined into boxes which could be played by a keyboard in the case of Moog, or by dials and switches in the case of Buchla. The new sounds, which could cover the full range of human hearing capacities, were early picked up by both movie makers (particularly science fiction and horror styles), but also by rock and other already electronically amplified music makers (including Frank Zappa and the Beatles).

And while the specialised use of synthesizers remained somewhat restricted, a second blink is illustrated in the sort of popular hybrid synthesizer, the electronic keyboard, which soon swept the industrialised world in sales and popularity. Every high school "band" playing in a garage had one. By hybrid, I mean that keyboards often utilized *recorded* sounds, for example from extant instruments, and these could be played by anyone skilled in keyboard skills. One could choose piano, harpsichord, koto ... on to drums, organs and the like in a built-in bricolage of possibilities. These hybrids are a form of "constructed" music, but such sounds which then are played, performed, in a new human-instrument practice. One might appreciate the disdain that skilled expressive piano players might feel since bodily skill could not produce nuanced sound differences on such machines. But that is not where the strength of this musical trajectory lies. Its strengths had to be discovered through both new bodily skills and the exploration of what new and transformed sounds could be produced.

The *digital synthesizer* takes this a step farther. As with the analog synthesizers, the digital variety uses electronic means of producing sounds, but in this case parallel to digital photography, each sound is itself open to manipulation. In our own Stony Brook "composition lab" the machines have both a visual display and audio play. One can literally display the sound wave one wants to create and "sculpt" it according to wish. And, in this case there are no "originals" which have been recorded – this is no longer a "recording" technology. And, it is a technology which can, through human-instrument created "programming" produce music which exceeds ordinary human performance capacities. I close with a very simple example: one of my son's composition hook-ups combined a digital keyboard with a composition program run on a desktop computer. One way of composing retained a traditional set of player-instrument relations. Mark could play his piece on the keyboard and the program would display it on the screen, and when ready after tinkering, he could save and print out a score. This was close to a traditional mode of composing except that the slow and painful process of inking in notes by hand was replaced by an immediate full staff scoring of anything played. But the process could also be reversed. Mark could produce a score with any number of notes on the staff, many more than the ten which one person could play with ten fingers, or even the twenty a duet of players could play, and moreover have them played at tempos too fast for any human to play! Is this, then, *posthuman* music? In phenomenological terms, this means again that the when and where of the human bodily actor may be changed.

7. Phenomenological reprise

But for one more step, I have finished my anthropological-archaeological-historical set of variations. And while I have usually referred to actual events, artifacts and technologies, I have been using these as concrete *phenomenological variations.* All the musics referred to imply roles involving *embodiment, experienced perceptions,* in relation to musical sounds. By casting my variations in the context of a technology of instrumentation, I have been suggesting that contemporary musical technologies introduce new elements and possibilities into the production of musics. For example, once recording technologies were invented, different variations upon human-technology relations were also introduced. With recording, the live performance while "causal" in the recording chain of events, once recorded recedes in experienced space-time. Then, with the capacity to manipulate the final result through studio-editing processes, a different set of roles for human actors enters the musical production. And, finally, with the variants upon synthesizers, note that yet a different set of variations obtains. The composer becomes, as it were, the player as well. By "playing" the programs, the electronic machines, and then when satisfied, fixing or "recording" the result, one returns in a new way to the embodied player-instrument relation.

I have hinted at the possibilities for lovers of "purities" to react to these new musical variations at any point. Nostalgias for older modes and instruments, elitist reactions to new social contexts for musics, resistances to adapting to technologies can and do occur all along the variant spectrum. Nor should one forget that many musics and instruments are, in fact, abandoned. In contrast, the musical relativism I have practiced here emphasises that creativity and innovation can in fact occur with and within each of the possibilities noted. I have also suggested that recorded musics are in some sense transitional, or at the least only one set of musical practices, and I will conclude with one final variation which is basically the most contemporary of all.

8. Musics from beyond hearing

Ancient Chinese acoustics long ago recognised that there was sound beyond human hearing. Touching bells when sound had disappeared still yielded tactile perception of vibrations continuous with previously heard vibrations. But they had no way of recovering these within human perception. In a visual analog, until the 20th century all astronomy was optical, i.e. light emitting, astronomy, but since first the invention of radio astronomy, since expanded from gamma waves to radio waves, astronomy can now *translate* the full frequencies of the microwave spectrum into visual images which are perceivable. And while the sciences tend to favour visual imaging, the same translation variations are possible for sound.

Digital and computer processes today may translate data into images, or reverse the process and reduce images to data. This is the same process which lays behind my previous composition program referred to above. Once noted, one can search for and produce musics of many phenomena. But to attain perceptible results a mediated technological transformation is needed, a new "musical instrument" as it were. In the variations I am pointing to, both ultra- and infra-sounds can be so translated. For example, biologists have recently discovered that just as whales produce changeable cycles of songs recorded only in the last few decades, songs which are mostly at infrasound frequencies, today now at ultra-sound levels, mice, too, sing courting songs to their ladies.[8] Both these examples are "near hearing" examples. Much more extreme examples can come from phenomena previously not at all associated with musics. One imaginative artist has hooked up a geosatellite device which detects the wobble of the satellite to a digital piano and "played" the wobble music – it sounds quite like a Philip Glass or Steve Reich minimalist music.[9] But here the embodied human is engaged only in the set up of the technology complex. A much more extreme example may be found in the work of Felix Hess, a Dutch physicist-turned-artist. He has recorded what he discovered to be the rhythms of high and low pressure storm systems off the Icelandic coasts, but which could be detected with infra-sound equipment over Holland. By time compression (24 hours reduced to 8 minutes) with the consequent raising of frequencies into human hearing range, he has recorded what I call "earth songs" (Hess 2003). The possibilities of musics not yet heard, within in some sense the possibilities of recorded musics, are far from exhaustion.

My narrative has been both historical and phenomenological insofar as the examples I have given are from concrete musical technologies and I take account

8. Male mice have long been known to emit ultrasonic sounds in the presence of females, but only recently were these sounds noted to be more complex than mere "squeaks", and instead function as a sort of courting song. See Timothy Holy and Zhongshen Guo reporting in *PloS Biology*, Vol. 3, Issue 12, 2005.

9. "Ground Station", by Daniel Joliffe and Jocelyn Robert, a CD which recorded a digital piano playing satellite signals at the Surrey Art Gallery 2003, for reference: artgallery@city.surrey.bc.ca

of different styles and forms of human embodiment. What complicates this situation is that there are multiple possibilities concerning where and when we fit into the multiplicity of musics, of instruments, and both social and technological contexts.

References

Heim, M. (1987). *Electronic Language: A Philosophical Study of Word Processing.* New Haven: Yale University Press.

Hess, F. (2003). *Light as Air.* Heidelberg: Keher Verlag.

Holy, T., & Guo, Z. (2005). Ultrasonic Songs of Male Mice, *PloS Biology, 3*(12), e386.

Ihde, D. (1979). *Technics and Praxis: A Philosophy of Technology.* Dordrecht: Reidl Publishers.

Ihde, D. (1990). *Technology and the Lifeworld: From Garden to Earth.* Bloomington: Indiana University Press.

Joliffe, D., & Robert, J. (1999–2003). *Ground Station.* http://www.danieljolliffe.ca/sdn/sdn.htm (Accessed October 2012)

Neandertals Lived Harmoniously, *The AAAS Science News Service*, April 3, 1997.

Pinch, T., & Bijsterveld, K. (2000). *Breaches and Boundaries in the Reception of New Technologies in Music.* Ithaca: Cornell working papers.

Pinch, T., & Trocco, F. (2000). *Analog Days: The Invention and Impact of the Moog Synthesizer.* Cambridge: Harvard University Press.

Is gesture knowledge? A philosophical approach to the epistemology of musical gestures

Michael Funk & Mark Coeckelbergh
Technische Universität Dresden and University of Twente

1. Introduction

With this chapter we want to provide a philosophical approach to the epistemology of *musical gestures* as a perspective to the discussion of *moving imagination*. Our basic question is: "Is gesture knowledge?"

In section two we want to clarify the context of studies on musical gestures in musical scholarship and its interdisciplinary implications. Definitions of musical gestures are introduced with respect to two basic assumptions: meaning and movement. The third section is on classical epistemology. We discuss the definition of propositional knowledge, its Platonic implications and we also focus on critiques. In the next step, and with respect to Michael Polanyi, we reconstruct the limits of propositional knowledge and the potentials of implicit knowledge for an epistemology of musical gestures. In the fifth section the notion of post-Cartesian thinking and gestures as critique on Cartesian dualism are discussed by taking into account the epistemology of Ludwig Wittgenstein and the enactive approach with its implications for sensorimotor knowledge and its embodiment. After these epistemological steps with respect to Bernhard Irrgang, Don Ihde, Marc Leman and Rolf Inge Godøy, we focus on technical mediation of gestural body movements and material, non-linguistic, hermeneutics. Section seven is on cultural and social aspects. We introduce three forms of knowledge, the concepts of dis-embodiment and re-embodiment and the cultural dependence of musical gestures with respect to Western score-oriented music(s) and Indian music(s). The results and thesis are summarised in the last section.

2. Musical gestures as subject of musical scholarship and interdisciplinary research

Currently, in musical scholarship interdisciplinary shaped discussions on musical gestures, respectively the relation between music and gestures develops increasingly.

These discussions are characteristic for methodological changes from score centered research to body oriented studies in musical scholarship at the beginning of the 21st century (Leman 2008, pp. 27–49, Godøy & Leman 2010, p. ix, Gritten & King 2006, p. ix). The "First International Conference on Music and Gesture [...] was held in August 2003" (Gritten & King 2006, p. xix). With respect to piano music, for Robert S. Hatten musical gestures became the main topic in his *Interpreting Musical Gestures, Topics, and Tropes* (Hatten 2004). This book is another important contribution to the systematic research of musical gestures (Mazzola & Cherlin 2009, p. 68).

The terminology and methodology in research on gestures depends on the academic context: "What can be said about the nature of gestures is very much dependent on the paradigm in which they are studied." (Ishino & Stam 2011, p. 6) Studying gestures and especially musical gestures means interdisciplinary research (Gritten & King 2011, pp. 1ff., Jensenius et al. 2010, p. 28, Leman & Godøy 2010, p. 10).

> Consequently, the field has attracted researchers from a number of different disciplines such as anthropology, cognitive science, communication, neuroscience, psycholinguistics, primatology, psychology, robotics, sociology and semiotics, and the number of modern gesture studies has grown. (Ishino & Stam 2011, p. 3)

With this chapter we want to add a philosophical perspective to the discussion. To clarify our academic background and the methodological paradigm it is important to indicate that philosophical research on musical gestures does not necessarily mean empirical studies of musical practice. We focus on conceptual analysis with respect to the history of philosophical thinking. Therefore we need a systematic starting point: a definition of musical gesture.

Definitions of gesture in terms of communication or control, and metaphors with respect to the recent discussions are summarised in Jensenius et al. (2010, p. 14–19). The approach of Hatten (2004) is interpreted as the metaphorical definition because of his crucial claim that gestural competency arises from physical, biological, cognitive, social, cultural and multi-stylistic experience. This definition is discussed in Jensenius et al. (2010, p. 18) insofar

> he seems not to refer to the body movement or the generating actions that create sound. [...] [And a] somewhat analogous definition to those of [...] Hatten is suggested in (Gritten & King 2006, xx) [...].

Hatten states: "I define human gesture rather inclusively as *any energetic shaping through time that may be interpreted as significant*." (Hatten 2006, p. 1) Anthony Gritten and Elaine King (2011, p. 1) furthermore are supporting him with this statement: "Hatten's definition of human gesture as 'any energetic shaping through time that may be interpreted as significant' (2006, p. 1) provides a central starting point for researchers." (Gritten & King 2011, p. 1) But most attempts to find a definition of musical gesture remain "vague to some extent" (Jensenius et al. 2010, p. 30, see also Ishino & Stam 2011, p. 4). There is no overarching and adequate definition. But explicitly or at least implicitly, and at first sight, movement (action) and meaning (significance) in relation to sound shape the roots of 21st century research on musical gestures. Rolf Inge Godøy and Marc Leman claim:

> We would go so far as to claim that music is basically a combination of sound and movement, and that music means something to us because of this combination. We use the expression "musical gesture" to denote this meaningful combination of sound and movement [...].
> (Godøy & Leman 2010, p. ix, see also Leman & Godøy 2010, p. 3)

Whether or not Hatten addresses the notion of body movement and action for studying musical gestures adequately (Jensenius et al. 2010, p. 18), even for Gritten and King movement and significance seems to be a "ground assumption":

> a gesture is movement or change in state that becomes marked as significant by an agent. This is to say that for movement or sound to be(come) gesture, it must be taken intentionally by an interpreter, who may or may not be involved in the actual sound production of a performance, in such a manner as to donate it with the trappings of human significance. (Gritten & King 2006, p. xx)

And in 2011 both authors highlight the significance of physical movement:

> Indeed, all of the chapters are grounded in the premise that musical gestures are cross-modal and that gestures include non-sounding physical movements as well as those that produce sound. (Gritten & King 2011, p. 6)

For Jensenius et al. (2010, p. 30) "most authors seem to agree that gestures involve both body movement and meaning." Guerino Mazzola and Paul Cherlin accept movement as an implicit aspect of what they call "hypergesture" in their *Flow, Gesture, and Spaces in Free Jazz*. Gestures are "complex configurations of curves" and thereby the abstract form of complex movements (Mazzola & Cherlin 2009, p. 80). "The problem is not only one of realistic representation of body movement." (Mazzola & Cherlin 2009, p. 82) But without body movement there would be no gesture at all. Another assumption of gestural action and meaning is formulated in Gale Stam and Mika Ishino's volume *Integrating Gestures, The interdisciplinary nature of gesture*:

> Nevertheless, the gestures that each author in this volume deals with are all visible bodily actions employed intentionally and meaningfully. This is a broad definition that covers the many different aspects of gestures. (Ishino & Stam 2011, p. 4)

One can argue that movement (action) and meaning (significance) are not only characteristic of musical gestures, but also for gestures in dance or in theatre, as well as for any other gesture in human life. From a philosophical point of view, we have the following reason to answer the question "Is gesture knowledge?" with respect to *musical* gestures: As Georg Mohr argues, for epistemological investigations, music is an interesting and outstanding topic. Music is a basic part of human everyday life as well as subject of specialised scientific investigations (Mohr 2011, p. 1318). Because of its peculiar combination between abstract symbols for example in musical scores and complex bodily and technical interpretations of music(s) we can illustrate the main epistemological theses in a paradigmatic way.

3. Classical epistemology and propositional knowledge

Epistêmê is the ancient Greek word for knowledge (Horn & Rapp 2002, pp. 146f.), and thus epistemology means philosophy of knowledge and knowing. Classical epistemology is specialised in investigations about certain terms and linguistic concepts. Thereby the notion of visual perception is often seen as more important than acoustical perception, and the meanings and understandings of music(s) are systematically blended out (Mohr 2011, p. 1317). This narrowing of classical epistemology is related to the concept of propositional knowledge.

The discussion of propositional knowledge shapes modern epistemology (Hardy & Meier-Oeser 2004, p. 855) and was strongly presented in the standard analytical epistemology of the 20th century by Edmund Gettier (Anacker 2004, p. 897). This epistemology, Gettier argues, attempts to

> state necessary and sufficient conditions for someone's knowing a given proposition [...] can be stated in a form similar to the following:
>
> S knows that P IFF
> (i) P is true,
> (ii) S believes that P, and
> (iii) S is justified in believing that P.
>
> (Gettier 1963, p. 121)

His basic assumption is that knowledge needs to be analysed as *justified true belief*. In analytical epistemology, knowledge is seen as a term with necessary and sufficient conditions: we can say what we know in strict and clear words and we can even explain in strict and clear words the necessary and sufficient conditions for what knowledge is (Baumann 2006, p. 2, Rehkämpfer & Wachtendorf 2009, pp. 79f.).

Edmund Gettier identifies Plato as the basic ancient root for this approach: "Plato seems to be considering some such definition at Theaetetus 201, and perhaps accepting one at Meno 98." (Gettier 1963, p. 121) In the philosophy of Plato we can find this classical understanding of knowledge as *justified ("anchored") true belief* (Hardy 2004, p. 861; Meixner 2007, p. 109). In Plato's words:

> The problem is that they [true beliefs] tend not to stay for long; they escape from the human soul and this reduces their value, unless they're anchored by working out the reason. And this anchoring is recollection [...]. When true beliefs are anchored, they become pieces of knowledge and they become stable. That's why knowledge is more valuable than true belief, and the difference between the two is that knowledge has been anchored.
>
> (Plato 2005, p. 139/Meno 98a)

To understand the implications of this statement, one needs to pay attention to the sentence: "And this anchoring is recollection". Justification (anchoring) turns true beliefs into knowledge. But justification in that sense is *recollecting* (remembering) bodiless *ideas* (Frede 2007, p. 142). A human body can die, but the soul lives on and gets to know all true beliefs (*ideas*) when it leaves the sensory and material human world. But once the soul is reborn in a human body, all ideas are forgotten. In a Platonic way, learning in the everyday live means *recollecting* forgotten *ideas* (*anamnesis*). Insofar, knowledge is a state of the non-material soul, but not a matter of the sensory human body (Seitschek 2007, p. 330). Sense-data could be a first impulse for starting recollecting knowledge, but never sufficient for learning new knowledge (Seitschek 2007, p. 331). Insofar, Plato develops an approach of the apriority of knowledge, meaning that knowing is separated from the empirical everyday life (Seitschek 2007, p. 332).

Since Plato's theory of knowledge is a theory of recollection and separateness between soul and body (Thurner 2007, p. 99), it is only if one accepts these two premises (as Edmund Gettier and the analytical epistemology in his tradition implicitly do) that you can say that knowledge is *justified true belief*.

Plato diminishes the epistemic dimension of human bodies and empirical perception (Borsche 1980b, p. 186; Brinker 2007, p. 254; Meixner 2007, p. 114; Thurner 2007, p. 99); an impact that characterised European philosophy until modernity and analytical epistemology till today (Böhme 2003, pp. 11ff., pp. 51ff., p. 224; Irrgang 2005, p. 7, pp. 29ff., p. 208; Irrgang 2009a, p. 109). The concept of propositional knowledge with its Platonic implications is, however, not sufficient for explaining physical, material or sensory body-movement (Perkams 2007, p. 56). Insofar, this approach is not sufficient for explaining knowledge of musical gestures and needs to be criticised and complemented.

Plato himself provides all aspects of the classical definition of propositional knowledge, but he also included strong critique of this concept in his philosophical work (Meixner 2007, p. 109). His far reaching insight into the inadequacy of the classical definition of knowledge has been forgotten until Gettier reactivated this insight in the mid-20th century (Meixner 2007, p. 116). He is criticizing propositional knowledge, because justification (I) of true (II) beliefs (III) seems not to be sufficient: a fourth (IV?) parameter needs to be added (Gettier 1963, p. 121ff.). A rich discussion on the missing parameter or alternative definitions shapes analytical investigations till today (e.g. the overviews in Baumann 2006, Rehkämpfer & Wachtendorf 2009). But alternative philosophical approaches exist.

4. Implicit knowledge

Every justification needs a starting point. A justification for a true belief needs to be supported by a knowledge basis. But is this unjustified knowledge at the beginning of one certain justification really knowledge (Meixner 2007, p. 110)? Plato formulates this problem in Meno 80:

> The claim is that it's impossible for a man to search either for what he knows or for what he doesn't know: he wouldn't be searching for what he knows, since he knows it and that makes the search unnecessary, and he can't search for what he doesn't know either, since he doesn't even know what it is he's going to search for.
> (Plato 2005, p. 113/Meno 80e)

Plato didn't find a final solution for this problem (Meixner 2007, p. 110). In the 1960s, nearly the same time when Gettier published his influential paper about propositional knowledge, Polanyi captured the paradox of Meno 80:

> He [Plato in the Meno] says that to search for the solution of a problem is an absurdity; for either you know what you are looking for, and then there is no problem; or you do not know what you are looking for, and then you cannot expect to find anything. (Polanyi 2009, p. 22)

Polanyi's solution is not an approach of propositional knowledge with respect to explicit, strict and true words or linguistic concepts. The basis of Polanyi's solution is implicit knowledge: "I shall reconsider human knowledge by starting from the fact that *we can know more than we can tell*." (Polanyi 2009, p. 4) Within this insight, Polanyi criticises one premise of Plato's epistemology: the assumption that recollecting (*anamnesis*) is remembering forgotten ideas by a separated, bodiless soul. Polanyi argues:

> The solution which Plato offered for this paradox was that all discovery is a remembering of past lives. This explanation has hardly ever been accepted, but neither has any other solution been offered for avoiding the contradiction. (Polanyi 2009, p. 22)

Polanyi's conclusion is that explicit knowledge is not sufficient for explaining human knowing. Moreover, we need to pay attention to silent intimations:

> For the *Meno* conclusively that if all knowledge is explicit, i.e. capable of being clearly stated, then we cannot know a problem or look for its solution. And the *Meno* also shows, therefore, that if problems nevertheless exist, and discoveries can be made by solving them, we can know things, and important things, that we cannot tell. The kind of tacit knowledge that solves the paradox of the *Meno* consists in the intimation of something hidden, which we may yet discover. (Polanyi 2009, pp. 22–23)

His basic insight is that "Knowledge is an activity which would be better described as a process of knowing" (Polanyi 1969, p. 132). This statement illustrates Polanyi's sensitivity for the non-propositional basis of human knowing and the limits of reasoning.

> This conception of knowledge as personal knowing departs two closely related respects from the ideal of a strictly justifiable knowledge. It accredits man's capacity to acquire knowledge even though he cannot specify the grounds of his knowing […]. (Polanyi 1969, pp. 133f.)

Implicit knowledge is a matter of meaningful human corporeality ("understanding physiognomies"), competent activities ("performance of skills"), successful sensory actions ("proper use of sensory organs") and successful handling of instruments ("mastery of tools"):

> We have now established analogous structures in several processes of knowing: namely, (1) the understanding of physiognomies, (2) the performance of skills, (3) the proper use of sensory organs, and (4) the mastery of tools and probes. (Polanyi 1969, pp. 128)

The bases for implicit knowledge are not bodiless Platonic ideas, but sensory activities in everyday life. "A peculiar combination of skilful doing and knowing is present in the working of our senses." (Polanyi 1969, p. 126).

Implicit knowledge is an adequate concept for describing the subsidiary dimension in performing musical gestures. This means that a musician has knowledge in realising meaningful body movements that are related to sound, but is not able to explain his knowledge in strict and true words.

If we start from the premise that musical gestures are meaningful (significant) movements (actions) with respect to sound and assume that these movements are body-movements with respect to physiognomies, performing skills, the use of sensory organs and the mastery of instruments, then implicit knowledge is the epistemological basis for musical gestures.

Polanyi's differentiation into explicit and implicit knowledge shows strong similarities to Gilbert Ryle's approach in the ordinary language philosophy and his differentiation into *knowing that* and *knowing how* (Anacker 2004, p. 897; Ryle 1946). But this is not the only similarity. 20th century philosophy is shaped by strong intellectual movements against the primacy of Cartesian mind-body-dualism and its implications on philosophy of consciousness and knowledge. In the tradition of the Platonic distinction between soul and body, René Descartes established an ontological version of the mind-body-dualism that influenced early modern and modern philosophy (Böhme 2003, p. 54; Borsche 1980b, p. 186). Within his dualistic approach, the *res extensa* (physical body, corpus) and *res cogitans* (soul, mind) are thought as two separated substances (Descartes 2009, pp. 79–97). Criticising this mind-body-dualism means going beyond Plato's and Descartes' belief, that the mind (soul) is separated from the human sensory body and its actions during everyday life.

Polanyi and Ryle are important authors in the tradition of post-Cartesian thinking (Irrgang 2009a, p. 215; Rentsch 1980, p. 201). The fundamental critique on the distinction between mind and body makes these philosophical approaches appropriate for a philosophical epistemology of musical gestures.

5. Gesture as critique on Cartesian dualism

Critiques on Descartes' dualism are central in current discussions on musical gestures in musical scholarship. "The main advantage of using the term gestures is that it surpasses the Cartesian divide between physics and the mind." (Jensenius et al. 2010, p. 19) In his book *Embodied Music Cognition and Mediating Technology* Marc Leman develops a post-Cartesian approach:

> In particular, neuroscience has provided compelling arguments that the Cartesian division between mind and matter can no longer be maintained and that a disembodied mind as such does not exist [...]. [...] From that perspective, the subjective world of mental representation is *not* an autonomous category but a result of an embodied interaction with the physical environment.
>
> (Leman 2008, p. 13)

And with respect to this methodological observation, Jensenius et al. (2010, p. 13) state:

> The notion of gesture somehow covers both aspects [movement and meaning] and therefore bypasses the Cartesian divide between matter and mind. […] The crossing of this boundary is at the core of the entire embodiment paradigm and it forms the strength of the current extension from disembodied music cognition to embodied music cognition […].

From a philosophical point of view, disembodied music cognition is related to analytical epistemology which focuses on propositional knowledge. Embodied music cognition is appropriate for research on musical gestures and close to post-Cartesian philosophies such as the approach of implicit knowledge.

Next to Michael Polanyi and Gilbert Ryle, other authors of 20th century philosophy like Ludwig Wittgenstein, Martin Heidegger or Maurice Merleau-Ponty could be added because of their contribution to post-Cartesian thinking and its epistemological implications. Exemplarily, we focus on Ludwig Wittgenstein. Like Michael Polanyi, he presented a concept of implicit knowledge (Funk 2010, pp. 78ff.; Gröbl-Steinbach 2000, p. 39), like Gilbert Ryle, he formulated his epistemology with respect to ordinary language (Anacker, HWP 12, p. 897) and like Martin Heidegger, his approach is characterised by highlighting the philosophical significance of everyday life and its implemented background-knowledge (Irrgang 2010, pp. 45ff.; Rentsch 2003, p. 15).

The *Philosophical Investigations* of Ludwig Wittgenstein are characterised in many passages by an extensive critique of Cartesian epistemology and the premise of a mind-body-dualism (Rentsch 1980, p. 202). Wittgenstein argues:

> 78. Compare knowing and saying:
> how many metres high Mont Blanc is –
> how the word "game" is used –
> how a clarinet sounds.
> Someone who is surprised that one can know something and not be able to say it is perhaps thinking on a case like the first. Certainly not of one like the third.
> (Wittgenstein et al. 2010, p. 41e)

"If one knows the use of the word, one can say something about it, but one cannot specify what one knows in the way one can specify one's knowledge about the height of Mont Blanc." (Lugg 2000, p. 137) Wittgenstein "draws attention to the fact that we cannot always state what we know […]." (Lugg 2000, p. 137, see also Rentsch 2003, p. 15). But this non-propositional knowledge is not the physical opposite of a *justified true belief* of the bodiless soul. There is no distinction at all and that is why Wittgenstein rejects a grammatical dualism between "conscious" and "unconscious" (Wittgenstein et al. 2010, p. 60^{e}ff.). Once the mind-body-dualism and its implications are philosophically overcome, the methodological basis for a perspective on non-propositional knowledge and its implications is reached:

> 150. The grammar of the word "know" is evidently closely related to the grammar of the words "can", "is able to". But also closely related to that of the word "understand". (To have 'mastered' a technique.) (Wittgenstein et al. 2010, p. 65[e])

Mastering a technique, we can also say "skill", and "understanding" are aspects of knowing, which are not detachable from human sensory and bodily life. Here we find the epistemological parallel to Polanyi's approach on implicit knowledge:

> Though we may prefer to speak of *understanding* a comprehensive object or situation and of *mastering* a skill, we do use the two words nearly as synonyms. [...] A peculiar combination of skillful doing and knowing is present in the working of our senses. (Polanyi 1969, p. 126)

Skills, mastering of techniques and understanding of objects are equal and closely associated processes of sensory knowing.

The paradigmatic movement from theory-centred observations to body-oriented research is not only characteristic of musical scholarship. The same could be said for the cognitive sciences (Jensenius et al. 2010, p. 12). Thereby, the close relation between action and perception constitutes the enactive approach and its impact on *sensorimotor knowledge*:

> In a nutshell, the enactive approach consists of two points: (1) perception consists in perceptually guided action and (2) cognitive structures emerge from the recurrent sensorimotor patterns that enable action to be perceptually guided. (Varela et al. 1997, p. 173)

The paradigm of embodied knowledge plays an important role in this approach. With respect to Johnson (1987) and Dreyfus (1979) Varela et al. introduce the term "embodiment" as epistemological category:

> By using the term *embodied* we mean to highlight two points: first, that cognition depends upon the kinds of experience that come from having a body with various sensorimotor capacities, and second, that these individual sensorimotor capacities are themselves embedded in a more encompassing biological, psychological, and cultural context. (Varela et al. 1997, pp. 172f.)

We will come to the cultural context later. In this section it is important to clarify in what sense sensorimotor knowledge is not propositional knowledge. Following Alva Noë,

> the mastery in question be purely practical and not a matter of the knowledge of propositions [...]. Instead of comparing perceiving to speech, we should instead compare it to gestural devices of communication. (Noë 2004, p. 120)

Propositional knowledge is somehow subordinate to the bodily movement and active perception. "Sensorimotor knowledge is basic." (Noë 2004, p. 120) As such, the enactive approach provides an epistemological basis for the adequate understanding of musical gestures in the tradition of post-Cartesian thinking. Sensorimotor movements and its meanings are not separable from biologically shaped body motions and its cultural forms of gestural communication. Performing free jazz for example is per se an active circle of perceiving and communicating significant movements:

> Listening to and understanding intelligent music is by no means a passive activity; a fortiori, a quality performance of free jazz requires an optimum of activity in order to be able to throw back the gestures one has received. This type of active listening, of course, is not exclusive to free jazz […]. (Mazzola & Cherlin 2009, p. 95)

Important roles, not only in free jazz, play musical instruments that influence sensorimotor knowledge and moving patterns.

6. Musical gestures and technologies

Implicit knowledge and the enactive approach are a methodological basis for Bernhard Irrgang's philosophical concept of technological development and his phenomenological-hermeneutical anthropology of the *Leib*. The term *Leib* (human lived body) does not include the assumption that the *Körper* (physical body) is separated from the mind, as is the case in the tradition of Platonic or Cartesian thinking (Borsche 1980a, p. 174).

Bernhard Irrgang has argued that "*Umgangswissen*" (knowing in handling) and remembering sequences of long sensorimotor movements, for example while playing piano, is a reason for the biological and cultural difference between human *Leib* and the body of apes (Irrgang 2009a, pp. 47ff., pp. 68 ff.). In other words: what makes humans become humans is not only propositional knowledge, but moreover the ability of corporeal understanding and remembering long sequences of body movements and its social meanings. Sensorimotor patterns are the basis for cognitive structures and the fundament for becoming a "being with abstract reason in adulthood" (Varela et al. 1997, p. 176, see also Piaget 1954). These patterns shape skills in handling technical tools or handcraft technologies and its historical development; they are the fundament for human societies and cultural traditions (Irrgang 2009a, pp. 109ff., Irrgang 2009b, pp. 7ff.). *Umgangswissen* is mostly related to implicit knowledge in using technical or scientific tools. This phenomenon is not new; it shapes in its basic structure human mankind since the first use of hand axes in the Stone Age and even earlier (Irrgang 2009b, pp. 91ff.).

For Don Ihde, music is a certain kind of embodied technical praxis. The role of scientific instruments "in the production of knowledge often could be seen in both comparison and contrast to the role of instruments in producing music." (Ihde 2007, p. xii) One lesson we can draw from music is that knowing crucially involves the body and the materiality of technologies:

> At the outset it can be seen that phenomenological epistemology is "materialist" at least insofar as it centers in actional, perceiving embodiment. And, on the other side, technologies are also material – at least as one component in the larger technological context. The "hardware" aspect of technology is its "bodily" characteristic. It is at this very point, in the analogization of human embodiment with artificial embodiment, that an *expanded hermeneutics* is called for.
> (Ihde 1998, p. 44)

In the tradition of 20th century phenomenological and hermeneutical philosophy Don Ihde develops an approach on expanding hermeneutics. Human understanding and interpreting is not only initialised by written texts or musical scores. It involves the material dimension of scientific tools, technical artifacts or musical instruments (Ihde 1998, p. 40; Irrgang 2009b, p. 102). In the trajectory of Martin Heidegger, technological mediation becomes a central aspect of our bodily praxis: we understand ourselves while understanding our environment by using certain tools (Ihde 1998, p. 42; Irrgang 2010, p. 50). We are what we are able to do. This insight even influenced the philosophical framework of Varela et al. (1997) and the enactive approach:

> We should note, however, that the philosophical source for this attitude is [...] based in the early work of Martin Heidegger [...]. The term *hermeneutics* originally referred to the discipline of interpreting ancient texts, but it has been extended to denote the entire phenomenon of interpretation, understood as the enactment or bringing forth of meaning from a background of understanding.
> (Varela et al. 1997, p. 149)

Music(s) are embedded in technical praxis, the use of and understanding through certain instruments: "as Heidegger had already noted in his tool analysis, so very much of our relation to an environment is *mediated through the use of tools or artifacts*." (Ihde 1998, p. 45) One can argue that singing is not a matter of using instruments. But at least singing "is directly *bodily expressive*" and "should also be expanded to variations on whole body movement such as dance, even self-percussion such as slapping oneself or other objects." (Ihde 2007, p. 254).

A similar approach is developed by Leman and Godøy, who claim that "[...] gesture can be defined as a pattern through which we structure our environment from the viewpoint of actions." (Leman & Godøy 2010, p. 8) And "embodied music cognition [...] conceives the musical mind as embodied, that is, as mediated by the human body." (Leman 2008, p. 235) For Marc Leman technical instruments and especially

> New media technologies call for a new theory for music research. [...] The suggestion is that an action-oriented approach, based on the notion of corporeality, provides a possible epistemological foundation for bridging the gap between musical mind and matter. (Leman 2008, p. 26)

Embodied music cognition and expanding hermeneutics in combination with the concept of implicit knowledge and the enactive approach provide a fruitful fundament for understanding the technical dimension of musical gestures: meaningful sensory movement in combination with bodily and technically mediated sound.

7. Musical gestures as cultural and social phenomenon

We cannot separate a philosophical epistemology of musical gestures from epistemological questions of technological mediation, its development and the cultural or social contexts: "technologies are always *culturally embedded*" (Ihde 1998, p. 48) and also musical gestures are often related to cultural and social meaning (Leman & Godøy 2010, pp. 9–10).

We can distinguish three forms of knowledge, which are strongly interrelated and shape musical understanding and cultural meaning (see also the pre-study Funk 2011). First, theoretical knowledge: notation, semantics and theory of harmonic structures, musical scores, musical tablatures. Second, sensorimotor knowledge: bodily skills (also in handling musical instruments). And third, perceptual knowledge: embodied skills in sensory interpretation of music.

The first form is the linguistic, score oriented aspect of musical knowledge. This explicit knowledge is related to musical theories. For example, we can say in clear and strict words: "I *know that* Beethoven composed the first movement of his Moonlight-Sonata in c-sharp minor." These words are true; this is *justified true belief*. Philosophically this can be explained by using the classical analytical methodology, which focuses on propositional knowledge. "The propositional character of a linguistic description of a musical experience implies symbolic communication." (Leman 2008, p. 15).

But as we have already seen, this form is not sufficient for developing a philosophical approach to the epistemology of musical gestures and gestural communication. How can we explain in strict and true words the meaningful movements of a pianist that *knows how* to play the Moonlight-Sonata? The second and third form of knowledge are implicit knowledge: more than we can say. Following the enactive approach, both are the sensorimotor embodied fundament of *knowing how* musical gestures. The second and third form are very close to one other: when we know how to execute a movement, we usually also know how to realise a sensory perception that belongs to it.

What we share is not only the theory of notation or scores (form 1) and the sequences and techniques of movement (form 2); we are also sharing knowledge in handling emotions and perceptions (form 3). That is why aural training is an independent subject in the academic education of music(s) (Kaiser 2009, p. xi ff.). The second and third form belong together but are not exactly congruent.

Following the enactive approach, sensorimotor movements and active perception are basic, and theoretical knowledge (words, notation, any kind of formalization or musical scores) is somehow subordinate to bodily knowledge. An appropriate philosophical understanding of musical gestures is related to implicit knowledge and non-linguistic understanding of interpreting body actions while handling instruments (hermeneutical approach). We are not able to explain the proper understanding of our human bodies and the piano in strict and true words, but we are able to perform it. While interpreting bodily and technically mediated movements, our implicit knowing of certain meanings and significances develops. We can try to make this implicit understanding explicit. But we cannot separate the genesis of meaning from sensory movement and active perception. In this context, the concepts of dis-embodiment and re-embodiment can be explained.

These concepts can be illustrated with respect to the cultural impact of score-oriented music(s). Rolf Inge Godøy explains:

> Western musical culture has been able to create highly complex organizations of musical sound with large-scale forms and large ensembles, thanks to the development of notation. But this has happened to the price of splitting music into a "score" part and a "performance" part, where the score part is essentially a set of symbols for discrete actions, [...]. (Godøy 2010, p. 109)

The score-part is related to theoretical knowledge, the performance-part to knowledge in terms of movement and perception. "Dis-embodiment" means bringing a performance-part into a score-part, thus translating embodied knowledge into dis-embodied knowledge. For example, if a piano player improvises a piece of music and is notating it afterwards, then this is a process of dis-embodiment: transforming movement and perception in a theoretical form. When another pianist reads this musical score and interprets it while playing the instrument, this is a process of re-embodiment: transforming symbols into movement and perception. And here we can see why musical gestures are related to technical mediation and non-linguistic hermeneutics: performance and sound would be different, if the musician(s) would interpret the same score while playing another set of instruments. This could be happen if, for example, a jazz-trio (bass, saxophone, drums) would interpret and translate the same piano-score into significant movements. Different musical instruments cause different technical mediations and musical gestures.

The split between score-part and performance-part in music(s) seems to correlate with the linguistic gap between theoretical knowledge and embodied knowledge. European philosophy, especially in the Platonic and Cartesian tradition, has been over-emphasising the importance of theoretical knowledge and often has been blind to the other forms, since "Western philosophy over-emphasizes propositional knowledge" (Irrgang 2009a, p. 109, translated by the authors). Varela et al. (1997, p. 149) claims "it is fair to say that analytic philosophy in general resists this notion of cognition as embodied understanding." And Don Ihde summarises, that positivistic and analytic philosophy of science "where largely linguistic or propositionally oriented and placed theory building at the center of their concerns." (Ihde 1998, p. 42) With respect to musical scholarship Rolf Inge Godøy continues:

> Western musical thought has not been well equipped for thinking the gestural-contextual inclusion of tone-events in music [...]. An embodied perspective on music could turn this around. (Godøy 2010, p. 110)

And here we can find the paradigmatic shift:

> For music research, this embodied perspective is a significant change of paradigm, as it shifts the focus away from more abstract symbols of music notation towards the holistic experience of continuous sound and movement in relation to our bodies. (Godøy & Leman 2010, p. ix)

The over-emphasising of theoretical knowledge in Western culture, before the paradigmatic shift in philosophy, cognitive sciences and musical scholarship, itself is one concrete cultural achievement. In classical music it seems that improvisation is the ideal in Indian music, whereas composition is the ideal in European music:

> If music can be understood as expression of culture, this contrast could be generalized in this way: classical Indian music mirrors the concept of improvisation as cultural ideal – classical European music mirrors the concept of composition as cultural ideal. (Kurt 2009, p. 184, translated by the authors)

In other words: in Indian culture, for example Raga-music(s), the bodily dimension (second and third form of knowledge) is more idealised. In contrast, the European culture highlighted the semantic dimension within complex compositions and score orientated notations. "And, as with so much late, or even postmodern scholarship, it was only by mid-twentieth century that the parochialism of

Eurocentrism concerning scores was broken." (Ihde 2007, p. 257) Free jazz is not the only one, but one example as Mazzola and Cherlin explain. Because

> the question of semiotics of gestures arises when we display the overall image of traditional Western musical performance [...]. This process starts from the score, which is a text of more or less analyzed symbols. [...] In other words, the semiotic approach to gestures in music is traditionally related to the score-driven production of music. But there are many musics that are not score-driven, and free jazz is one of them [...]. (Mazzola & Cherlin 2009, p. 69)

It is important to see that theoretical knowledge is not only related to musical scores in Western highly educated music culture, but also to tablatures or other visualisations of many music(s) in many social and cultural contexts. But the score-orientation and over-emphasising of theoretical knowledge in classical Western culture has an impact on musical gestures. Since musical gestures are shaped by all three forms of knowledge, in classical European culture the gestural performances of musicians are embedded in a highly developed theoretical context that is score and notation oriented.

In other cultural contexts, like classical Indian music(s) or free jazz, the theoretical embedding of musical gestures is different and not so complex. Musical gestures in a score oriented culture are not similar to musical gestures in cultures that highlight improvisation. The peculiar idealisation and emphasis of the three forms in relation to each other are different. In other words: it is not possible to understand musical gestures adequately by investigating meaningful movements in relation to harmonic theories, linguistic concepts, or semiotics, if the gestures are performed in a cultural context where scores do not or less influence musicians.

8. Conclusion

Is gesture knowledge? Movement of a bodiless soul is seen as knowledge in the tradition of dualistic Platonic and Cartesian thinking. Following analytical philosophy, propositional knowledge is linguistic-oriented and we can make this knowledge explicit by using strict and true words. *Moving imagination* in that sense could mean the ideas of a bodiless soul. But because of its dualistic Platonic and Cartesian premises, this concept is not sufficient for developing a philosophical approach to the epistemology of musical gestures.

When it comes to knowledge, mind and body cannot be separated. As we have seen, current paradigmatic turns in post-Cartesian philosophy, musical scholarship and the cognitive sciences illustrate this fundamental insight. Knowing means sensory activity in everyday life and bodily movement: more than we are able to tell. Therefore gestural movement is *sensorimotor knowledge* and *perceptual knowledge* that is bodily and technical mediated. *Moving imagination* in that sense means human embodied sensory activities. There is no passive and bodiless imagination, even in classical Western culture that idealises propositional knowledge and musical scores.

References

Anacker, M. (2004). Wissen. 19. Und 20. Jh. In J. Ritter, K. Gründer, & G. Gabriel (Eds.), *Historisches Wörterbuch der Philosophie. Band 12* (pp. 891–900). Basel: Schwabe.

Böhme, G. (2003). *Leibsein als Aufgabe. Leibphilosophie in pragmatischer Hinsicht*. Kusterdingen: SFG.

Baumann, P. (2006). *Erkenntnistheorie* (2 Aufl.). Stuttgart & Weimar: Metzler.

Borsche, T. (1980a). Leib, Körper. Begriff. Antike und Mittelalter. In J. Ritter, & K. Gründer (Eds.), *Historisches Wörterbuch der Philosophie. Band 5* (pp. 174–179). Basel: Schwabe.

Borsche, T. (1980b). Leib-Seele-Verhältnis. Problemstellung. In J. Ritter, & K. Gründer (Eds.), *Historisches Wörterbuch der Philosophie. Band 5* (pp. 186–187). Basel: Schwabe.

Brinker, W. (2007). Seele (psychê). In Ch. Schäfer (Ed). *Platon-Lexikon. Begriffswörterbuch zu Platon und der platonischen Tradition* (pp. 253–258). Darmstadt: WBG.

Descartes, R. (2009). *Meditationen. Mit sämtlichen Einwänden und Erwiederungen*. Hamburg: Meiner.

Dreyfus, H. (1979). *What Computers Can't Do* (Revised edition). New York: Harper and Row.

Frede, D. (2007). Grund/Begründung/Ursache (aition/synaition, aitia usw.). In Ch. Schäfer (Ed). *Platon-Lexikon. Begriffswörterbuch zu Platon und der platonischen Tradition* (pp. 141–145). Darmstadt: WBG.

Funk, M. (2010). Verstehen und Wissen. Ludwig Wittgensteins Philosophie der Technik. In L. Leidl, & D. Pinzer (Eds.), *Technikhermeneutik. Technik zwischen Verstehen und Gestalten* (pp. 75–88). Frankfurt am Main a.o.: Peter Lang.

Funk, M. (2011). Vom Blick zum Klang – Was wissen die Noten über mein Klavierspiel? In T. Hug, & A. Kriwak (Eds.), *Visuelle Kompetenz. Beiträge des interfakultären Forums Innsbruck Media Studies* (pp. 270–284). Innsbruck: Innsbruck University Press.

Gettier, E. (1963). Is Justified True Belief Knowledge?, *Analysis, 23*(6), 121–123.

Godøy, R.I. (2010). Gestural Affordances of Musical Sound. In R. I. Godøy, & M. Leman (Eds.), *Musical Gestures. Sound, Movement, and Meaning*, (pp. 103–125). New York/ Oxon: Routledge.

Godøy, R.I., & Leman, M. (2010). Editor's Preface. In R. I. Godøy, & M. Leman (Eds.), *Musical Gestures. Sound, Movement, and Meaning*, (pp. ix–xi). New York/ Oxon: Routledge.

Gritten, A., & King, E. (2006). Introduction. In A. Gritten, & E. King (Eds.), *Music and Gesture*, (pp. xix–xxv). Burlington/Hampshire: Ashgate.

Gritten, A., & King, E. (2011). Introduction. In A. Gritten, & E. King, (Eds.), *New Perspectives on Music and Gestures* (pp. 1–9). Farnham/Burlington: Ashgate.

Gröbl-Steinbach, E. (2000). Wissen und Praxis in der pragmatischen Sprachphilosophie Wittgensteins. In G. H. Neuweg (Ed.), *Wissen – Können – Reflexion. Ausgewählte Verhältnisbestimmungen* (pp. 27–43). Innsbruck a.o.: Studien-Verlag.

Hardy, J. (2004). Wissen. Antike. In J. Ritter, K. Gründer, & G. Gabriel (Eds.), *Historisches Wörterbuch der Philosophie. Band 12* (pp. 857–868). Basel: Schwabe.

Hardy, J., & Meier-Oeser, S. (2004). Wissen. Terminologie. In J. Ritter, K. Gründer, & G. Gabriel (Eds.), *Historisches Wörterbuch der Philosophie. Band 12* (pp. 855–857). Basel: Schwabe.

Hatten, R.S. (2004). *Interpreting musical gestures, Topics, and Tropes: Mozart, Beethoven, Schubert*. Bloomington: Indiana University Press.

Hatten, R.S. (2006). A Theory of Musical Gesture and its Application to Beethoven and Schubert. In A. Gritten, & E. King (Eds.), *Music and Gesture* (pp. 1–23). Burlington/Hampshire: Ashgate.

Horn, Ch., & Rapp, Ch. (Eds.). (2002). *Wörterbuch der antiken Philosophie*. München: C.H. Beck.

Ihde, D. (1998). *Expanding Hermeneutics. Visualism in Science*. Evanston: NU Press.

Ihde, D. (2007). *Listening and Voice. Phenomenologies of Sound* (Second edition). New York: SUNY Press.

Irrgang, B. (2005). *Posthumanes Menschsein? Künstliche Intelligenz, Cyberspace, Roboter, Cyborgs und Designer-Menschen – Anthropologie des künstlichen Menschen im 21. Jahrhundert*. Stuttgart: Franz Steiner Verlag.

Irrgang, B. (2009a). *Der Leib des Menschen. Grundriss einer phänomenologisch-hermeneutischen Anthropologie*. Stuttgart: Steiner Verlag.

Irrgang, B. (2009b). *Grundriss der Technikphilosophie. Hermeneutisch-phänomenologische Perspektiven*. Würzburg: Königshausen & Neumann.

Irrgang, B. (2010). Martin Heideggers Technikphilosophie. Vom Umgehen-Können zum Entbergen. In L. Leidl, & D. Pinzer (Eds.), *Technikhermeneutik. Technik zwischen Verstehen und Gestalten* (pp. 45–590). Frankfurt am Main a.o.: Peter Lang.

Ishino, M., & Stam, G. (2011). Introduction. In G. Stam, & M. Ishino (Eds.), *Integrating Gestures, The interdisciplinary nature of gesture* (pp. 3–13). Amsterdam/Philadelphia: John Benjamins Publishing Company.

Jensenius, A.R., Wanderley, M.M., Godøy, R.I., & Leman, M. (2010). Musical Gestures. Concepts and Methods in Research. In R. I. Godøy, & M. Leman (Eds.), *Musical Gestures. Sound, Movement, and Meaning* (pp. 12–35). New York/Oxon: Routledge.

Johnson, M. (1987). *The Body in the Mind: The Bodily Basis of Imagination, Reason, and Meaning*. Chicago: University of Chicago Press.

Kaiser, U. (2009). *Gehörbildung. Satzlehre – Improvisation – Höranalyse. Ein Lehrgang mit historischen Beispielen. Grundkurs* (5. Auflage). Kassel: Bärenreiter.

Kurt, R. (2009). *Indien und Europa: Ein kultur- und musiksoziologischer Verstehensversuch*. Bielefeld: Transcript.

Leman, M. (2008). *Embodied Music Cognition and Mediating Technology*. Cambridge/London: MIT Press.

Leman, M., & Godøy, R.I. (2010). Why Study Musical Gestures? In R. I. Godøy, & M. Leman (Eds.), *Musical Gestures. Sound, Movement, and Meaning* (pp. 3–11). New York/Oxon: Routledge.

Lugg, A. (2000). *Wittgenstein's Investigations 1–133. A Guide and Interpretation*. London/New York: Routledge.

Mazzola, G., & Cherlin, P.B. (in collaboration with Rissi, M. & Kennedy, N.) (2009). *Flow, Gesture, and Spaces in Free Jazz*. Berlin and Heidelberg: Springer-Verlag.

Meixner, U. (2007). Erkenntnis (epistêmê, noêsis, nous, gnôsis, phronêsis, mathêsis). In Ch. Schäfer (Ed). *Platon-Lexikon. Begriffswörterbuch zu Platon und der platonischen Tradition* (pp. 109–116). Darmstadt: WBG.

Mohr, G. (2011). Einführung: Musikphilosophie – Musikästhetik. In C. F. Gethmann (Ed.), *Lebenswelt und Wissenschaft XXI. Deutscher Kongress für Philosophie. 15.-19. September 2008. an der Universität Duisburg-Essen. Kolloquiumsbeiträge* (pp. 1317–1326). Hamburg: Meiner.

Noë, A. (2004). *Action in Perception*. Cambridge, Ma.: MIT Press.

Perkams, M. (2007). Bewegung (kinêsis). In Ch. Schäfer (Ed). *Platon-Lexikon. Begriffswörterbuch zu Platon und der platonischen Tradition* (pp. 55–57). Darmstadt: WBG.

Piaget, J. (1954). *The Construction of Reality in the Child*. New York: Basic Books.

Plato (2005). *Meno and Other Dialogues. A new translation by Robin Waterfield*. Oxford: OUP.

Polanyi, M. (1969). *Knowing and Being. Essays by Michael Polanyi* (Ed. by Marjorie Grene). Chicago: University of Chicago Press.

Polanyi, M. (2009). *The tacit Dimension. With a new foreword by Amartya Sen*. Chicago/London: The University of Chicago Press.

Rehkämper, K., & Wachtendorf, T. (2009). Analytische Erkenntnistheorie. In H. Leerhoff, K. Rehkämper, & T. Wachtendorf (Eds.), *Analytische Philosophie* (pp. 79–91). Darmstadt: WBG.

Rentsch, Th. (1980). Leib-Seele-Verhältnis. Gegenwärtige Sprachphilosophie. In J. Ritter, & K. Gründer (Eds.), *Historisches Wörterbuch der Philosophie. Band 5* (pp. 201–206). Basel: Schwabe.

Rentsch, Th. (2003). *Heidegger und Wittgenstein. Existential- und Sprachanalysen zu den Grundlagen philosophischer Anthropologie*. Stuttgart: Klett-Cotta.

Ryle, G. (1946). Knowing how and knowing that. *Proceedings of the Aristotelian Society, 46 (1945/46)*, 1–16.

Seitschek, H.O. (2007). Wiedererinnerung/Anamnesis (anamnêsis). In Ch. Schäfer (Ed). *Platon-Lexikon. Begriffswörterbuch zu Platon und der platonischen Tradition* (pp. 330–333). Darmstadt: WBG.

Thurner, M. (2007). Dualismus (Leib-Seele-Verhältnis). In Ch. Schäfer (Ed.), *Platon-Lexikon. Begriffswörterbuch zu Platon und der platonischen Tradition* (pp. 99–101). Darmstadt: WBG.

Varela, F.J., Thompson, E., & Rosch, E. (1997). *The Embodied Mind. Cognitive Science and Human Experience* (Sixth printing). Cambridge/London: MIT Press.

Wittgenstein, L., Hacker, P.M. S., & Schulte, J. (2010). *Philosophical Investigations*. Hoboken: Wiley-Blackwell.

Sound in film as an inner movement

Towards embodied listening strategies

Martine Huvenne
School of Arts, University College Ghent

1. Introduction

In most film theories, the dominant position of the visual image is taken for granted. However, when transmitting an experience in film, sound plays a crucial role. To enable a discussion on sound as an inner movement in the transmission of an experience in film, I propose a phenomenological approach. In this chapter I discuss listening to sound in film from the perspective of motor imagery and listening as an (embodied) act, in order to question the role of the imagination which emerges from sound in film.

Focussing on sound and listening in film, the ways in which the experience of sound in film invites us to use both perception and imagination are investigated. The investigation of film sound starts from the "movement experience" of sound which enables both a pre-reflective "thinking in movement" and the reflective intentional act in which meaningful intentional objects are constituted. The focus on an embodied way of listening to sound in terms of energetic movement and bodily resonance allows us to discuss a pre-reflective experience of sound which we are all familiar with. It is this pre-reflective experience which plays a crucial role in evoking attention and establishing meaning.

In accordance with Edmund Husserl's analysis of intentional acts motivated by kinaesthetic and pre-reflective experiences and Maurice Merleau-Ponty's definition of abstract movement in relation to a situated body, I analyse the experience of a recorded sound in an (imagined) visual context. I investigate the way in which sound evokes motor imagery in combination with, but also independent of the image.

2. Existing views on sound in film

When studying sound in film two opposite views are common. One can be introduced by the sound theory of Michel Chion, the other by the film theory of Gilles Deleuze. Chion defines sound in the audiovisual perception of film as 'added value' to the image (Chion1994 [1990]) and Deleuze defines sound in film as a heautonomous sonorous image, equivalent to the visual image (Deleuze 2008 [1985], p. 241). To contextualise my research, I briefly introduce both views.

According to Chion, sound in film is an added value to the visual image rather than intertwined with it.

> By added value I mean the expressive and informative value with which a sound enriches a given image so as to create the definite impression, in the immediate or remembered experience one has of it, that this information or expression "naturally" comes from what is seen, and is already contained in the image itself. (Chion 1994, p. 5)

Consequently, the contribution of sound and listening independent of the perception of the given image is not investigated in his film sound theory. Chion denies an autonomous auditory field existing in film as an audiovisual medium. In his view, the auditory field is always defined in function of the visual image.

> In cinema the notion of the auditory field is completely a function of what appears on the screen. In other words, in film there is no autonomous auditory field; its real and imaginary dimensions are created in collaboration with the image, and at the same time sound is always overflowing and transgressing it. It is in this double movement that film sound operates. (Chion 2009, p. 249)

Chion's view, based on the film image and the frame, corresponds to film theories that start from visual perception in order to analyse audiovisual perception and thus to investigate sound in film.[1] Chion's thinking is clearly illustrated in his description of the topography of the prison Fort Montluc (Lyon) in *A man escaped* (1956) by Robert Bresson. In this film, a prisoner, Fontaine, has the intention to escape. With him, the audience discovers through the sound what is happening outside of the prison cell of Fontaine. On the basis of those sounds Fontaine tries to understand the map of the prison. In his listening to the sounds of the city he also stays connected to the exterior world outside of the prison. In his analysis of the soundtrack of the film, Chion invites us to listen to the different sounds positioned

1. In the first chapter of *Film theorie* (2010), Thomas Elsaesser and Malte Hagener present theories based on a visual primacy in film perception: "For constructivists as well as for realists, perception is limited to the visual dimension, the sense and data processing are thought of as highly rational while the primary goal is to consciously work through what is being perceived. In this respect Balazs and Bazin, Eisenstein and Kracauer all conceptualize the spectator-film relationship along similar lines, even though Kracauer and Eisenstein were sensitive to the 'shock' value and somatic dimension of the film experience." (Elsaesser & Hagener 2010, p.15)

according to a visual, imagined plan in which he distinguishes different 'zones': the prison cell of Fontaine, the inside of the prison, the city, the world beyond the city (Chion 2009, p. 255). Chion's notion of sound as added value can be understood in two different ways: on the one hand Bresson's film gives us an example of the fact that it is possible that both the audience and the character Fontaine in the film are informed through sound about situations they are not able to see.

> ...we see that Bresson tightly framed the shots of corridors, walls, and stairs through which characters move – so that he could shoot in an extremely reduced space. It's the reverberation of the whistles, the footsteps, and the noise of keys and locks that etched these imaginary spaces into my memory. This observation, which struck me in 1980, at the beginning of my work on film sound, led eventually to my idea of added value. (Chion 2009, p. 255)

On the other hand the added values can also be described as the way sound informs us in a complementary way about visible actions: when a sound is produced simultaneously with a visible action, the brain correlates the visible and the audible actions in a single audiovisual perception. Chion calls this *synchresis* (synchronisation+synthesis) and concludes that the sound is added to the image.

In his foreword to the English version of Chion's book *Audio-vision* (1994), sound designer Walter Murch adds from his practice-based perspective a nuance to Chion's way of thinking:

> In much the same way, the mental effort of fusing image and sound in a film produces a "dimensionality" that the mind projects back onto the image *as if* it had come from the image in the first place.
>
> (Murch in Chion 1994, p. xxi, italics added)

Instead of emphasising the "audiovisual illusion", Murch draws attention to the act of perception and imagination in an audiovisual context. Emphasising the *acts* of perception and imagination, Murch expands Chion's concept of synchresis. This expansion points to a particular characteristic of the illusion, namely that the image onscreen is experienced as the source of the sound *(as if)* when a sound sounds simultaneously with the image. Thus, whereas Chion emphasises that the recorded sound is an added value to the recorded image in the construction of an audiovisual image, Murch emphasises that visual and auditory perception are co-constitutive of film experience. This indicates that the common idea of the primacy of vision is misleading, and, consequently that sound is not just added value to the image. Concerning visible and auditory actions, I interpret Murch's remark as an introduction to the role of motor imagery in audiovisual perception, emphasising the act of perception. Motor imagery can be defined as a dynamic state during which an individual mentally simulates a given action.

Starting from the perspective of the audience, Deleuze opens a radically different way of investigating sound in film (Deleuze 1989 [1985]). Deleuze disconnects sound from image and argues that image and sound in film exist independently and are characterised by an interstice: "Two heautonomous images, one visual image and one sound image, with a fault, an interstice, and irrational cut between them" (Deleuze 2008 [1985], p. 241). Defining sound as a 'sound image' in his film theory, Deleuze nonetheless seldom writes about sound as sound (in contrast to sound as music or spoken word). Moreover, and although he starts from the perspective of the audience, he does not really explore the act of listening to sound. In her critique on Deleuze's film theory, Vivian Sobchack explains that Deleuze ignores the central position of the spectator in film perception: "He neglects the embodied situation of the spectator and of the film" (Sobchack 1992, p. 31). In her phenomenology of film perception, Sobchack introduces an embodied approach of film perception. It can be said that she also introduces an enactive approach of film perception, in which emotions and motor actions in the world are taken into account (Varela, Thompson & Rosch 1991; Thompson 2007).

In this embodied approach, the Husserlian idea of passive genesis, underlying active synthesis, becomes crucial in an account of experience and perception. Central in this approach are movement and the embodied sense of movement. Husserl argues that the intentional act is motivated by kinaesthetic experience, preceding a thematic experience. The active genesis of the intentional object presupposes in other words always a degree of passivity, meaning that the subject does not decide that he or she is affected by something.

The thought behind active/passive distinction is that our active orientation toward things in practical and theoretical reason, or artistic creation, presupposes a deeper and more fundamental openness to the world. It is an openness to being sensuously affected and solicited by the world through the medium of our living body, and responding by the attraction and repulsion. Investigating these sensorimotor and affective depths of experience leads phenomenology to the notion of passive genesis. (cf. Thompson 2007, pp. 29–30)

3. Sound in film as an audible dynamic energetic movement

In audiovisual perception, sound seems neither dependent, nor independent of the image. Starting from a bodily felt sound, sound 'resonates' in our body. Mostly the felt sound is described by 'transmodal' characteristics (descriptions of movement, intensity, rhythm, ...). They are not specific to any of the senses, but can be transposed from one sense to another (Petitmengin et al. 2009, pp. 268–269). Since the experience of sound can be transmodal, the act of listening is experientially also correlated with visual perception. But depending on the listening strategy, the experience of sound can evoke visual, tactile, olfactory or kinaesthetic resonances (Petitmengin et al. 2009, p. 277). In research on sound in film and the experience of it, it turns out that the concepts of 'visual image' and 'audiovisual image' are too narrow and too visually conceived. One must not forget that sound is essentially an audible movement that can never be grasped in a static moment. It is therefore in the course of the act of listening that a sound is constituted. Listening to a sound includes the reception or the perception of an audible movement. This brings us to fundamentally different concepts to analyse sound in film, which are connected with the perception of visible and audible movements (and actions) rather than with the perception of a visual image on screen. Coming back to Chion's concept of 'synchresis', the 'synthesis' leads to a kind of encoded sound: through the connection with images, we 'understand' the sound. The sound becomes part of an 'audiovisual object'. In a similar way, Christian Metz, who tried to give sound as an 'aural object' a status similar to the 'visual object' in film, emphasises the visual source of the sound as basic element in the identification of a sound. But at the same time he points out that at a certain moment the real characteristics of sounds have to be described.

> As soon as the source of the sound is recognized, the taxonomies of the sound itself (buzzing, whistling, etc.) can only provide at least in our era and geographic location, supplementary precisions, which are felt to be dispensable, of a basically adjectival nature, even when linguistically they are expressed by nouns. At the discursive level, we are no longer naming, but already describing to a certain extent. Ideologically, the aural sound is an object, the sound itself is a "characteristic". (Metz in Weis 1985, p. 156)

It is Véronique Campan (1999) who takes a radically different angle to study film sound. She starts her thinking consequently from the auditory aspect of film instead of the relation image-sound. She describes the listening to a film as a sensible, perceptive and cognitive conduct which attaches to the sonorous and emphasises the mobile and the variable nature of the qualities of movement (Campan 1999, p. 9). Following her approach of filmic listening, the embodied perception of movement becomes central, and with this a "thinking in movement" as described by Maxine Sheets-Johnstone:

> Thinking in movement is thus clearly not the work of a symbol-making body, a body mediating its way through the world by means of a language, for example; it is the work of an existentially resonant body. An existentially resonant body creates a particular dynamic world not an immutable or factitious world, but a protean world created moment by moment [...] In short, *to have meaning is not necessarily to refer and neither is it necessarily to have a verbal label.* (Sheets-Johnstone 2009, p. 35)

In what follows, I start from the interpretation of sound as a dynamic energetic movement in correlation with an embodied listening. This entails that sound does not exist in a so-called "objective" way as an equivalent of a visual image ("sound-image", cf. Deleuze, or "aural object", cf. Metz). Since sounds arise in the act of listening by a subject, the subject-object correlation needs to be taken into account. Moreover, it should be mentioned that the listener is always at the centre of her or his listening. Post-phenomenologist Don Ihde introduces the term 'surroundability' of the auditory field. This field is copresent with the often quite precise and definite directionality of sound presence (Ihde 2007, p. 77). Consequently, the description of listening asks for a description from a first-person perspective. With this I emphasise the intimate link between the sound as an experiential phenomenon and the first-personal givenness.

When I listen to a sound, I actively make choices. Even if I have the impression that I am moved by the sounds in a passive way, there is also an active component in the act of listening. I do not undergo a chaos of vibrations, but I actively distinguish, e.g. sounds from voices, or from music. Listening from a first-person perspective, I make these choices in the act of listening itself, without reflecting neither on the listening, nor on the sound.

In *Ideeen II*, Husserl makes the difference between "inner perception" as a reflection and "inner consciousness" with a non-thematic kind of self-awareness that precedes reflection. In Husserl's view the subjective or first-personal givenness of the experience is something that essentially characterises experiential life.

> … In contrast to physical objects, which can exist regardless of whether or not they *de facto* appear for a subject, experiences are essentially characterized by their subjective givenness, by the fact that there is a subjective "feel" to them. To undergo an experience necessarily means that there is something "it is like" for the subject to have that experience.
>
> On Husserl's account, an act of reflection is a *founded* form of self-awareness in the sense that it relies upon a prior, tacit form of self-awareness. To utilize a terminological distinction between perceiving (*Wahrnehmen*) and experiencing (*Erleben*) dating back to the *Logische Untersuchungen*: Prior to reflection one perceives the intentional object, but one experiences [*erlebt*] the intentional act. Although I am not intentionally directed at the act (this only happens in the subsequent reflection, where the act is thematized), it is not unconscious but conscious (Hua III, 162, 168, 251, 349, IX, 29), that is, given in an implicit and pre-reflective manner (Hua IV, 118). … However, in order to explain the occurrence of reflection it is necessary that that which is to be disclosed and thematized is (unthematically) present, otherwise there would be nothing to motivate and call forth the act of reflection. As Husserl points out, it is in the nature of reflection to grasp something which was already given prior to the grasping. Reflection is characterized by disclosing, not by producing its theme.
> (Zahavi 2010, pp. 325–327)

According to Dan Zahavi's interpretation of the later Husserl, I can say that I am listening on a pre-reflective conscious level to distinguish sounds by "feeling" the sounds. In other words: it is possible that I am aware of different kinds of sounds without the sounds being intentional objects. This awareness in the act of listening is pre-reflective and starts in the resonance with the sound as an energetic movement.

4. Different listening strategies provoking different kinds of imagination

In investigating the correlation of listening and sound, different strategies of listening are possible, such as listening to the meaning of a sound, listening to the source of sound in combination with the act producing the sound, listening to the position of a sound in space, listening to the relation between the sound recording and the original position of sound in space (versus the position of the recorded sound in the diegetic, filmed space) and an embodied resonating listening to a sound without attending to the meaning or the source of the sound.

In what follows, I first focus on listening strategies connected with the perception or imagination of images in order to understand better how listening finds a place in audiovisual perception. Next, I discuss recorded sound independent from a given audiovisual context.

We start with a film fragment from *A man escaped* (1956) by Robert Bresson (34′12″–35′12″). The fragment begins at the moment when Fontaine (the prisoner) is able to 'open' his door for the first time. We hear subdued little sounds produced by the actions of Fontaine himself that sound very nearby and present. We can see where they originate from. We see that Fontaine is busy dismantling the door of his cell. Suddenly, we hear the footsteps of a jailer in the corridor. He is opening and closing doors. With Fontaine we are hearing how the distance of his steps is changing. But we do not see the jailer. In this fragment sound gives a different kind of information from what we, the audience, see onscreen.

Apart from the voice-over, we hear in this fragment two types of sounds, mentioned higher (cf. Chion's concept of added value) in relation to the image onscreen: sound in connection with what is shown onscreen (the source is visible) and offscreen sounds with an invisible source. In his film sound theory Chion distinguishes *onscreen* sounds as sounds with a source visible onscreen and *offscreen* sounds as sounds connected to the image onscreen, but with an invisible source. For example, the sounds in the garden or on the street, connected with an interior onscreen, are interpreted as offscreen sounds (Chion 2009, p. 251).

The public imagines that the sounds without a visible source are nonetheless related to the situation onscreen. We imagine that Fontaine is listening to the sounds and with him we imagine the sources of those sounds. At a certain point, the offscreen sounds of the steps of the jailer evoke an image. We can 'imagine' the source of these sounds and can explore different kinds of images evoked by different ways of listening to the sounds. This means that visual images are but one possibility.

5. Different kinds of images evoked by listening to sound

I propose to distinguish four different strategies of listening in this fragment, evoking different kinds of "images", which can co-exist simultaneously and can be interpreted as different elements and levels in the constitution of the scene. In the descriptions that follow, I use the phenomenological first-person perspective not to describe my subjective interpretations or experiences, but because listening inevitably starts from a first-person perspective (see supra).

On a first level I can imagine the visual image of the jailer: a man walking on staircases through a big corridor, opening and closing doors. Through the sounds I receive information regarding the acoustics of the corridors, the sounds of the actions with the keys, I can hear that he is ascending and descending staircases… I recognise the situation because earlier in the film I saw the visual image of jailers onscreen in connection with similar sounds. With the information given by the sounds and the memory of these images I can imagine in a fairly precise way the visual image of the man.

On a second level, I can focus on the way the man is moving: the use of his weight in his steps, small accelerations, the resolute way in which he is walking… Instead of a visual image being evoked, we listen first and foremost to the dynamic qualities of the movement and the physical efforts in the steps. Rather than a visual image, a "motor image" is evoked: an "impression" of the way the man is moving which can described reflectively focussing on the qualities of his movement, more than on what he looks like. This listening to the qualities of movement implies "thinking in movement" which Sheets-Johnstone defines as our primary way of making sense of the world (Sheets-Johnstone 2009, p. 43).

The "listening to qualities of movement" refers also, as mentioned higher, to the filmic listening of Campan. This listening strategy is a pre-reflective way of listening which can be reflectively described, focussing on the qualities of movement. This listening is a resonating pre-reflective embodied way experiencing the dynamic forms of the sound as an energetic movement. To say something about this listening strategy we have to reflect on the dynamics forms of the sound event.

But the point is that the language used to reflect on the dynamic forms of a movement is not well elaborated. As beginners of this language we can follow the suggestions by Maxine Sheets-Johnstone to focus on the qualities of movement, the Effort Theory (1947) of the dancer Rudolf von Laban and the term "forms of vitality" (2009), suggested by developmental psychologist, Daniel Stern.

> Exploding, surging, accelerating, fading, drawn out, fleeting, forceful, powerful, feeble, cresting, pulsing, tentative, pulling, pushing, relaxing, floating, fluttering, effortful, easy, tense, gliding and many more. [...] They are dynamic forms of vitality. [...] They describe a separate kind of experience that structures the pre-reflexive. (Stern in Petitmengin et al. 2009, pp. 313–314)

According to Stern, forms of vitality are experienced as the dynamics of a happening (its movement, force, temporal profile, directionality, spatial excursion) (Stern 2009, p. 308). Stern explains the concept of dynamic forms as a holistic unit borrowing the words of Einstein answering the question whether he thinks in words or in pictures: "Neither, I think in terms of forces and volumes moving in time and space" (Stern 2009, p. 311).

Stern argues that the experience of a human regardless of whether the action is real, virtual, anticipated, or imagined, or whether it is visually, auditorily, tactually or otherwise perceived, or even whether it is performed by oneself or observed in another is key in interpersonal and intersubjective interactions (Stern 2009). This means that the body of a perceiving subject resonates with someone else's movements he or she is observing. This leads us also to Merleau-Ponty's idea of synchronising modulation.

Just as the sense-giving intention which has set in motion the other person's speech is not an explicit thought, but a certain lack which is asking to be made good, so my taking up of his intention is not a process of thinking on my part, but a synchronizing change of my own existence, a transformation of my being. (Merleau-Ponty 1945, p. 213)

In the film fragment, the body of the listener is "modulated" by resonating, through the act of listening, with the movements of the jailer walking in the corridor. There is a dynamic correlation between the body producing the sound and the body of someone listening to the sound. This announces a fourth kind of listening strategy (see below).

To summarise so far, applying an embodied way of listening to the film fragment of Bresson, in this second listening strategy, I engage my whole phenomenal body to resonate with the efforts in the movements of the jailer. At this level I am moving along with the man. This means that, in the act of listening, and resonating with the movements of the jailer walking in the corridor, my body is 'modulated'. There is thus a dynamic correlation between the body producing the sound and the body of the person listening to this sound. At this second level, we focus on the listening of the audience to the movements of the jailer and not yet on the 'listening' to the listening of Fontaine as character in the film, whom we understand is also listening to the steps of the jailer.

Does this embodied way of listening necessarily evoke an image? What exactly do we imagine in listening to these qualities of movement? Does this way of listening evoke a visual image in the sense of Daniel Deshays' "sonorous image", an image that is evoked in the listener through the sound and constituted through the experience or personal memories of the listener (*l'image sonore*) (Deshays 2010, p. 13)? I claim that what is evoked by the way the jailer is walking, is a 'motor image.' The more I listen to the details in the sound, the more I am able to experience and to replay his movements and gestures in my own body.

As mentioned by Stern and Sheets-Johnstone, at this level I am not analysing the movements of the jailer in a reflective way. In this strategy of listening, I rather feel how he is moving by the way my own body resonates with his movements. In phenomenological terms, I can say that I am primarily listening in a pre-reflective way to the audible actions of the jailer. Listening to actions brings us also into the domain of the mirror neurons (see also De Preester 2008). Gallese and colleagues conclude in their research that we recognise the action in a sound we hear, because of the coupling of our inner representation of the action through the mirror neuronal system (Gallese et al. 1996). Audiovisual mirror neurons would play a crucial role in the evocation of an action through sound. In a more recent article, Gallese suggests that the mirror neuronal system and automatic embodied simulation are responsible for an active attunement or a congruent response in the perception of movement.

> We suggest that the term [mirroring] be replaced with such locutions as attunement or congruent response... What makes active attunement possible and what constitutes the biological basis for such attunement, we propose, is the existence of the mirror neuronal system and automatic embodied simulation. (2005, p. 152)

This brings us back to the remark of Stern concerning the importance of pre-reflective experience of a human action as key in interpersonal and intersubjective interactions and the concept of synchronising modulation of Merleau-Ponty. Thus, in listening to the "efforts" of the steps of the jailer, a motor image is evoked rather than a visual image. Acting ourselves we "understand his way of walking". Listening to the steps in combination with their context, we can understand how the acoustics of the hall, the surfaces of the floor on which he is walking, the distances, et cetera are constitutive elements in the constitution of a motor image.

On a third level, I focus on the experience and the perception of the composition of the different sounds in the film fragment. I focus on the fact that the experience I am going through, resonating now with Fontaine, happens in time, and that the scene is situated in the totality of the film. I hear the little sounds Fontaine is producing when dismantling his door. These sounds not only bear witness to his actions, but also to the way he is reacting to the situation in the corridor. In his listening, the steps of the jailer become meaningful: since Fontaine is trying to escape, the steps of the jailer can be interpreted as "dangerous". When he is approaching the cell of Fontaine, a potentially harmful confrontation becomes more likely. To fully grasp this level I introduce the view on film sound of Campan and the genetic phenomenology of Husserl that focuses on the intentional act instead of the intentional object. Husserl distinguishes between sensory data transmitted through the senses and the intentional object we perceive. This intentional object is constituted in the intentional act, for example the sounds of the steps of the jailer are constituted in our listening to these steps. Dependent on our 'listening strategy', other intentional objects can be constituted in the listening. It is possible to focus on the identity of the jailer, or on the way he is walking through the prison, or on the space exterior to the cell. The question is: how is a particular intentional act initiated? How do we "decide" to listen in a certain way (listening strategy) to a certain sound? According to Husserl, to be motivated for an intentional act is to be affected by something and then to respond to it.

> Whenever I reflect, I find myself 'in relation' to something as affected or active. That to which I am related is experientially conscious – it is already there for me as a 'lived-experience' in order for me to be able to relate myself to it.
>
> (Husserl, quoted in Zahavi 2003, p. 89)

For Husserl the concrete and full structure of all lived experience is structured by the temporality of inner time consciousness, more in particular by the structure of protention, primal impression and retention. This means that the primal impression is always co-existing with a future-oriented temporal context and a past-directed temporal context (Zahavi 2010, p. 321). The primal impression is narrowly directed toward the strictly circumscribed now-phase of the object and is accompanied with a retentional aspect. This provides us with a consciousness of the just-elapsed phase of the object. At the other side the primal impression is accompanied with a protentional aspect, which in a more-or-less indefinite way intends the phase of the object about to occur.

In her essay on filmic listening Campan develops the concept of 'listening to the filmic sound as a trace', based on Husserl's structure of inner time consciousness. For Campan the meaning of a sound in film is progressively worked out by the fact that this sound forms a trace through the lived time of the film. By trace Campan means that what is happening at a certain moment is more than the moment in itself. Sound as a trace is different from an encoded sound: the meaning is established through a process. This gives the possibility to expound the virtual moments which are included in the process. Different layers of meaning penetrate in each other without losing their autonomy (Campan 1999, pp. 16–23). The way Bresson introduces the music in *A man escaped*, is a good example of Campan's idea of "sound as a trace" (Huvenne 2012, p. 83).

From this perspective, the discussed film fragment cannot be isolated from the film as a whole. The moment Fontaine opens his door correlates with previous moments in the film and previous confrontations of Fontaine with jailors, which are playing a role in the constitution of the meaning of this moment. This creates a tension for both Fontaine as a character, and for the audience that is resonating with the different situations of Fontaine. As an audience we are engaged in an alert listening,[2] waiting in a very active way for what will happen next. In this way, the scene can be described as an example of the way the temporal structure of consciousness plays a role in the perception of a film scene or film sounds as temporal objects.

On the fourth level I want to focus on the fact that a sound in film is always a recorded sound and that the recording gives the listener a certain position in relation to this sound. In the film by Bresson I am primarily listening along with Fontaine to the sounds. The sounds are recorded from *his* point of audition, and it is his body which is situated in time and space. This means that I am not merely resonating with the sounds I hear, but with the embodied listening of Fontaine as a situated body in the virtual diegetic space of the film. I do not just see his reaction and do not just hear what he is doing, but I can co-experience what is happening. With Fontaine I am going through a very delicate moment. In this feeling the visual imagery of the jailer is not so important. I am able to listen to the relation of Fontaine vis-à-vis the steps of the jailer by the sound he is producing. The sounds produced by the jailer in the film are situated in relation to Fontaine, and the corporeal reaction of Fontaine, expressed in the sounds he is producing and which are recorded.

Through the way the sound is recorded, in this strategy I am listening along with Fontaine. In this listening strategy two factors are play a role: on the one hand the intersubjective way of listing in which my listening body it attuned to the listening body of Fontaine (cf. the synchronising modulation of Merleau-Ponty), and on the other hand the fact that through the sound recording not only a positioned (in space), but also a situated listening is presented. Instead of giving the sound source a position in the virtual space of the diegetic space through the

2. In his article on *Listening* (*L'écoute* 1976), Roland Barthes distinguishes three modes of listening: an alert listening which is connected with a survival attitude in the world, a listening that is seeking to understand and is searching to discover the meaning of sound and a third mode of listening which he calls "panic listening", an open mode of listening that can be compared to a pre-reflective way of listening.

recording, the sound can also be recorded in function of the way the listener is invited by the sound to react. Merleau-Ponty defines the word "here" in function of a situated body rather than a body positioned in space.

> The word "here" applied to my body does not refer to a determinate position in relation to other positions or to external coordinates, but the laying down of the first co-ordinates, the anchoring of the active body in an object, the situation of the body in face of its task. (Merleau-Ponty 2002, p. 115)

As part of the audience I resonate with the steps of the jailer, to understand what is happening, I resonate with the actions of Fontaine and I am reacting myself to the whole situation. This reaction is, in this case, also guided by the voice-over, which gives me the inner thoughts of Fontaine in meaningful words. In the process of constituting audiovisual images, I receive through the recording of the sound a point of audition which can differ from the point of view and I receive also the qualities of movement, expressed in the acoustic nuances of the sound.

6. Listening to a recorded sound as such

In this section I consider listening to a recorded sound as such. The question is then to what degree listening without an image or a character onscreen evokes visual or motor images. I propose to listen to the sound of a dying crow, recorded by Daniel Deshays (cf. *Battements d'ailes*, www.silenceradio.org/grid.php). I hear the environment and the cries of a bird approaching to a level where the sounds become almost touchable. When I listen to this sound, my body is situated in space through the sound. The distance between the bird and my body changes and I can hear the change in distance. At a given moment I feel the sound (and the bird) very close. In daily life I have never heard the sound of crow so near. I have the feeling that the bird is sitting on my shoulder and cries into my ear. Something is happening in my body: I am affected by the sound and even without expressing it, I react. I am listening as an embodied person, situated in a virtual (non-visible) space. As a listener, my body is anchored in the sound. At this point my consciousness is not reflective, but pre-reflective.

The situation of the listener can be compared to Merleau-Ponty's discussion of the bodily "here" (see supra), and the recorded sound with the way he describes abstract movements.

> The abstract movement carves out within that plenum of the world in which concrete movement took place a zone of reflection and subjectivity; it superimposes upon physical space a virtual or human space. ... The [concrete movement] occurs in the realm of being or of the actual, the [abstract movement] on the other hand

> in that of the virtual or the non-existent; the first adheres to a given background, the second throws out its own background. The normal function which makes abstract movement possible is one of 'projection' whereby the subject of movement keeps in front of him an area of free space in which what does not naturally exist may take on a semblance of existence. (Merleau-Ponty 2002, p. 128)

In the recorded sound as an abstract movement, the experience of the concrete movement is nonetheless playing a role. We hear the recorded sound at a distance defined in the position of the recording microphone and we hear the qualities of the (original) sound movement. At the same time, a virtual or human space is superimposed onto physical space.

As in the case of the example of the film fragment, different listening strategies again provoke different images. Even if the sound is not part of an "audiovisual image", listening to a sound can provoke a visual image.

This is well expressed in the reaction of the South-African anthropologist Edgar Siernaert to this sound. "When I was listening to the cries of the crow 'with my body', I have re-SEEN (j'ai reVU) a pan of my childhood in the North of France" (Siernaert, personal communication).

But unlike the sound in an audiovisual context, the image was not given in a previous audiovisual image. The evoking of the memory of his childhood images by the sounds of the crow in embodied listening, is in this case procured from a lived experience of Sienaert in the past. For him it is through the listening experience to the transmodal features of the qualities of the sounding movement that a lived experience from childhood became actual.

7. Conclusion

Starting from sound and the way sound evokes images, it is not so easy to distinguish imagination from perception. From a first-person perspective, embodied listening strategies evoke visual and motor images which implement the lived experiences of the listener. Listening to a sound implies not necessarily a reflective way of listening. Focus on a pre-reflective way of listening enables an enactive approach of sound perception in film, expressed in an embodied "thinking in movement".

With the example of the film fragment from *A man escaped* by Bresson, I described four different strategies of listening, procuring four different ways of evoking images. Through remembrance of a visual image I saw before in connection with similar sounds, a visual image is evoked. Through the resonation of my body with the efforts of the movement procuring the sounds, a motor image is evoked. By listening to the time composition of sounds in relation to the time composition of the film fragment, I can imagine what is happening, how the different elements are related to each other. Hence an experienced image is evoked.

By focussing on the way the recorded sound, as an abstract movement, situates the body of the listener in a virtual diegetic space, the listener is situated in a double experience and perception of sound. Resonating with the point of audition produced by the recorded sound, and situated as a phenomenological body in the concrete space in which the sound is distributed, the listener is not only resonating with the character or the bodies procuring sound in the film but he is also kinaesthetically reacting to the sound in correlation with his own lived body.

Starting from sound and the way sound evokes images, it is not so easy to distinguish imagination from perception. This has to be investigated further, but it becomes clear that the filter of visual imagery to study sound in film or to reduce sound in film to an added value to image, fails to capture the essence of film as an audio-visual medium. Introducing the listener as a phenomenologically situated body in time and space and resonating with a recorded sound, sound is able to evoke both visual and motor imagery. In this approach, sound plays a crucial role in the transmission of an experience in film.

References

Barthes, R. (1976). L'écoute. In *L'obvie et l'obtus* (1982) (pp. 217–230). Paris: Les éditions Seuil.

Campan, V. (1999). *L'écoute filmique: écho du son en image.* Saint-Denis: Presses universitaires de Vincennes.

Chion, M. (1994). *Audio-vision: sound onscreen* (transl. by C. Gorbman, with a preface of W. Murch). New York: Columbia University Press.

Chion, M. (2009). *Film, a Sound Art* (transl. by C. Gorbman). New York: Columbia University Press.

De Preester, H. (2008). From ego to alter ego: Husserl, Merleau-Ponty and a layered approach to intersubjectivity, *Phenomenology and the cognitive sciences, 7*(1), 133–142.

Deshays, D. (2010). *Entendre le cinema.* Paris: Klinksieck.

Deshays, D. (sound recording). Battements d'ailes. http://www.silenceradio.org/grid.php, May 25 1985 – 5′23. Accessed 6/13/12.

Deleuze, G. (2008 [1989]). *Cinema 2: Time Image.* London: Continuum.

Elsaesser, Th., & Hagener, M. (2010). *Filmtheory: an introduction through the senses.* New York: Routledge.

Gallese, V., Fadiga, L., Fogassi, L. & Rizzolatti, G. (1996). Action recognition in the premotor cortex. *Brain, 119,* 593–609.

Huvenne, M. (2012). Het geluid als een innerlijke beweging in de overdracht van een ervaring in film: een phenomenologische benadering. Amsterdam: Amsterdam University Press.

Ihde, D. (2007). *Listening and Voice: Phenomenologies of Sound.* New York: State University of New York Press.

Laban, R. (1947). *Effort. Economy of Human Movement.* Plymouth: MacDonald & Evens.
Merleau-Ponty, M. (2002). *Phenomenology of Perception.* London/New York: Routledge.
Metz, Ch. (1985). Aural Objects. In E. Weis, & J. Belton (Eds.), *Film Sound: theory and Practice* (pp. 154–161). New York: Columbia University Press.
Petitmengin, C., Bitbol, M., Nissou, J.M., Pachoud, M., Curalluci, H., Cermolace, M., & Vion-Dury J. (2009). Listening from within. In C. Petitmengin (Ed.), *Ten Years of Viewing from Within. The Legacy of Francisco Varela* (pp. 252–284). Exeter: Imprint Academic.
Sheets-Johnstone, M. (2009). *The corporeal turn: an interdisciplinary reader.* Exeter: Imprint Academic.
Sobchack, V. (1992). *The Address of the Eye.* Princeton: Princeton University Press.
Stern, D.N. (2009). Pre-reflexive Experience and its Passage to Reflexive Experience. In C. Petitmengin (Ed.), *Ten Years of Viewing from Within. The Legacy of Francisco Varela* (pp. 307–331). Exeter: Imprint Academic.
Thompson, E. (2007). *Mind in life: biology, phenomenology and the sciences of mind.* Cambridge/London: The Belknap Press.
Varela, F., Thompson, E., & Rosch, E. (1991) *The Embodied Mind: Cognitive Science and Human Experience.* London/Cambridge (MA): The MIT Press.
Zahavi, D. (2003). *Husserl's Phenomenology.* Stanford, California: Stanford University Press.
Zahavi, D. (2010). *Inner (time-)consciousness.* In D. Lohmar, & I. Yamaguchi (Eds.), *On Time – New Contributions to the Husserlian Phenomenology of Time (Phaenomenologica 197)* (pp. 319–339). Springer: Dordrecht.

Body English

Kinaesthetic empathy, dance and the art of Len Lye

Michael Parmenter
University of Auckland, New Zealand and L'Université de Paris-1 (Panthéon / Sorbonne)

1. Len Lye and the dance

The idea of dance occupies a place of particular importance in the work and writings of New Zealand-born artist Len Lye (1901–1980). On numerous occasions, in texts and recorded commentary, Lye makes explicit mention of the connections between his filmic and sculptural "figures of motion" and the art of dance (Lye 1984, p. 76, p. 81, p. 84). From child-hood Lye was attracted to images of dance in Pacific and Asian culture, and has noted (Curnow 1980, p. 56) the early influence of the dance element in Frank Hurley's 1921 anthropological film *Pearls and Savages*. In 20s and 30s London, where his first wife was a dance teacher and in New York, where he lived from the 50s till his death in 1980 and where he participated in dance "events" with his friends Merce Cunningham and John Cage, Lye was an informed enthusiast of the developing forms of modern dance. Lye acknowledged that before the invention of art that moves, the dance was the only art form to traffic in movement itself, and he continually referred to his process of creating movement in his sculptures as "choreography" (Lye 1984, pp. 75–76). It is certainly not difficult, when witnessing the rhythms of Lye's animated films and observing the twists, turns and shakings of his agitated sculptures, to imagine that their creator had decamped from the sturdy sculptural domain traditionally presided over by Athena and taken up with the less decorous devotees of Terpsichore.

This identification with dance is not however unproblematic, for nearly the entirety of Len Lye's work, and certainly the catalogue of his most significant creations, is devoid of that seemingly indispensible ingredient, representations of the human body. Len Lye's work consists for the most part of either abstract films of lines, patches and fields of colour or abstract polished steel sculptures. The dancing body, literally depicted, is with one exception, conspicuous by its absence.[1]

1. The actor and dancer Rupert Doone appears in the 1936 film *Rainbow Dance*.

To further complicate this problematic, numerous statements by the artist indicate that Lye saw the particularity of his art to involve freedom from the constraints and limitations of the human body: "Kinetic art has freed us from the restricted anatomical range of dance movements" (Lye 1984, p. 81). Not only did Len Lye avoid the human body as a subject in his art works, but he was consciously occupied in realising manifestations of dance that transcended the body's capabilities.

And yet it would be hard to find either a film-maker or a sculptor from within the whole panorama of 20th century art, for whom the body played a more pivotal role in both the act of creation and the reception of work of art. The whole *body* of Len Lye's work is premised on the primacy of the bodily-felt experience of movement. For Len Lye, between the movement of the world and the kinaesthetic experience of inner movement, there is an intimate complicity, and his art is the manifestation of this intimacy.

Long before he had discovered his unique calling in the world of art – to imagine and create figures of movement – Len Lye had instituted for himself a game, a discipline, of recognising and experiencing in his own body the sensuous dimension of the world. As a child, each day he awoke, the first thing that struck his senses would determine whether it would be a colour day, a sound day, a pattern day, a taste day. He would pay as much attention as possible to this aspect of the world, record it in diaries and before falling asleep, recall through the remaining echoes in his own body, the experiences of the day (Horrocks 2010, p. 99).

Very soon Lye noticed that the days that gave him the most pleasure, the most excitement, were movement days, and soon these began to dominate his personal practice: "I could remember difficult things like a special sea wave or cloud or some silvery shape in the water; but climbing and smiles and any good shots with stones and watching seagulls flying were things I'd go over the most" (Lye 2002, p. 15). Lye soon become adept at experiencing – as he would later become articulate in describing – the process of taking into his own body, the movement of the world: "I was agog with the notion that I was getting a toe-hold on the fleet-footed feeling of motion" (Lye 2002, p. 31). He was still a teenager when he had his aesthetic epiphany:

> I was looking over Wellington from the best view I knew. Up came the sun and the clouds were bowling along. Then it hit me: if movement is the important thing why not keep it the thing, and really make objects move. I had my idea – to compose movement as movement. It grew: I could change movement in actual motion as a cloud does [...] create a shape, compose its motion, and keep it going in a figure of motion. (Lye 2002, p. 9)

While Lye never deviated from this commitment to making art that moves, he was no less insistent in specifying that it was not the representation of movement in the world that was his primary concern but how that movement of the world was experienced in his own body: "One day in my diver's suit I was full fathoming the five depths of my Know Thyself, and farther for good measure, when I tumbled to the idea that my very body was the plumb-bob hook-line-and-sinker I was trying to fathom the sea of life with" (Lye 2009, p. 3). The body would be the prism through which the movement of the world would be cast: "I suppose the mind's refining process is like the honing the poet gives to the edge of his image; and through my more or less continuous practice of empathy with motion, I felt that my body is a great refiner too" (Lye 2002, p. 40).

While observable movement in the world around him was no doubt the source of much of his art, it was movement, not as a visual, but as a kinaesthetic phenomenon that was to be his quarry:[2]

> I eventually came to look at the way things moved mainly to try to feel movement, and only feel it. This is what dancers do; but instead, I wanted to put the feeling of a figure of motion outside of myself to see what I'd got. I came to realise that this feeling had to come out of myself, not out of streams, swaying grasses, soaring birds; so, instead of sketching line and accents described by things in motion, I now tried to tie and plait their particular motion characteristics into my sinews – to attach an inner kind of echo of them to my bones. (Lye 1984, p. 82)

Lye uses various images and expressions to denote this empathy between the body and movement in the world, but having stumbled on one in particular, "Who hasn't seen the purposeful *body english* of the putter who attempts to squirm his ball into the hole by remote control as it rolls towards it" (Lye 2009, p. 38) he sticks with it, and "body-english" becomes his catch-phrase for this notion of kinaesthetic empathy.

It is certainly this important corporeal element, one that could lead us to consider Lye not so much as a kinetic, but a *kinaesthetic* artist, that separates his work from many of the contemporaneous filmmakers in the 30s and kinetic sculptors of the 60s with whose work his creations are often compared. Despite the desire to go beyond literal representations and restrictions of the human body, Lye was at all times creating from the perspective of his own felt experience. Of his first film *Tulsalava* (1929), he notes that "to get the spirit of the imagery, I […] imagined I was myself an Australian aboriginal who was making this animated tribal dance film" (Quoted in Lye 1984, p. iii). In his great films of the 30s Lye pioneered the technique, later taken up by artists such as Norman McLaren, of painting and

2. It seems hard here to go beyond Maxine Sheets-Johnstone's articulate definition of kinaesthesia: "The sense we have of our own movement and its spatio-temporal energetic dynamics" (Sheets-Johnstone 2011, p. 387).

inscribing directly onto the film stock. In this way he was physically involved with the medium throughout the process of creation and the films can therefore be seen as traces of his corporeal gestures. The jittery and flickering images merely replicate the irregular firing of the neuro-muscular system.

Lye also developed a method of synchronising the images to the soundtrack of his films, but where contemporaneous film artists such as Oskar Fischinger and Hans Richter chose mostly abstract modernist concert music – a device by which they sought to take their productions into the realm of the transcendental and the sublime – Lye turned to the stamping ground or the dance-hall, choreographing his images to music that was created for or arose out of specific dance environments, thus anchoring his images in the every-day world of corporeal life. In his conference presentation "Len Lye: The Vital Body of Cinema" (Smythe, in preparation), Luke Smythe points out that the reason Lye's first hand-painted film *A Colour Box* was booed and condemned at the Venice Film Festival in 1936, was because its celebration of unruly and spontaneous movement was directly opposed to the regimented and formalised corporeal logic of the fascist regimes under whose purview the festival was staged.[3]

Similarly, when Lye turned to kinetic sculpture in the late 50s he was following a course that, if not in direct opposition, was at least only tangentially related to the concerns of other artists in the field. While many of the kinetic sculptors of the 60s were drawn to the medium by the endeavour to capture the frenetic pace and confusion of life in contemporary industrial and technological society, Lye was staging a defence of a much more primitive sense of bodily movement. Lye's theory of the "old-brain" (Horrocks 2010, p. 114–18), though ostensibly built on Freudian and Jungian ideas of the "unconscious", can, because of its strongly corporeal and kinetic dimension, be much more readily aligned with contemporaneous formulations derived from Jakob Von Uexküll's notion of the relation between animal and *Umwelt* (von Uexküll 2010). From this perspective, the life of the animal is understood to be one with its particular environmental surroundings and its specific movement capabilities a response to the unique demands and needs that allow the animal to function in that locale. Movement for Lye was the expression of a primordial unity between the living being and the world rather than a more recent sense of dis-location.

In accordance with this participatory notion of movement, Lye approached his work as an artisan rather than a technician or an engineer; he would play with strips of steel, dancing with them, feeling their acceptance of the movement that

3. Presented at a symposium for the Len Lye exhibition *All Soul's Carnival*, New Plymouth, New Zealand, 10th Sept., 2011.

he would provoke in them and sensing with his own body either their compliance or their resistance. His sculptures started out as duets – tangos of tension and release – in which his own role would eventually be taken over by either an electronic motor or a natural moving element such as the wind. Lye's process of creation was at every stage anchored in his own bodily experience of movement, and the works themselves attempt, not so much to transcribe the movement of the world, but to create figures of that movement as transformed through the prism of the artist's body.

If Len Lye was completely focused on discovering the means of creating out of his own corporeal experience of movement, how did he understand the process by which the films and sculptures that he made would communicate with those witnessing them? Since these works are largely devoid of representations of the body, by what means could the felt sense of movement so integral to their creation be conveyed to those largely stationary observers?

Given the degree to which Len Lye drew on his own corporeal experience of movement in the creation of his art works, it is not surprising that the notion of kinaesthesia should figure prominently in his understanding of how we experience movement in the world and by extrapolation, in the movement of the works that he himself has made. In "The Art That Moves", perhaps Lye's most influential essay, after a brief etymological explication of the term "kinesthesia" and the affirmation that "Aesthetic Kinesthesia" (Lye 1984, p. 78) is the "muse" of the new art form, the artist provides a phenomenological description that offers some clues as to how the chasm between corporeal experience and abstract movement might be traversed:

> From time immemorial the Muse of Motion has promoted not only humanity's most simple pleasures but also some of its most poetic feelings […]. It [Aesthetic Kinesthesia] is our sense of bodily weight which stirs when we see a mighty missile slowly lift off the pad. I feel a kinesthetic touch on my shoulder when I see the porpoise hump its back down in the deep. It's Kinesthesia's presence which seeps into my bones when I relax on the beach. She is by my side when I watch the big comber break, or when my eye follows the white crests travelling along the long lines of the incoming waves. From our earliest days we've all basked in the pleasures which this muse offers. (Lye 1984, p. 79)

In this description Lye uses a number of in-animate images – a missile at lift-off, rolling waves at the beach – which invoke a sense of kinaesthetic resonance in the observer, and though in this essay Lye is still primarily concerned with the experience of the artist himself, we can perhaps develop from these insights a means of understanding the affective power of the artist's work. Given the specific role that kinaesthesia played in Lye's explanations of his own creative practice and the close association that he made between his own work and dance, and it seems appropriate to turn to the idea of kinaesthetic empathy as it has been deployed in the world of dance, particularly over the period when Lye was active as an artist, to endeavour to understand more precisely the process of aesthetic reception of his films and kinetic sculptures.

2. Kinaesthetic empathy in dance

The history of the concept of "empathy" has been so widely recounted (Foster 2010; Reason & Reynolds 2010) that it is necessary here to indicate only a couple of salient features. We are all, no doubt, familiar with the story of how the concept arose in 19th century German aesthetic theory with the coinage in 1873 by Robert Vischer of the term *Einfühlung* – in-feeling – to describe the capacity of viewers of aesthetic objects, or even landscapes, to feel them-selves *into* the dimensions, the qualities, of the objects under surveillance. Equally familiar is the story of Edward Titchener's invention of the term "empathy" in 1909 as a translation of Vischer's notion into English. Considering that the term *kinaesthesia* presents itself with an almost contemporaneous history – the coining of the term in 1880 being the culmination of a series of discoveries throughout the century revealing the various element of the proprioceptive system – it is not surprising to discover that from the beginning the notion of empathy contained a strong somatic element.

One might insist – in a manner comparable to Michel Foucault's claim (Foucault 1976) that homosexual identities did not exist before the coining of the term "homosexual" in 1868 – that empathy as a phenomenon was unknown before the late 19th century. However, there is certainly no denying that notions comparable to "empathy" predated the development of the term. Theorists have given various descriptions of the relationship between empathy and "sympathy" – the most widely used prior expression to describe the phenomenon we are addressing – but the strong physical component of empathy can be seen as one aspect that differentiates it from the earlier more psychological or imaginative notion.

Another feature of differentiation might involve a more complex play of dimensional perspectives at stake in empathy than is drawn upon by the notion of sympathy. Alain Berthoz (Berthoz & Jorland 2004) in his characterisations of empathy and sympathy, suggests that sympathy is more of an emotional resonance, a feeling for the other's situation, whereas empathy requires a change in spatial perspective, demands that we both see the world from the other's position whilst at the same time maintaining our own somatic grounding in the world. Certainly Edith Stein in her classic 1916 study of empathy, while acknowledging that empathy involves a degree of participation in the feeling-state of the other, also affirms that, as a result of the power of one's own primordial experience, fusion in any real sense is impossible. Referring to the experience of observing an acrobat, she notes that "I am not one with the acrobat, but 'at' him" (Stein 1970, p. 16). In truth, for empathy to have any real meaning a separation must be maintained otherwise the experience of self and other would be indistinguishable. In empathy, notes Stein, "there is a split between our own actual experience and the empathic experience" (Stein 1970, p. 15). With both Stein and Berthoz there is a complex overlay of the other's experience and of one's own.

Einfühlung or empathy continued to play a significant role in art theory through the transition into the 20th century until the appearance of Wilhelm Worringer's influential 1908 study *Abstraktion und Einfühlung* (*Abstraction and Empathy*) (1963). Empathy, argued Worringer, is seen as being complicit with aesthetic naturalism and realism and therefore with a complacent accommodation with the current climate and environment. The new aesthetic worlds of abstraction and primitivism however, with their concern for the more transcendental experience of abstract spiritual form had no use for the comfortable identifications of empathy. In due course, empathy migrated from the field of aesthetics to psychology. Ironically, it was the very pursuit of modernist purity, the movement towards abstraction, but this time in the field of dance, that gave the theory of empathy a second wind in aesthetic philosophy.

It was John Martin, dance critic New York Times from 1927–1962 who brought the notions of kinaesthesia and empathy together for the first time (Martin 1933). Defending the emergent form of modern dance and justifying its position in relation to both the ballet of the 19th century and the popular expression of dance in burlesque, Martin needed a principle of interpretation that aligned with the new dance form's more narrowly defined parameters.

Modern dance had largely severed the connection with the narrative element in classical ballet, and to a lesser extent with the associated notion of characterization. Aligned with these as well was the liberation from the dependence on emotionally charged or programmatic music. Martin viewed Isadora Duncan as a transitional figure who, though she had liberated the creative movement potential of the body, had not yet made the separation from romantic music. The new form of modern dance, in contrast, often used very minimal musical means: the drum was omnipresent, although silence itself was not uncommon. Modern dance was modernist to the extent that it was endeavouring to isolate the particular aesthetic field that differentiated it from the other arts, and this unique element was identified as expressive movement. With modern dance, Martin wrote: "the dance became for the first time an independent art [...] completely self contained, related directly to life, subject to infinite variety" (Martin 1933, p. 6). If dance though, could not depend on the dramatic trajectory of narration, the psychological underpinning of characterisation and the emotional sweep of music, how in fact did dance create meaning; how was dance supposed to make sense to its audience?[4]

In order to overcome this difficulty, Martin put forward the thesis that a process named *metakinesis* was the means by which meaning is made available in dance. The emotional or intentional motivation of the dancer was perceived, even experienced by viewers, through their sympathetic participation in the actual movements of the performer: "you have no difficulty in following their meaning because you have often done them yourself, or you can easily picture yourself as doing them [...]. Instantaneously, through a sympathetic muscular memory you associate the movement with its purpose" (Martin 1933, p. 12).

There are actually two parts to Martin's theory. Firstly, the idea that observed movement is experienced by the viewer. Here Martin uses a variety of terms like "muscular" and "kinaesthetic" sympathy to describe the process by which the observer of human movement transposes herself into the physical action of the mover. Secondly, the idea that this kinaesthetic identification is a vehicle for perceiving the intention of the dancer: "a medium for the transference of an aesthetic and emotional concept from the consciousness of one individual to that of another (Martin 1933, p. 13). Martin rejects the notion that sensual satisfaction alone is sufficient justification for dance as an art form and notes that it is "extremely important that we see in the dance the relation that exists between physical movement and mental – or psychical if you will – intention" (Martin 1933, p. 13–14).

Martin's theory, though only lightly sketched in his work, went on to become a corner-stone of much theorising concerning the communicative power of contemporary dance (see essays by Katherine Everett Gilbert, Selma Jean Cohen & Roger Copeland in Copeland & Sahlins 1983). The theory moved beyond modern and contemporary dance into dance anthropology with Joann Kealiinohomoku (Kealiinohomoku 1970) and Deirdre Sklar (Sklar 1994), and even beyond dance itself with Annette Michelson writing about the drawings of film-maker Eisenstein (Michelson 2001) from the perspective of kinaesthetic empathy.

A further step in the departure from representational movement, one that indeed challenged a significant component of Martin's theory, presented itself in the 1950s and 60s when first Merce Cunningham and then the Judson Church innovators brought the modernist dream of purification to full realisation by questioning the imperative of the psychological or emotional underpinning of movement. Dance now stood on the foundation of nothing but the moving body: choreography was less about emotional or psychological expression than it was

4. The problem that Martin encounters here might be seen as representing a significant step, if not the first, towards the degree of kinetic abstraction that will ultimately lead, with artists such as Len Lye, to the complete separation of movement from the dancing body.

about corporeal possibilities. Martin's assertion therefore that kinaesthetic empathy gave us direct access to the dancer's emotions and intentions was considered irrelevant since the very connection between movement and emotion had been called into question. But even at this juncture, the mainstay of Martin's theory, the notion of kinaesthetic empathy, still held significant influence. Merce Cunningham and John Cage, both friends and peers of sculptor Len Lye, continued to use the notion of kinaesthetic empathy to explain the communicative power of the dancing body. In his influential book *Silence,* Cage describes the choreography of his friend Merce Cunningham:

> We are in the presence of a dance which utilises the entire body, requiring for its enjoyment the use of your faculty of kinesthetic sympathy. It is this faculty we employ when seeing the flight of birds, we ourselves, by identification, fly up, glide, soar. (Cage 1961, p. 94)

Carrie Lambert (Lambert 2003) has shown how the notion of kinaesthetic empathy continued to be an important element in the radical aesthetic of perhaps the most important of the Judson Church artists, Yvonne Rainer. One of the principal motivations behind Rainer's classic 1965 work *Trio A*, with its non-performative, everyday movement, was to develop a gestural vocabulary with which viewers could more easily identify and therefore empathically participate in the movement of the dance, thus challenging that pervasive active/passive dancer/ audience opposition.

By the 80s however, the notion of dance's supposed purity was beginning to wear thin. Over the ensuing decades, Martin's theory of *metakinesis* underwent a strong critical challenge from a number of dance theorists such as Susan Foster (Foster 1988), Mark Franko (Franko 1995), Sally Gardner (Gardner 1997) and Hanna Järvinen (Järvinen 2006), who had been influenced by post-structuralist theory. Dance could never be a pure art form, these theorists argued; movement never was, nor could it ever be, the only aesthetic element in dance. There would always be a sound component – a dance without music is never a silent dance; and a design element – even nudity is a costume choice; and due to its being a performative art, there is always a social environment in which the work is being experienced. Dance was now to be viewed from a social/historical perspective involving a whole nexus of aesthetic and social parameters.

From this perspective the theory of *metakinesis* was understood to be too dependant on a notion of universal corporeal and psychological experience. Eliding uncritically "we" and "any human body" (Martin 1968, p. 117), and coupling these to the notion that "the irreducible minimum of equipment demanded of a spectator [...] is a kinaesthetic sense in working condition" (Martin 1968, p. 117), Martin presupposes that the kinaesthetic and emotional modalities are experienced in the same manner across different temporal or social situations; that any person observing a particular series of movements will have exactly the same kinaesthetic experience as the dancer, and consequently as other viewers.

In response, Mark Franko points to a "historical and historically bounded self" (Franko 2002, p. 53) and Hanna Järvinen particularises the notion of kinaesthesia when she notes that "bodies and bodily experience are historically specific rather than universally alike" (Järvinen 2007, p. 145). Sally Gardner notes that the "whole notion of empathy begs the question of how one can enter into the (bodily) experience of another across difference" (Quoted in Järvinen 2006, p. 76) and Järvinen again clarifies, suggesting that "sympathy actually has to claim that gestures are a language the meaning of which is rather simple and straightforward: if you are attuned to the bodies you see, you can "read" them correctly" (Järvinen 2006, p. 77). Drawing on a prior analysis by Graham McFee (McFee 1992) Järvinen goes so far as to suggest that "the logic of kinesthetic sympathy aims to exclude all analyses of dance not made by dance practitioners, since it assumes a universal meaning for dance based on personal experience of the act of creating a dance" (Järvinen 2006, p. 76). While Martin's theory continued to have its supporters, these could not often be found in the halls of academia. In the flourishing area of university dance studies, such notions of dance were dismissed as romantic and consigned to the world of the dance studio.

The notion of kinaesthetic empathy was dismissed due to its complicity with universalist and essentialist notions often associated with transcendental phenomenology, whereas the new critical climate of post-structuralism and cultural studies demanded that choreographic meaning be sought by analysing dance from socio-political, historical and cultural perspectives. When Järvinen claims that dance gains its significance as an art-form from the plurality and flexibility of meanings attached to it "regardless of whether the people constructing these meanings have actually seen the work or not" (Järvinen 2006, p. 77), and when Graham McFee, in his most recent contribution to dance aesthetics (McFee 2011) asserts that "all-in-all there is no real case for a proprioceptive sensory modality" (McFee 2011, p. 189) and that "even were the argument against the existence (or the possibility) of something like a sensory modality here set aside, we should still insist [...] that this is not explanatory of our interest in dance" (McFee 2011, p. 189), it would seem that the theory of kinaesthetic empathy had been well and truly laid to rest.

With the emergence of the field of mirror neuron theory however in the mid-1990s, Martin's theory of kinaesthetic sympathy seemed to receive scientific support. The notion that an observer of movement mentally rehearses, at least on a neurological level, the movement observed, immediately drew the attention of dancers, and the name of John Martin once again started to appear in academic bibliographies. As mirror neuron theory has developed, it has taken on the same bi-partite structure of Martin's exposition of *metakinesis.* While the original theories focused mainly on the notion of corporeal or kinaesthetic empathy, some researchers, like Vittorio Gallese (Gallese 2003), have gone on to suggest that the mirror neuron process also gives access to the intentions and the desires behind those actions. Not surprisingly there has been a flurry of new research projects and writings around the notion of kinaesthetic empathy in dance: the two most significant contributions being Susan Foster's comprehensive, *Choreographing Empathy: Kinesthesia in Performance* (Foster 2010) and the "Watching Dance Project" in the U.K. which has hosted the important conference in 2010, "Kinesthetic Empathy: Concepts and Contexts", and sponsored the publication of the papers from that conference, *Kinesthetic Empathy in Creative and Cultural Practices* (Reynolds & Reason 2012).

While the dialogue between dance and mirror neuron theory seems to a certain degree to offer a vindication of the insights of John Martin, it provides supporting evidence as well for the idea of cultural specificity championed by recent dance theorists and thus the possibility of reconciliation between the two perspectives. For while the neurological studies do indeed provide scientific underpinning to the notion of kinaesthetic empathy, a significant dimension of many of these studies suggests that though mirror imaging is identified as a biological given, it finds itself actualised and realised differently in different cultural environments (Calvo-Merino, Jola, Glaser & Haggard 2008). The understanding of this dimension of cultural relativity is supported by Susan Foster's historical analysis (2010) that shows that notions of kinaesthesia and empathy are dependant on changing vocabularies, frameworks and experiences of corporeal life. Kinaesthetic empathy cannot be simply understood as a universal language, but must always be located in a particular cultural and historical climate.

Perhaps the clearest explication of this aspect of the recent studies can be found in Alain Berthoz's utilisation of Von Uexküll's notion of *Umwelt* to explain how even something as fundamental as perception takes places within a world of context and meaning. As noted above, Von Uexküll's original notion of *Umwelt* (von Uexküll 2010) describes how each animal is tied to its own distinctive environment by means of its specific biological tasks and its activities in that environment. Most importantly though, notes Berthoz, "it includes the significance or meaning of things for each animal, in that they are potentially participating in the survival and social relations of the animal" (Berthoz 2009, p. 18). According to Berthoz, the brain of the living being imposes a structure or rules of interpretation upon perceptual encounters with its *Umwelt.* It does not just passively receive, but predicts, anticipates and tries to solve ambiguities according the structure of its own meaningful world. "Each species" notes Berthoz "has a repertoire of canonical forms that it can recognise rapidly according to the meaning of that form for each species" (Berthoz 2009, p. 22).

Berthoz's deployment of the notion of *Umwelt* takes on new significance in the light of recent neuroscience, since it places movement at the heart of perception, highlighting the fact that mirror neurons are merely the mechanism of a more fundamental relationship, the movement response of the living being to its environment.[5] The discovery of mirror neurons, notes Berthoz "calls for a repertoire of perceptions linked with the repertoire of actions of each individual" (Berthoz 2009, p. 22). Mirror neurons respond to specific actions depending on how they accord with the signifying world of the perceiving subject. As Christian Keysers notes in his book *The Empathic Brain,* the term "mirror neurons" has almost been supplanted since the mirror system does not so much "mirror" as "*translate* and *reinterpret* what we see into the language of what we would have done or felt in that situation" (Keysers 2011, p. 123). In an influential study directed by Calvo-Merino (Calvo-Merino et al. 2008), subjects with previous participatory experience in ballet and subjects with previous participatory experience of Capoeira both responded to presentations of both ballet and Capoeira, but the ballet dancers responded more to the ballet and the capoeiristas more to the Capoeira. Physical activity is perceived by the observer within a meaningful kinetic world, and the observer will extract from what is presented, those aspects that accord with that world. Kinaesthetic empathy can be understood therefore as an innate dimension of perceptual life that nonetheless finds itself differently realised according to changing cultural and temporal parameters.

3. Len Lye's conception of aesthetic reception

We can now return to the writings and practice of Len Lye in order to discover whether his particular understanding of the role of empathy in aesthetic reception is compatible with this more nuanced contextual understanding of the phenomenon of kinaesthetic empathy as it has emerged through the refiner's fire of dance theory.

5. A point that Maxine-Sheets Johnstone makes well in her essay "Movement and mirror neurons: a challenging and choice conversation" (Sheets-Johnstone 2011). However, where Sheets-Johnstone focuses on self-movement, self-apprenticeship, somewhat removed from environmental and social circumstances – "we are indeed [...] first challenged to learn our bodies and learn to move ourselves – all without an owner's manual or instruction from others" (n.p.), I follow Berthoz in seeing this apprenticeship as taking place and being shaped by the meanings inherent in a historically and culturally specific environmental context.

There is no doubt, that along with other representatives of the modernist movement in art like Wassily Kandinsky and Constantin Brancusi, Lye embraced certain universalist notions of aesthetic communication and his conception of kinaesthetic empathy seems aligned to the understanding of movement as a universal language. "Movement is strictly the language of life," he writes, almost mimicking John Martin, "it expresses nothing but the initial living connotations of life. It is the earliest language" (Lye 1984, p. 39). Lye seems to adhere to a notion of direct communion that works below the level of symbolic or semiotic specificity: "We all speak body to body in a dialogue that goes on under the skin of art" (Lye 2009, p. 6).

And yet we recall that in choosing to name the phenomenon of corporeal empathy "body *english*", Lye quite specifically avoids the clichéd generalities of a term such as "body language" and instead acknowledges the fact that the kinaesthetic entails a degree of regional particularity. In his own descriptions of the experience of moments of "body english", Lye is very explicit that he is interpreting observed movement from the context of his own corporeal schema. Describing how he rose early one morning to study the way porpoises dive, he notes:

> I practiced some empathy of motion by watching them hump their shoulders, while I felt in my mind the way I served tennis with mine. I started to feel the way the fish humped their backs to hit the deep. And when the fish had gone I felt my right shoulder turn into a waterwheel. (Lye 2002, p. 36)

Kinaesthetic empathy for Len Lye is both a taking up of the other's position – "for a moment I know what it felt like to live in the sea" (Lye 2002, p. 6) – and yet an acknowledgement that the empathic experience can only ever be partial for it is always experienced through a particular body/world relationship. In a more theoretical modality, Len Lye, this time seeming to anticipate the somatic/spatial language of Berthoz, notes that "Empathy prances blatantly into the picture when that world is given space and dimension, for dimension and space are but ideas dragged out of the organism's own sense of its neuromuscular and spatially motor functioning body" (Quoted in Horrocks 2010, p. 111).

It is because the body is so imbricated into the phenomenon of perception that appreciation of work of art must always be primarily a corporeal experience. Even as a child, Len Lye would deploy a form of naïve phenomenology, bracketing out conceptual information to allow art works to speak directly to his own corporeal experience: "with the big art books I would use a piece of paper to cover up the titles and captions under the paintings to get only the feeling of how they looked. I learned that this feeling was called 'aesthetic emotion'" (Lye 2002, p. 28). It is precisely because all bodies are different and each living being has its own particular world of experience, that each aesthetic response will have its own unique texture and qualities: "our own moments [of body english] are different from other people's moments, but we all get them" (Lye 2002, pp. 1–2).

In fact it is precisely this projective nature of perception that allows us to understand how Len Lye's films and sculptures, primarily devoid as they are of representations of the body, can still transmit to their viewers an empathic experience of embodied movement. Alain Berthoz (2012) describes how the brain simplifies perceptual information and re-interprets it in terms of a predetermined vocabulary of gestures and kinetic figures. Surely the film animator's and puppet master's art rests on the fact that the human perceptual system has need of only the barest sketch of animal or human movement for this figure to be empathically filled in as a living entity (Kourtsi & Shiffrar 1999; Thornton et.al. 2003). Mirror neuron research shows us that even inanimate objects provoke the mirror neuron response in human observers (Gazzola, Rizzolatti, Canessa, Wicker & Keysers 2007). The movement of non-representational and non-organic figures invites the projection of the observer's experience onto the object observed. Long-time users of complex prosthetic limbs report the development of sensation in their non-organic limbs: the brain projects the sensation of touch from a naturally functioning limb, onto the prosthesis. The brain is essentially anthropomorphic and reads the world, particularly movement in the world, in terms of its own experience.

The same projective dynamic of human perception comes into play when we remember that Len Lye's films and sculptures are not movement loops. They do not merely repeat the same movement pattern, but are choreographed to perform gestural phrases that go through periods of stability, tension, relaxation, development and sometimes ecstatic release. In the same way that our perceptual system reads movement in terms of known vocabularies, the temporal journey of Len Lye's works is understood by a process that can be described as "teleological apperception" (Ferencz-Flatz 2011), in which non-representative movement figures are read in terms of familiar temporal structures. Whether we read the figure as having a consciousness of its own, or as clearly representing the intentions of its maker, we understand and experience the kinetic melody of the work in terms of the intentional trajectory of our own corporeal actions and expectations.

Given the projective nature of the human perceptual system, it is not at all surprising that abstract film images and kinetic sculpture partake of the tendency to take on the characteristics of living entities, and that we as observers empathically experience these movement events in our own bodies. As with the observers at a dancer event, it is not unusual at a Len Lye exhibition for a round of applause to break out when one of his sculptures has completed its performance.

4. The double movement of introjection and projection

Not only are Lye's filmic images and kinetic sculptural figures created out of an intimate duet with the artist's body, retaining in their movements traces of his kinetic gestures, but they are perceived and understood by a perceptual system that reads and translates movements in the world according to the observer's personal repertoire of movement experiences.

These films and sculptures, though constituted largely of abstract filmic and sculptural forms, are intricately interwoven with experiences of corporeal inner movement. Out of the rich kinaesthetic experiences of his own life, Len Lye created, through a process of tactile conversation with the elements of film and metal, wind and water, his figures of motion. These vibrant kinetic works are witnessed in turn, in a manner comparable to the experience of observers of a dance performance, through a process of kinaesthetic empathy, such that each observer, according to his or her own kinetic history and movement repertoire, will participate sympathetically with the dynamic tensions and narrative structures contained in the kinetic vocabularies of the works themselves. Implicit within this cycle of movement in the world and inner corporeal movement – this double movement of "introjection" and "projection" – is an understanding of dance as the tensional relation between the living being and the world, the movement of one is inconceivable without the movement of the other. The living being and the world participate together in a perpetual reconnaissance through movement and Len Lye's dance-films and dancing sculptures are the celebration of this shared life of animation.

References

Berthoz, A. (2009). The Human Brain "Projects" upon the World, Simplifying Principles and Rules for Perception. In A. Berthoz & Y. Christen (Eds.), *Neurobiology of "Umwelt": How Living beings perceive the World* (pp. 17–27). Heidelberg: Springer-Verlag.

Berthoz, A. (2012). *Simplexity. Simplifying Principles for a Complex World.* New Haven/London: Yale University Press.

Berthoz, A., & Jorland, G. (2004). *L'empathie.* Paris: Odile Jacob.

Cage, J. (1961). *Silence.* Middleton, Conecticut: Wesleyan University Press.

Calvo-Merino, B., Jola, C., Glaser, D.E., & Haggard, P. (2008). Towards a sensorimotor aesthetics of performing art. *Consciousness and Cognition, 17*, 911–922.

Copeland, R., & Sahlins, M. (Eds.). (1983). *What is Dance?* New York: Oxford University Press.

Curnow, W. (1980). An Interview with Len Lye. *Art New Zealand, 17,* 52–60.

Ferencz-Flatz, C. (2011). The Empathic Apprehension of Artifacts: A Husserlian Approach to Non-figurative Art. *Research in Phenomenology, 41*, 358–373.

Foster, S.L. (1988). *Reading Dancing: Bodies and Subjects in Contemporary American Dance.* Berkeley and Los Angeles: University of California Press.

Foster, S.L. (2010). *Choreographing Empathy: Kinesthesia in Performance.* New York: Routledge.

Foucault, M. (1976). *Histoire de la sexualité, 1: La volonté de savoir.* Paris: Gallimard.

Franko, M. (1995). *Dancing Modernism/Performing Politics.* Bloomington: Indiana University Press.

Franko, M. (2002). *The Work of Dance: Labour, Movement and Identity in the 1930s.* Middletown, C.T.: Wesleyan University Press.

Gallese, V. (2003). The Roots of Empathy: The Shared Manifold Hypothesis and the Neural Basis of Intersubjectivity. *Psychopathology, 36*, 171–180.

Gardner, S. (1997). *Lying Down in the Air: Feminism, (New) Dance, and Representation.* Monash University, Melbourne.

Gazzola, G., Rizzolatti, G., Canessa, N., Wicker, B., & Keysers, C. (2007). The anthropomorphic brain: the mirror neuron system responds to human and robotic actions. *Neuroimage, 35*, 1674–1684.

Horrocks, R. (2010). *Art That Moves: The work of Len Lye.* Auckland: Auckland University Press.

Järvinen, H. (2006). Kinesthesia, Synesthesia and Le Sacre du Printemps: Responses to Dance Modernism. *Senses & Society, 1*(1), 71–99.

Järvinen, H. (2007). Some steps towards a historical epistemology of corporeality. *Proceedings of the* 30th *Annual Conference of the Society for Dance History Scholars, Paris, 21–24 June 2007* (pp. 145–148): CORD.

Kealiinohomoku, J. (1970). An anthropologist looks at ballet as a form of ethnic dance. *Impulse, 1969–1970*, 24–33.

Keysers, C. (2011). *The Empathic Brain*: Kindle e-book.

Kourtsi, Z., & Shiffrar, M. (1999). Dynamic representations of Human Body Movement. *Perception, 28*, 49–62.

Lambert, C. (2003). On Being Moved: Rainer and the Aesthetics of Empathy In S. Sachs (Ed.), *Radical Juxtapositions: Yvonne Rainer 1961–2003* (pp. 41–63). Philadelphia: Rosenwald-Wolf Gallery, University of the Arts.

Lye, L. (1984). *Figures of Motion: Len Lye/Selected Writings.* Auckland: Auckland University Press.

Lye, L. (2002). *Happy moments: Text & images by Len Lye.* Auckland: Holloway Press.

Lye, L. (2009). *Body English: Text & images by Len Lye.* Auckland: Holloway Press.

Martin, J. (1933). *The Modern Dance.* New York: A.S. Barnes.

Martin, J. (1968). *America Dancing: The Background and Personalities of the Modern Dance.* New York: Dance Horizon.

McFee, G. (1992). *Understanding Dance.* London/New York: Routledge.

McFee, G. (2011). *The Philosophical Aesthetics of Dance: identity, performance and understanding.* Alton: Hampshire: Dance Books.

Michelson, A. (2001). A World Embodied in the Dancing Line. *OCTOBER, 96*, 3–16.

Reason, M., & Reynolds, D. (2010). Kinesthesia, Empathy, and Related Pleasures: An Inquiry into Audience Experiences of Watching Dance. *Dance Research Journal, 42*(2), 49–75.

Reynolds, D., & Reason, M. (2012). *Kinesthetic Empathy in Creative and Cultural Practices.* Bristol, UK/Chicago, USA: Intellect.

Sheets-Johnstone, M. (2011). Movement and Mirror Neurons: A Challenge and Choice Conversation. *Phenomenology and the Cognitive Sciences, 11*(3), 385–401.

Sklar, D. (1994). Can Bodylore Be Brought to Its Senses? *Journal of American Folklore, 107*(423), 9–22.

Smythe, L. (in preparation). Len Lye: The Vital Body of Cinema. *October*.
Stein, E. (1970). *On the problem of empathy*. The Hague: Martinus Nijhoff.
Thornton, E., & Vuong, Q.C., & Bülthoff, H.H. (2003). A Chimeric Point-light Walker. *Perception, 23*, 377–383.
von Uexküll, J. (2010). *A Foray into the Worlds of Animals and Humans, with A Theory of Meaning* (transl. by J. D. O'Neil.). Minneapolis: University of Minnesota Press.
Worringer, W. (1963). *Abstraction and Empathy* (transl. by M. Bullock). London: Routledge and Kegan Paul.

The somatic in kinetic sculpture

From Len Lye to an introverted kinetic sculpture (via Donna Haraway's cyborg)

Laura Woodward
Faculty of the Victorian College of the Arts and Melbourne Conservatorium of Music, University of Melbourne

1. Introduction

The nineteen-fifties and sixties were a pivotal time for those artists practising within the field of kinetic sculpture. Artists such as Alexander Calder, Jean Tinguely, George Rickey and Len Lye, amongst others, focused on the potential of motion within the sculptural realm. However, this "movement movement", as it was referred to by artist Hans Richter (Selz 1966, p. 10), petered out towards the end of the sixties; the last texts offering serious surveys of the kinetic field were Gyorgy Kepes' *The Nature and Art of Motion* in 1965, Michael Compton's brief *Optical and Kinetic Art* in 1967, Guy Brett's *Kinetic Art: the Language of Movement* in 1968, and Frank Popper's through *Origins and Development of Kinetic Art* in 1968. Since then, those artists who have practised as kinetic sculptors tend to function individually; contemporarily, there is no "movement movement". There are, however, kinetic sculptors within whose work we can find similar focuses. Aided by the internet which allows an awareness of other practitioners across the globe, these sculptors may be loosely grouped into fields.

The field of interest here is defined by: a focus on motion as a material rather than as subject matter; the creation of systems; and a tendency to create works in a space of co-agency – that is, the artist and the material co-create the work of art through developmental processes and experimentation. Artists of particular note currently practising within this field are Arthur Ganson from the United States, and Dutch engineer-turned-artist Theo Jansen. *Introverted kinetic sculpture*, the focus of my current practice-led doctorate of philosophy, is positioned within this field.

This chapter focuses on the introverted kinetic sculpture in relation to the pivotal essay *The Art that Moves*, written in 1964 by New Zealand artist Len Lye. In doing so, it will propose that, through his writing, Lye touched on considerations that can be seen as precursors to the field under discussion, effectively laying the groundwork for a space in which the introverted kinetic sculpture could emerge.

Lye spent his career focussing on motion. He practised across disciplines, producing serious bodies of work in film, sculpture, poetry and essays. Lye's writings and philosophical musings were always closely linked to his ongoing practice, and thus there is no single essay which could be considered a final statement on his foremost concerns. However, it is in his 1964 essay *The Art that Moves* that he comes closest to providing a complete statement of his artistic intentions and position (Horrocks 2009, p. 88).

The Art that Moves is a distinct, contained discussion of Lye's thoughts around what he calls "motion sculpture", written at a time of significant import to the historical arc of kinetic art. It is due to this specific consideration of "motion sculpture", and the way in which the body is taken into particular account, that it has been selected as the focus of this paper. Lye's writings allow somewhat rare access to the thoughts, considerations and musings of an artist who worked with kinetics at the core of his practice. A close reading of *The Art that Moves*, undertaken almost half a century later, allows an opportunity to develop, refine and consider the emerging concept of an introverted kinetic sculpture, and its relation to the body.

This chapter commences with an overview of *The Art that Moves*. It then provides a brief explanation of the development and qualities of the introverted kinetic sculpture. The final section involves a reading of *The Art that Moves* in relation to the introverted kinetic sculpture and its field. This discussion proposes that, though Lye pre-empted certain directions in kinetic sculpture, two important shifts were to occur between *The Art that Moves* and now which would allow both the artistic and theoretical spaces in which an introverted kinetic sculpture and other practices within this field could emerge.

2. The art that Moves

The Art that Moves is not an academic paper. Rather, it slips between various voices; whilst on the most part it reads as an extended artist statement, it also reads, in part, as a manifesto in defence of "motion sculpture" and, more broadly, kinetic art. In other sections it becomes both historically and poetically descriptive of Lye's personal experiences with his "muse of motion", his "Aesthetic Kinesthesia" (Lye 1984, p. 78).

The Art that Moves has a haphazard flow; certain elements are discussed or described in lengthy detail, whilst other statements are blithely asserted with a distinct lack of supporting argument. This structure and writing style, however, does not detract from the content, but instead reinforces it; the frenetic, tangential tone is not dissimilar to the motion within many of Lye's sculptural and film works, a correlation which fits particularly well with Lye's very conscious attempts to embody his own kinaesthetic experiences within his work.

The Art that Moves is divided into four sections. The first, *The Muse of Motion*, asserts that "kinetic art is the first new category of art since prehistory" (Lye 1984, p. 78). Lye acknowledges similarities in the aesthetics of motion sculpture and film, but separates them for the sake of the paper due to society's conditioning to film as "an adjunct to drama and literature [...] virtues [which are] absolutely secondary to the kinetic fine art end of motion composition"; a statement for which no supporting argument is offered (Lye 1984, p. 78). He then goes on to title the fine art composition of motion "The Art of Kinetics", and its muse "Aesthetic Kinesthesia" (Lye 1984, p. 78). According to Lye, "Aesthetic Kinesthesia" is due a temple to house her "portents of a great future"; a future which is, in Lye's mind, "built on the bones of our anatomy" (Lye 1984, p. 79).

It is at this point that the tone of the paper shifts from manifesto to artist statement. Lye goes on to explain that the future, as based on "the bones of our anatomy", is an acknowledgement that our sense of motion, our "neuro-motor" or "nerve-muscle sense", is anchored in our unconscious experience of bodily weight, and that through this sense comes both a power over movement and a freedom implicit in this power: "the organic source of our psychological sense of freedom" (Lye 1984, p. 79). He goes on to describe in poetic detail the impact that this sense of bodily weight (or, in other words, a kinaesthetic response) has upon him when witnessing motion: "I feel a kinesthetic touch on my shoulder when I see the porpoise hump its back down to the deep [...] it was she [Aesthetic Kinesthesia] who first got me to wiggle my toes" (Lye 1984, p. 79).

He then ties his description back to kinetic art by stating that "this kind of kinetic imagery can now be transposed into formal figures of motion by the kinetic artist. He does it in a similar vein to the composer transposing sound into musical figures" (Lye 1984, p. 79).

Lye claims that our inherent bodily skills in timing and emotion are vital to our existence, in that it allows us to coordinate action for the control of weight, energy and motion. He believes that empathic response is impacted upon by scale, comparing a fallen shrub to a fallen redwood tree: " [...] our lack of response to the smaller object is in marked contrast to the feeling we get from the larger" (Lye 1984, p. 80). He then sums up this section:

> We've seen how the Muse of Motion not only permeates the physical actuality of our lives, but, also, how she most affects the sensuousness and the empathic kicks we get out of life. In art we are beginning to take her value seriously – by impressing it with the mark of creative individuality. (Lye 1984, p. 80)

In the second section, *The Static and the Kinetic*, Lye discusses the differences between the static and the kinetic sense of imagery in pictorial art. He touches on the fact that the merit of kinetic art might be undermined by the idea that everything is, at base, "held together by countless electrons in motion", but feels this is unjustified due to the fact that in art we are more interested in aesthetic experience than an object's atomic nature. He then asserts, somewhat unnecessarily, that "both the *static* and *kinetic* forms of art can have equal aesthetic merit" (Lye 1984, p. 80). He highlights that the static is associated with durability, whilst the "image of motion" is transient; and therefore, that the static perhaps allows an identification of "the essential self with some durable man-made quality of individuality" (Lye 1984, p. 81).

He goes on to claim that "no-one exists without some form of rhythm and motion occurring", and that "our sense of motion is so ingrained that it permeates our lives more consistently than any other single sensory phenomenon". He asserts that, until recently, "the only art form which expressed this all-embracing sense of individual being was dance" and that "kinetic art has freed us from the restricted anatomical range of dance movements" (Lye 1984, p. 81).

In the third section, *The Practice*, Lye describes aspects of his making processes. In doing so, he raises his concern that kinetic art often draws comments that are "made to smack of the analytical brain's intellect, rather than the sensory body's heart and rump." He argues against this by stating that, "of all forms of art, the imagery of motion best describes itself [...] [that is,] the object defines its own action" (Lye 1984, p. 81). The logic of his argument is somewhat obscure here, however it seems that he is suggesting that, to subvert intellectualised discussions of kinetics, the artist must embody his own somatic experiences within the work: "[getting] the bodily senses into the act" (Lye 1984, p. 81).

Somewhat tellingly, Lye specifically decides that he will discuss his own bodily experiences rather than particular works of art. Over several pages he describes his somatic experience and its relation to his work:

> I wanted to put the figure of motion outside of myself to see what I'd got. I came to realise that this feeling had to come out of myself, not out of streams, swaying grasses, soaring birds; so, instead of sketching lines and accents described by things in motion, I now tried to tie and plait their particular motion characteristics into my sinews – to attach an inner kind of echo of them to my bones. (Lye 1984, p. 82)

He considers these acts of embodiment as a form of "practising empathy", going on to offer several examples.

In his brief mention of the studio amongst discussions of his own bodily experiences, Lye talks of the need for a motion to fascinate him in order to pursue its potential in a work: "I go on with the work only while this magical mystery lasts – while it seductively preoccupies me above all else" (Lye 1984, p. 83). At another point, he discusses his belief that these exercises in practising the "feel" of motion, and in tracing and identifying kinaesthetic response in his own body, are the most important means "to keep fit for [his] kinetic activities" (Lye 1984, p. 83).

In the fourth section, *The Image of Energy*, Lye draws a parallel between the ways in which the human body directs energy to "end-effects of value" and the way in which a motorised kinetic sculpture "programmes" energy. He correlates the reciprocal action in his work *Rotating Harmonic* (1959) with the bodily act of breathing, and also with the "anatomical feedback system", or "negative feedback", directly involved in the making of the work (such as reaching for a wrench without over-reaching). He then asks himself "does the [motion] which goes on in my work serve to isolate an image which portrays the fundamental force of nature – energy?" (Lye 1984, p. 85). He feels that anything beyond this singular portrayal would be embellishment, but that embellishment or allusion to other objects may have another purpose, in allowing a viewer to "feel at home [...] long enough to dig deeper – and perhaps come to respond unconsciously to their underlying significance in relation to energy" (Lye 1984, p. 86).

This discussion of energy then allows Lye to speak briefly of the "directional force" of evolution – a force which he believes is the same force that drives the creative imagination. The creative imagination, for Lye, is not a "purely brain-generated, brain-held thing." Instead, he believes that it results from a combination of individuality, gene-patterns and bodily senses, all of which he considers as carried within the body (Lye 1984, p. 86). He continues this discussion by describing his own experiences in making one of his film works, the sound-track of which, with its African drum music, "required literal body action to enable one to retain its bodily appeal" (Lye 1984, p. 86). Though this point is not expanded upon further, it is particularly fascinating; that an ongoing bodily responsiveness is required to maintain connection with a work. Lye describes his experience of viewing this particular film with its soundtrack as "a vicarious experience on an "old" brain or sensory level of aesthetic emotion" (Lye 1984, p. 86).

Lye finishes this section, and the paper, by stating that kinetic art will, in its new position alongside disciplines such as sculpture, painting, dance and theatre, enlarge the range of expression in the Arts; and that, "of all things ever made by man, the Arts alone give lasting evidence of the uniqueness of humanity in *essence of itself*" (Lye 1984, p. 87).

3. The Introverted Kinetic Sculpture

The practice-led project *The Introverted Kinetic Sculpture* has developed over the past two years. *The Introverted Kinetic Sculpture* is the title of my current research project, whilst introverted kinetic sculpture is the body of work that has developed throughout this project.

Introversion in the kinetic sculpture is the sense that the work functions inwardly; that is, that the logic within which it functions and is understood is found only within the sculpture itself. This logic is not placed upon the work of art by the artist, but instead develops during the in-studio making of the work, where materials, systems, tools, movements and other factors not only feed into the work but drive its emergence. In this way, the logic has been practice-led; the ideas that are under investigation have come through the in-studio processes of experimentation, making and refinement. The project commenced with no clear outlines. The first introverted kinetic sculpture, *Shallows* (see Figures 1 to 3) did not emerge through an active decision to enact co-agency (a space in which the artist and the material co-create the work of art through developmental processes and experimentation), but rather through a process in which the artist's attempts were consistently frustrated and altered by the material's qualities; in the end, it seemed that the work of art itself had asserted its own manifestation. The pieces and subsequent manifestations directed the emerging anatomy of the project, whilst also driving a developing in-studio methodology which has come to frame the project.

One of the challenges in this project, in being practice-led, is that as new works of art emerge from the studio, they interact with assumptions and concepts previously developed within the project. Ideas which previously felt certain become slippery, difficult to maintain a grip upon; others emerge to confuse and contradict. Ideas of introversion cannot be forced onto the emerging work of art, as doing so undermines the very basis of introversion in the work – co-agency – and thus immediately removes any introverted potentials or possibilities. For this reason, the introverted kinetic sculpture itself is forever in a state of flux, of motion – developing, changing – and therefore any discussions attempting to define it must hold this state as one of the few consistent factors.

It is for this reason that the introverted kinetic sculpture cannot be specifically "defined". Instead, discussion throughout the next section will construct a framework of qualities which become apparent in introverted kinetic sculpture, and within which the introverted kinetic sculpture may function. The primary quality of the introverted kinetic sculpture, in that this quality allows the introverted kinetic sculpture to emerge in the first place, is the role that in-studio processes play in the development of the work. Each process is specific to each individual work of art and the set of conditions and problems inherent to that work. However, they each require the artist to work very much in conversation with the materials; it is through this conversation that the work may emerge as introverted.

4. From Len Lye to an Introverted Kinetic Sculpture

This section considers *The Art that Moves* in relation to the introverted kinetic sculpture. In doing so, it will propose that in many of his assertions, Lye pre-empted certain directions in kinetic sculpture which have manifested in the field under

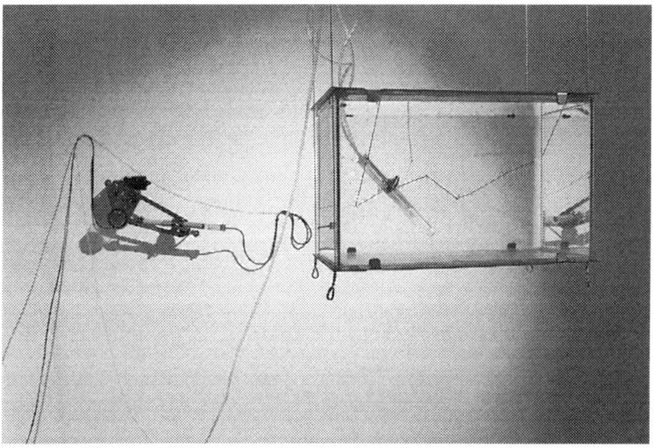

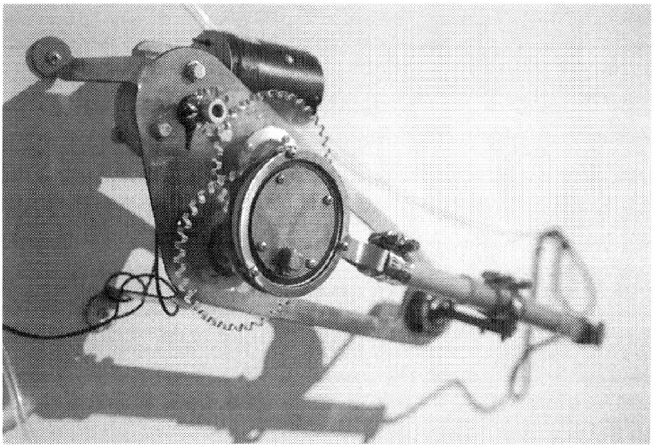

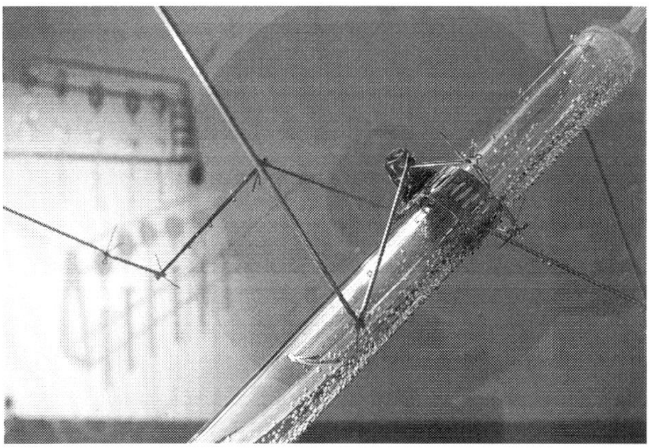

Figures 1 to 3. *Shallows* 2010. Stainless steel, acrylic, water, air, glass, pvc pipe, motor. Dimensions variable. Images by the author. Photographed at Place Gallery, Richmond, Melbourne, Australia. Footage of *Shallows* in motion can be seen at laurawoodward.com.au discussion. It then proposes that despite this pre-emption by Lye, two important shifts were to occur before the introverted kinetic sculpture could emerge.

As discussed earlier, Lye's writing in *The Art that Moves* is haphazard. Some sections appear to contradict others, whilst certain statements are made without significant supporting argument. Whilst Lye's sculptures tend to be focused investigations into a singular motive quality, his writings carry a multiplicity of ideas. It is in this energetic and complicated writing that Lye's pre-emption of the field under discussion becomes apparent.

We shall start this discussion by considering the way in which Lye discusses motion. Throughout *The Art that Moves* Lye refers to "the image of motion" or "kinetic imagery" as that which he transposes into his work. Lye considers his motion sculptures a means of externalising his own bodily experiences: he then transposes these "kinetic images" onto the work, with the movement essentially sitting as subject. However, seemingly unintentionally, Lye does actually touch on the potential of motion as a material, and thus co-agency within the kinetic sculpture.

In claiming the kinetic artist as a composer – "the kinetic artist does it in a similar vein to the composer transposing sound into musical figures" (Lye 1984, p. 79) – Lye insinuates a precursor to artistic practices which we may consider as based in co-agency. Whereas the composer-as-auteur would create music from nothing, Lye's composer is plucking an already existing sound and forming it into musical figures. The sound already exists – and thus must inherently carry its own qualities with which the composer then works. In the same analogy, the kinetic sculptor would not begin with nothing, but instead has motion (and, we may extrapolate, other materials) at hand, the qualities of which will impact upon the work. Within a single sentence, Lye has acknowledged the fledgling idea which would not come to the fore of artistic thinking for some years to come.

The shift that has occurred since, pre-empted by Lye, posits motion not as subject but as material in the work. Considering the work of other kinetic artists such as Arthur Ganson and Theo Jansen, we see motion dealt with as a material. Within this project, those works that have evolved as introverted have been those in which motion is truly used as a material rather than as a subject or effect.

This shift from motion-as-subject to motion-as-material is significant in the ways in which empathy is considered by Lye and within the introverted kinetic sculpture. In both respects, empathy is bodily; for Lye, the motor response of the body – that which he considers kinaesthetic experience, or empathy – is part of the "old brain". The "new brain" is intellectual, analytical. For Lye, empathy is seated in the "old brain" – that is, in the motor-body response elicited through observation. Empathy is also considered as a bodily response in the introverted kinetic sculpture, however the way in which it is positioned differs significantly.

For Lye, motion in the work of art was representational of kinaesthetic experience, and empathic response was something that he experienced and then transposed into his work. The body – his body – is of most import, and descriptions of his bodily experiences paramount to his discussion of work. This is apparent in the volume of such descriptions in *The Art that Moves*. Early on in the essay, he speaks of the impact that one's sense of bodily weight (as experienced through what he calls the "neuro-motor" or "nerve-muscle sense") has on empathic response. Lye's discussion of empathy revolves around his own body and experiences – his own response to witnessing (usually) naturally occurring movements, which he then attempts to translate, as "images" or "figures" of motion, into his sculptural works.

This is not, however, direct transposing of a movement from one medium (such as the swaying grasses) to another medium (such as a film or sculpture). Rather, Lye undertakes what could be considered a "transmutation" of motion. In this respect, his actions go beyond empathetic ones; he is not simply identifying or understanding the "feeling" of grasses in motion, but taking this experience and embedding it within his own body. In this way, the empathic response shifts from vicarious to embodied – an act which, for Lye, physically alters his body: "I now tried to tie and plait their particular motion characteristics into my sinews – to attach an inner kind of echo to my bones" (Lye 1984, p. 82). For Lye, practising empathy goes beyond a mere response. Instead empathy is an act that, through imaginative transmutation, physically alters his bodily state.

This focus on the empathic site as situated within the artist differs to the position of empathy within the introverted kinetic sculpture, due to the way in which the introverted kinetic sculpture develops in-studio. For Lye, empathy was something to be practised, a physical exercising of a bodily response to motion, which he then transmuted into his work. However, Lye also asserts that "no-one exists without some form of rhythm and motion occurring", and that "our sense of motion is so ingrained that it permeates our lives more consistently than any other single sensory phenomenon" (Lye 1984, p. 81). It is with this conception of the interconnectedness of motion and body that empathy is considered within the introverted kinetic sculpture. In contrast to Lye's very active pursuits to transmute an empathic response into his work, the introverted kinetic sculpture relies upon each body's embedded motive experiences, and the empathically somatic responses that may then be elicited by tapping into this universally experienced motion, via the sensorial, somatosensorial and imaginative realms. In the introverted kinetic sculpture, empathy is not focused upon as actively transmuted by the artist, but is instead considered as a potential response from the viewer.

In this way, the act of empathy within the introverted kinetic sculpture is also an act of co-agency: the empathic response does not solely occur in the viewer's own body, but is co-generated between the work of art and the body of the viewer. The work of art, generated through co-agency with the artist, must literally move in order to be fully manifest; thus, the work must be in motion for the viewer to experience a sensorial or somatosensorial empathic response to the work of art in its fully realised state. In doing so, the viewer's empathic response acknowledges the work of art as *another body*. In this respect, empathy is not an after-image, or simply a one-way reaction to the work, but is instead a generative, ongoing and active element that is produced between and within the moving bodies of artist, work of art, and viewer.

With the transition that has occurred from motion-as-subject to motion-as-material, and the shift in how empathy manifests through works of art in the field under discussion, what comes to the fore is the interplay between various materials and elements. Whilst Lye's sculptural works tended to be transmutations of his empathic responses to a singular motion, the interplay mentioned here results not in singular outcomes but in systems. The logic and form of each system develops through the in-studio processes, both generating the work of art and defining it. The systems manifest in the introverted kinetic sculpture embody circular causality; in cybernetic definitions, they can be considered as autopoietic systems (see Maturana & Varela 1980, pp. 80–81). In both the introverted kinetic sculpture and in the field under discussion, the system as both concept and as actual manifestation is at the core of the work.

So, what has allowed such emergences within the realms of kinetic sculpture? How did the shift occur from motion-as-subject to motion-as-material, from artist-as-auteur to co-agency, from Lye's take on empathy to the interconnected co-empathic space of the introverted kinetic sculpture, and from a focus on a singular motive outcome to a system both conceptually and literally driving the work?

What is needed here to contextualise these evolutions is a consideration of two important shifts that have occurred within our artistic and theoretical thinking: the emergence in contemporary artistic practice of ideas to do with co-agency between artist and material,[1] and developments of our considerations of technology through the emergence of the cyborg. This discussion will take Donna Haraway's cyborg, as presented in *A Manifesto for Cyborgs: Science, Technology and Socialist Feminism in the 1980s* (first published in 1985) as a signifier to consider these shifts.

For Haraway, late twentieth century machines have "made thoroughly ambiguous the difference between natural and artificial, mind and body, self-developing and externally designed" (Haraway 2004, p. 11). Her cyborg,

1. Studies in "New Materialism" have been approached across multiple fields by authors such as Jane Bennett, Karen Barad, Manuel DeLanda, Rick Dolphijn and Iris van der Tuin; for studies that focus on artistic approaches and responses to the topic, see texts such as Barrett and Bolt 2013.

existing within these ambiguities, is important to the introverted kinetic sculpture in several ways: in considering systems; in the breaking down of dichotomous dualities; in a reconsideration of the role of technology; and in particular in its discussion of multi-generative, techno-human relationships.

Lye touched on the idea of a cyborg in *The Art that Moves*, discussing similarities between organisms and motorised motion sculptures. However, his musing remained fixed upon a human domination over machine. He garnered experience and took ideas to the studio to make examples of his experiences. Even his descriptions of the "imagery of motion" posited the kinetic sculpture as the dumb conduit between what the artist perceived and then expressed. His discussion is rarely of actual works of art, but instead it is of his own position as creator.

Haraway's cyborg disputes such a position. Her cyborg is evoked as a challenge to those traditional Western positions which function upon dichotomies. Her cyborgs are "creatures simultaneously animal and machine, who populate worlds ambiguously natural and crafted [...] a condensed image both of imagination and materiality" (Haraway 2004, p. 8). Haraway sees these dichotomies as border wars, as means of oppression, and as sites for an individual creator to stand autonomous, symptomatic of an origin story spawned in dust and Eden. However, for Haraway, the end of the twentieth century signalled a time when three crucial boundaries had been breached: human/animal; animal-human/machine; and physical/non-physical. The cyborg transgresses these boundaries, resulting in a site where the "difference between machine and organism is thoroughly blurred; mind, body and tool are on very intimate terms" (Haraway 2004, p. 24).

Haraway's cyborg (taken here as a signifier of the ways in which boundaries have been reconsidered since Lye's essay) seeks an embracing of complexity and ambiguity, a turning-away from our perception of ourselves as separate, entire, and impenetrable bodies. Haraway's cyborg allows a consideration of human and machine not as opposites, but instead a co-generative and blurred: "It is not clear who makes and who is made in the relation between human and machine [...] there is no fundamental, ontological separation in our formal knowledge of machine and organism, of technical and organic" (Haraway 2004, p. 35).

It is in the space of co-generated works of art and empathy that "behaviours" can emerge in the work. These "behaviours", impossible to foresee before the work exists, often form the basis for an empathetic response to the work, and for introversion.

An example of this behavioural emergence was a motive quality that appeared in three works of art over the course of a year. From a material and system perspective, this quality developed from different sources in each instance. In each of these works, a particular action akin to "twitching" became apparent.

The first twitching action appeared during the creation of *Underwing* in 2010. A large water-driver work, *Underwing* relied on seven peristaltic pumps to push water through meters of white hosing between vessels. The nature of a peristaltic pump causes fluid to be moved through the hose in a pulsing rhythm. With the lightweight hose hanging loosely over several meters, this pulsing caused the hose to jerk rhythmically, at a speed akin to a heartbeat. This twitching action across fourteen lengths of hose became the most significant factor in the "bodiliness" of the work (see Figures 4 and 5).

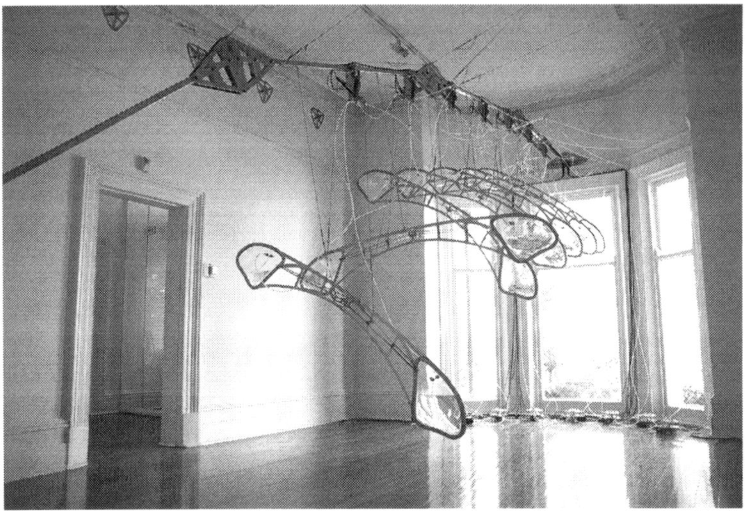

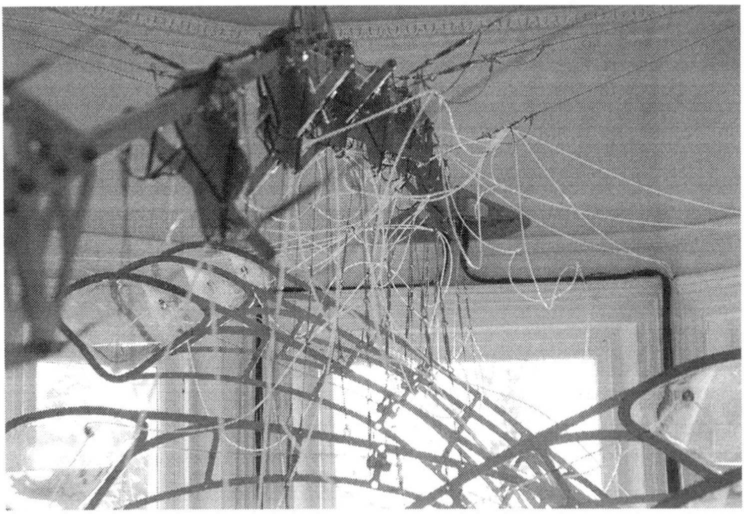

Figures 4 and 5. *Underwing*, 2010. Stainless steel, polycarbonate, fasteners, santoprene hose, nylon hose, electronic components, motors. Dimensions variable. Images by the author and Jem Selig Freeman. Photographed at Linden Centre for Contemporary Arts, St Kilda, Melbourne, Australia. Footage of *Underwing* in motion can be seen at laurawoodward.com.au

The second work in which a twitch emerged was a small work *Untitled (ripples)*, 2011 (see Figures 6 and 7) in which a motor mounted under a tank caused a magnet within the tank to move. The magnet, attached to a small steel arm and sitting in a few millimetres of clear oil, did not move in a smooth circular arc, but instead jerked from one position to the next. By the time it was complete, this twitching had become the primary characteristic of the work.

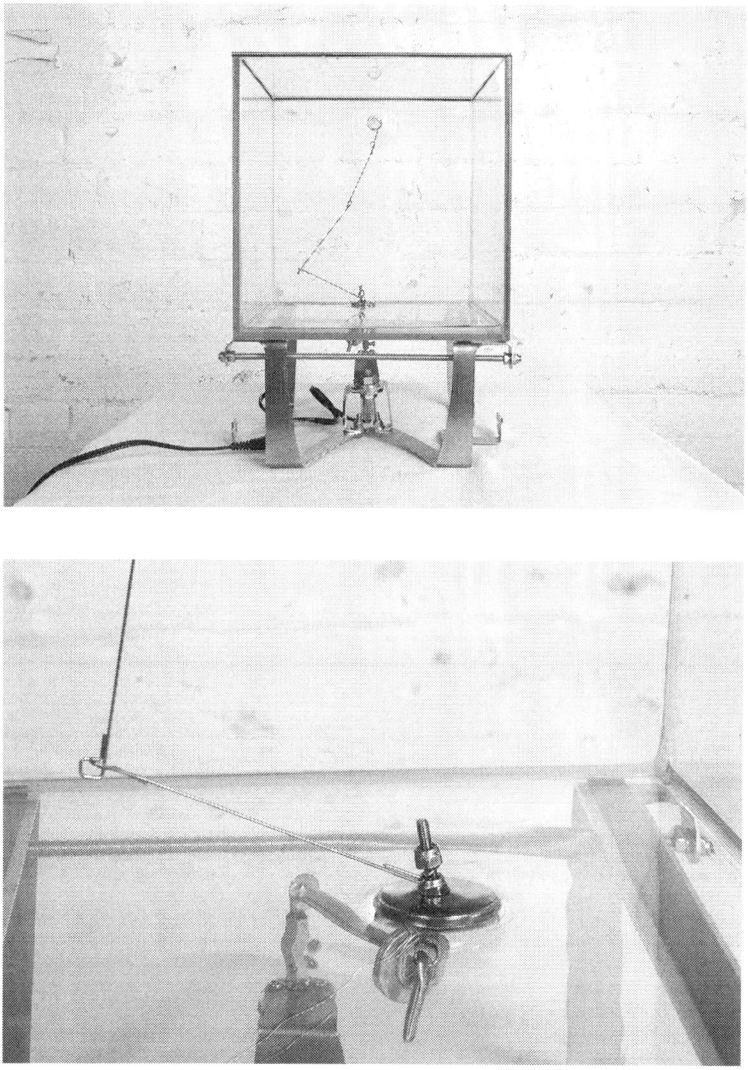

Figures 6 and 7. *Untitled (ripples)*, 2011. Stainless steel, mild steel, magnet, motor, fasteners, glass, mineral oil. 30cm × 30cm × 30cm. Images by Jem Selig Freeman. Photographed in the author's studio at Ironside Studios, Kensington, Melbourne, Australia. Footage of *Untitled (ripples)* in motion can be seen at laurawoodward.com.au

The third appearance of a twitching came to the work through a different means. Experiments in-studio began around the idea of using mechanical means to transfer physical 'signals'. The resulting work, *The Saltus* (2011) incorporated silicone hosing along which a mechanical pulse would run, causing a jerking action at the other end, whilst also closing a circuit which allowed a brief moment of current to reach another motor – which also jerked. Within this work, each twitching action was both responsive and generative, with the twitching contributing to an ongoing loop of motion where start and end was indefinable.

The realisation of the re-occurrence of a twitching prompted a questioning of what the twitch was *doing*. What is twitching? It is an involuntary action of the body. We experience it as a jolt, a jerk, an interruption. It can happen whilst we are awake, asleep or unconscious. It can even occur once the body has died, as the scientist Luigi Galvani discovered in the mid eighteenth century when he applied electrical impulses to the leg muscles of dead frogs – a response that Bruce Mazlish later named the "galvanic twitch" (Mazlish 1993, p. 40).

"To twitch", however, has two meanings. The first, as described above, denotes the involuntary action of a muscle spasm. The other understanding of "to twitch" is carried out actively: to tug, pull at, or jerk, with a quick, short movement. Considering both understandings of twitching may assist in comprehending the role that this twitching has in the introverted kinetic sculpture. The twitching suggestive of a muscle spasm may, when experienced by a viewer, be causing a "tugging" action – or in other words, an empathic response. When it appears in the introverted kinetic sculpture, it seems that the twitching has a dual action: that which the work of art is doing within itself, and that which (if it elicits an empathic response from the viewer) it causes outside of itself.

But it is perhaps the first kind of twitching – that which is suggestive of involuntary muscle spasm and internal processes such as the heart pumping blood – which actually allows the second understanding of a twitch – an empathic "pull" – to occur. The twitching actions, if experienced, are somatosensory – that is, they pertain to sensations that involve parts of the body not associated with the primary sense organs. In this way, an empathic response, experienced as somatosensorial, could be considered the recognition of a body by a body.

Haraway's cyborg, however, allows this consideration to be taken one step further, in ceasing to consider the body of machine and body of the human as separate at all. She asks: "Why should our bodies end at the skin, or include at best other things encapsulated by skin? [...] these machine/organism relationships are obsolete, unnecessary" (Haraway 2004, p. 36). She then goes on to further embed this relationship within a multiple body: "The machine is not an *it* to be animated, worshipped and dominated. The machine is us, our processes, an aspect of our embodiment" (Haraway 2004, p. 38).

This assertion, applied to the introverted kinetic sculpture, posits work of art, the artist and the viewer in relation to each other not as separate bodies, but in co-embodied existences. In the introverted kinetic sculpture, these sites of co-embodiment are generated through both co-agency and somatosensorial empathy; an empathy which emerges due to the nature of the seemingly bodily motions which developed within the sculpture.

Another example of emergent behaviour is a responsive-generative system, as discussed above in relation to *The Saltus*. This shift of motion from a position of subject/outcome/output of the work, to a position in which, enabled through co-agency, motion is both responsive and generative, highlights one of the biggest evolutions between Lye's work and the introverted kinetic sculpture and its field. The potential of a responsive-generative system was alluded to by Lye in his discussion of his work *Rotating Harmonic* (1959), in which:

> [...] electrical force is imparted to the bright, shiny, upright, springy rod [...] it whips back and forth [...] the point is, when the energy generated by the springiness of the rod feeds back to where it is held in the whipping device at its foot, it acts as a brake and slows the motorised force; whereupon the braking effect is diminished, allowing the motor to speed up again and repeat the feedback cycle. This results in an expansion and contraction of the upright elliptical shape, in a continuous, breathing sort of motion. (Lye 1984, p. 85)

The resistant action of the material caused the form to alter visually. He then ties this concept into the feedback system inherent in human movement, which, to Lye, involves muscles "expend[ing] energy backwards [...] [which] put[s] on the brakes so that he wouldn't overreach the tool he was aiming for" (Lye 1984, p. 85).

It is questionable however whether Lye's feedback, as apparent in *Rotating Harmonic*, is synonymous with those responsive-generative systems which thus far have appeared in two of the introverted kinetic sculptures – *Underwing* and *The Saltus*. It is perhaps in the role of the system in the introverted kinetic sculpture that we can clarify this distinction. Lye's works, overall, tended towards a singular vision for a sculpture which embodied a "figure (or form) of motion" – that is, a singular input generating a singular output. The introverted kinetic sculpture and other works within the field, in contrast, embody systems; often systems in which it is impossible to distinguish cause from effect, or response from production.

These developmental behaviours, emerging through co-generated systems, lie at the core of the introverted kinetic sculpture and other works within its field. In considering Haraway's cyborg as a signifier of shifts in thinking about material agency and techno-human relationships, it is possible to see how kinetic sculpture has developed since Lye wrote *The Art that Moves*. Haraway's cyborg allows a consideration of the shifts in conceptions of the body, processes, and dichotomies, and how these shifts impact on kinetic sculpture both bodily and empathetically, through its creation and reception.

5. In conclusion

Through his intimate practise of bodily empathy, and his lifelong quests to bring this kinaesthetic experience into his work and to have motion taken seriously within the aesthetic realm, Lye began, along with other artists of note, to lay the field in which an introverted kinetic sculpture might grow. However, it is in the theoretical space enabled by Haraway's cyborg that the introverted kinetic sculpture could emerge, with Lye's legacy as evolutionary ancestor.

This shift has not only allowed the emergence of the introverted kinetic sculpture, but of other practices which lay the field in which the introverted kinetic sculpture exists, most notably the work of Arthur Ganson and Theo Jansen. Though the work is aesthetically different, the language with which these artists describe their processes is that of the cyborg: where the artist and machine co-create the work, and where interconnection – and therefore systems – are crucial.

In the introverted kinetic sculpture, these concepts merge with those of material agency and co-responsibility in the work of art; the introverted kinetic sculpture is the product of a cyborgistic coupling between artist and machine, artist and material, artist and viewer, viewer and work of art. In this space, where artist, material, machine, viewer and motion co-create, the work of art embodies a logic which both *produce*s and *is generated by* the introverted kinetic sculpture. When it appears, the introverted kinetic sculpture is a site where dualities collapse: there is no longer the clarity of human and machine, artist as creator and audience as receiver, artist as creator and work of art as created, dumb material versus genius artist. Instead, behavioural and systematic developments in the work – those qualities which are crucial to the introverted kinetic sculpture – emerge, as co-developed somatic resonances. The bodily pull – that is, the "twitch" – of these qualities, frames the empathic space of the introverted kinetic sculpture as somatosensorial, responsive, generative and techno-human.

References

Barrett, E., & Bolt, B. (2013). *Carnal Knowledge: Towards a 'New Materialism' through the Arts.* London: I.B. Tauris.

Brett, G. (1968). *Kinetic Art, the Language of Movement.* London: Studio-Vista/New York: Rienhold Book Corporation.

Compton, M. (1967). *Optical and Kinetic Art*. London: Tate Gallery Publications.
Haraway, D. (2004). *The Haraway Reader*. New York: Routledge.
Horrocks, R. (2009). *Art that Moves: The work of Len Lye*. Auckland: Auckland University Press.
Kepes, G. (1965). *The Nature and Art of Motion*. New York: G. Braziller.
Lye, L. (1984). The Art that Moves. In W. Curnow, & R. Horrocks (Eds.), *Figures of Motion: Len Lye, selected writings* (pp. 78–87). Auckland: Oxford University Press.
Maturana, H.R., & Varela, F.J. (1980). *Autopoiesis and Cognition: the Realization of the Living*. Dordrecht, Holland: D. Reidel Publishing Company.
Mazlish, B. (1993). *The Fourth Discontinuity: The Co-Evolution of Humans and Machines*. London: Yale University Press.
Popper, F. (1968). *Origins and Development of Kinetic Art*. Greenwich: New York Graphic Society.
Selz, P. (1966). *Directions in Kinetic Sculpture*. Berkeley: University Art Museum, University of California.

Edgar Degas

Modelling movement. Being in the body

Boris Wiseman & Jonathan Cole
University of Copenhagen and University of Bournemouth / Poole Hospital

Edgar Degas's (1834–1917) representation of movement and, indeed, posture was revolutionary and has influenced artists and others since. Surprisingly, this topic has received comparatively little attention from Degas specialists. It has been discussed in relation to stylistic and formal considerations (for example Jamot 1924, pp. 93–95; Armstrong 1991, pp. 75–76, p. 126; Marques 2002), but the question of what is unique about Degas's way of reconstructing movement, and making us look at the body in action and in repose, remains largely unanswered. We focus on this question by looking, in particular, at Degas's work as a sculptor and its relationship to his paintings and drawings, a relationship that has been a much debated topic in the art historical literature on Degas.[1] We know that Degas made his wax and clay figures all through his career and that the ones that were cast in bronze posthumously were but the fragments of a private collection the extent of which will probably never be known. None was intended to be displayed. Degas essentially sculpted to prepare for work in other media. For this reason his sculptures provide a valuable document of Degas's thought processes, in particular when it comes to rendering movement, the almost exclusive concern of his sculptures. Degas's wax and clay figures were experiments of sorts, the means by which Degas modelled movement, in the scientific sense of the phrase as well as the art historical. This obsession with movement was very much of his times. Pierre-Auguste Renoir says about his epoch that it has "la bougeote" (it can't stop moving). The second half of the 19th century saw the development of new technologies that captured movement in new ways and lastingly altered perceptions, among the main film and photography. In this context, we will try to grasp something of the specificity of Degas's way of reconstructing movement. We will try to bring to light an unprecedented drive to see movement from the inside.

Our own interests are different but convergent. One of us is a clinical neuroscientist, whose day job is to diagnose neurological syndromes. But he also

1. For a recent discussion of it, see Czestochowski and Pingeot 2002.

writes on the first-person experience of what it is like to live without sensation, or with spinal cord injury, or pain or a facial problem. Such an approach goes beyond the usual clinical approach of delineating a deficit to ask what it is to be another person from the inside. This quasi phenomenological approach, from the outside in and from the experience to an understanding, does, we suggest, have a resonance with Degas's work. The other is a researcher in a French Studies department, with a particular interest in the 19th and 20th centuries, but who has often strayed into neighbouring disciplines, in particular anthropology and aesthetics. He has worked on the question of the image, and on issues of sensory perception.

Together, we would like to take up the question of Degas's reconstruction of movement and also through it, explore how we are defined by movement and by our bodies. For, we should ask not only what an understanding of movement can tell us about Degas's art but what Degas's art can tell us about movement. We look at Degas' explorations of movement, its unfolding in time, at his grappling with the representation of the body's mass and weight, and his attempts to capture the experience of the body in movement and in repose in new ways, trying to use clinical and scientific knowledge to extend and take into new domains the views of art critics. Previously neuroscience has ventured into aesthetics in what some may view as rather reductionist ways, for good or ill. Our approach has been and is to be more informed by a richer, phenomenological tradition and by the clinic. Our aim is, therefore, not to shoehorn an artist's work into a neuroscientific or evolutionary theory, but to explore more deeply, and to try to reveal something of the analysis of movement immanent to Degas's works, an analysis that we take to be as original in aesthetic terms as it was culturally and historically.

1. Freezing movement

The Degas exhibition at the Royal Academy, London, ("Degas and the Ballet: Picturing Movement", 17 September–11 December 2011) and the accompanying catalogue by Richard Kendall and Jill DeVonyar (Kendall & DeVonyar 2011), were the first to systematically examine how Degas used the motif of the dance to explore movement. It related Degas's work to parallel developments in photography and, to a lesser extent, early film. These new technologies extended our understanding of movement and provided new means of capturing it; this is the context in which Degas worked. He used photography in his artistic practices, had his paintings photographed, and even based some of his paintings and drawings on well known photographs – those by English photographer Eadweard Muybridge, for example. But, we suggest, he always saw beyond their frozen plates of time and was never constrained by the new medium.[2] He immediately saw that freezing parts of a movement through a photograph was very different to the experience of holding or stopping a movement. Some of the dance moves Degas captured in his paintings of the 1870's, those which made him famous, and his private, experimental drawings of the same period, show fleeting postures so unstable that they could not have been captured by the artist's untrained naked eye. The famous oil painting *Dancer on Pointe* (c.1877–78 [collection of Diane B. Wilsey]) is a good example. But neither could they be captured by the cameras of the day which needed long exposure, especially in low lighting (Kendall & DeVonyar 2011, pp. 56–9). As Kendall and DeVonyar show (ibid.), Degas's unique way of freezing a single moment in time cannot be attributed to the influence of photography. Degas in fact studied dance obsessively, and spent countless hours at the Opera Garnier in Paris, watching ballets, attending both classes and practise sessions.[3] He had professional dancers from the Garnier troupe model for him repeatedly in his studio and, on the basis of his meticulous observations, he built up a veritable archive of images of moving figures which he used to compose his larger works. Degas also used the modelling of wax and clay as a working tool for better understanding the movements and postures he wanted to depict, and at times substituted his hand made figures in the place of living models. Even if he wasn't modelling, the sketches he took of postures often presented multiple view points on the same movement. We also know from Edmond de Goncourt's diary that Degas sometimes took on himself the postures of his dancers while painting them, allowing him to experience the dance and posture within himself, as best he could, as well as observing it from the outside.

In short, Degas's representations of figures in motion were arrived at after a long process of analysis and his compositions built up slowly over time. This lengthy process of reconstruction, inspired by the techniques of European old masters, allowed him to ally an intimate understanding of movement with the

2. Muybridge was the first to visually record the correct attitude of a galloping horse. Degas integrated the lessons of Muybridge's famous images of horses after the publication of *Animal Locomotion* in 1887, although these images had been published earlier in France and probably seen by Degas. What is perhaps more revealing is his later return to the *incorrect* attitudes, for example in the key work, *Fallen Jockey* (c. 1996–8; oil, Oeffentliche Kunstmuseum Basel), in which the horse has all four hoofs off the ground. What this reworking of one of Degas's earliest images of a jokey, *The Steeplechase* (c.1866; Oil on canvas, Paul Mellon Collection) seems to be saying is that, ultimately, artistic truth is more important than realism.

3. He probably attended these sessions from around 1886 as he didn't have backstage access at the Opéra rue Le Peletier (Boggs 1988, p. 175).

artistic translation of observed reality. Rather than see his images in slavishly mimetic terms, these techniques suggest a strong use of memory and imaginative reconstruction. This allowed Degas, adopting something of the anthropologist's gaze, to situate his approach to the moving and indeed the stationary body in the deeper terrain of what the professor of neurophysiology Charles Phillips described as 'the internal brain models of our bodies and of visual space, built up by learning […]' (cited in Cole 1995, p. 32). These brain models not only filter immediate sensory information relating to, say, preceding postures but are also, as Jonathan Cole puts it, 'the product of movement patterns developed throughout life' (ibid.). It is these patterns, *and their subject's relationship to them*, that we find time and time again at the heart of Degas's works.

What we also learn from Degas's method of capturing movement is that initially photography was inferior to his own minute and prolonged observation and then representation of dance. The new medium needed intense light and long exposure times, both conspiring against the fragile yet beautiful unfolding of a dancer's grace. He assimilated and learnt from photography but soon saw both its strengths and limitations, and was always looking beyond its flat, though revelatory, decomposition of movement towards how he could communicate not just the frozen fragments of movement but its very essence.

From the mid 1870's Muybridge had developed photographic techniques that allowed him to break down sequences of movements into their component parts. He famously used a series of cameras rigged to trip wires to identify the attitudes and postures of a galloping horse. These images were first published in France in an article in the popular science journal *Nature* in 1878. Taking Muybridge's experiment one step further, the renowned Collège de France scientist and movement specialist Etienne-Jules Marey, who had already been inventing instruments for graphically transcribing movement patterns, created a photographic gun capable of taking a series of exposures at intervals of a 1/12 of a second. He used it to reveal, amongst other things, the mechanisms of the flight of various birds as well as to decompose human movement.

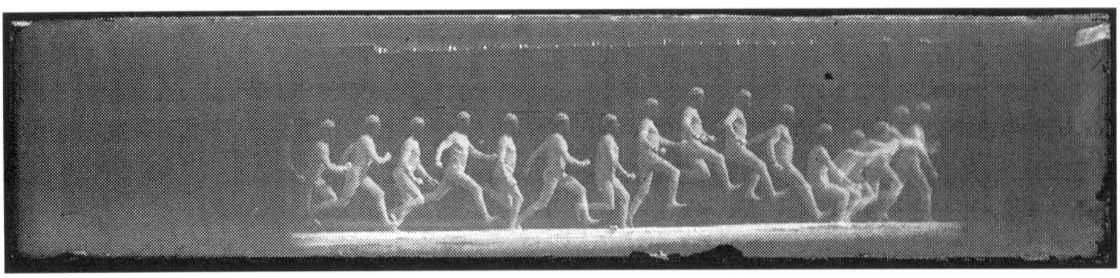

Etienne-Jules Marey. Saut en longueur précédé d'une course, chronphotographie, sujet Demenÿ. 1883. Chronophotograph on fixed plate. Negative. H 2.8cm, L 13 cm. Collège de France archives

He also used his photographs to construct time lapse sculptures of movement sequences which remain stunning. Unlike Muybridge's stop-action photography, which requires the assembly of multiple images into a kind of storyboard, Marey's techniques involved the repeated exposure of a single photographic plate. The resulting accordion effects often provide a striking visual translation of changes in velocity.

Part of the aim of the Royal Academy exhibition was to situate Degas's way of depicting moving figures in relation to chronophotography in general and Marey's sequences in particular. It identifies sequentially decomposed movements in Degas's painted and sculpted works, linking for example Etienne-Jules Marey, *Analysis of the Flight of a Seagul*, 1887[4] and Degas's *Four Dancers*, c. 1899.[5] The exhibition's hypothesis is that Degas used several figures to show the phases of a single Marey-like sequence or one figure represented several times to convey the idea of a movement unfolding through time and space.

2. Moments of being

We suggest, however, that what Degas did, even if inspired in part by Marey or Muybridge-like sequences, was quite different. Marey and Muybridge stayed on the outside of the animals and humans whose movements they analysed. Photography allowed them to assemble the moments of a particular movement into a sequence, so capturing its phases. Marey's photographs tell a story, with a beginning, middle and an end; that of a completed movement, sometime showing a series of cycles in a repeated movement. The images were startlingly original at the time and are as beautiful as they are astonishing, even to this day. For the first time, people were able to see a movement frozen in its parts to make a whole and thus how movements flowed and were constructed.

Degas saw these images and their revelatory power, but developed a very different, almost incompatible, approach to the decomposition and reconstruction of movement sequences. With his dancers, he often sampled a movement over a very small part of its life. What typically seems to interest him is a single moment, equivalent to one of the figures in the image of a

4. Available at: http://www.telegraph.co.uk/culture/culturepicturegalleries/7073785/On-the-Move-Visualising-Action-at-the-Estorick-Collection-of-Modern-Italian-Art.html?image=2

5. See respectively: http://www.newscientist.com/blogs/culturelab/2010/01/art-and-science-in-motion.html and http://www.nga.gov/collection/gallery/gg89/gg89-46597.html

jumping man above [P044], and what comes a few moments before it and/or a few momts after it – i.e. a group made up of no more than two or three attitudes extracted from the above Marey sequence. Degas seems to have intuited what neuroscience later demonstrated, namely that 'every recognisable [bodily] change enters consciousness already charged with its relation to something that has gone before, just as on a taximeter the distance is presented to us already transformed into shillings and pence.' (Henry Head cited in Cole 1995, p. 32). And indeed, one could add, already charged with its relation to something that comes after (the golfer knows he has miss-hit before he completes his swing). It is what occurs in this interval that most often or most distinctively seems to retain Degas's attention. His sequences, unlike those of Marey, are not strictly bound by chronology. They don't occur in an external, measurable time. Their temporal unity is *psychological and neuro-physiological*. The units he samples closely correspond to the way in which we experience movement in the first person, which involves a sort of toing and froing between the present moment, what has just occurred and what is about to occur. This artistic reconstruction of temporality is visible, for example, in Degas's pentimenti. The corrections to the feet of the dancer in the charcoal drawing 'Dancer (Préparation en dedans)' (c.1880–1885, Trinity House)[6] may be read as two states of the same drawing but also as the image of a dancer caught with her feet in two different moments. Similarly, the figures in the bronzes *Woman seated in an armchair wiping her left armpit* (c.1895–1900, The Art Institute of Chicago [Kendall 1996, p. 247]) and *Seated woman wiping her left side* (c.1900–5, Detroit Institute of Art [ibid, p. 239]) capture a moment whose extent is difficult to define perhaps precisely because it is made up of two or more moments. The first figure is *about* to get up, or at least that is what the position of her back is suggesting, but her arms seem to tell a different story. The second is simultaneously rising from her chair and straining to see a part of her back which lies outside of her field of vision, merging what one might otherwise think of as phases in a sequence of movements.

Occasionally, this interval is explored over successive works, as is the case with the famous sequence of sculptures, *Grande Arabesque, First Time, Second Time* and *Third Time* (1885–90).

6. Available at: http://www.trinityhousepaintings.com/DesktopDefault.aspx?tabid=6&tabindex=5&objectid=302984

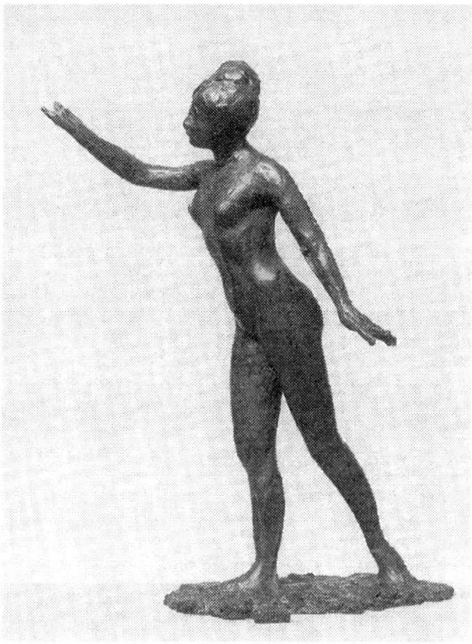

Edgar Degas. Grande Arabesque, First Time. C. 1885–1890. Bronze. Ny Carlsberg Glyptotek, Copenhagen, photographer: Ole Haupt

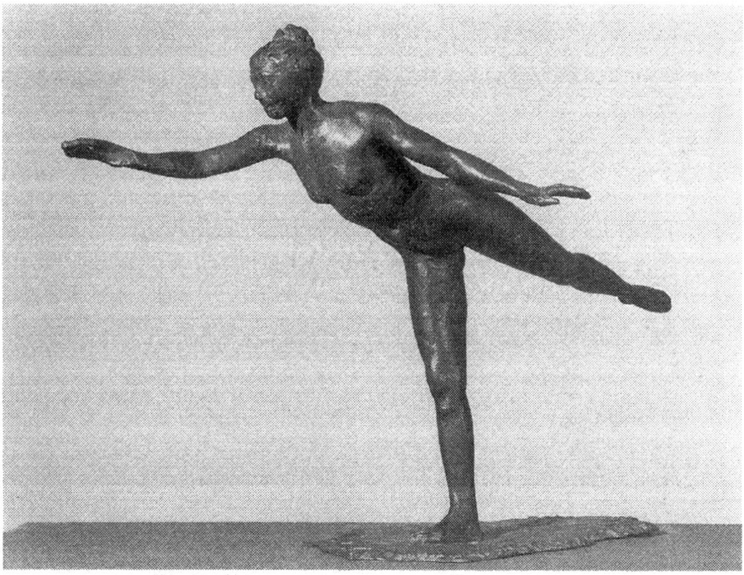

51 Grande Arabesque, Second Time

Edgar Degas. Grande Arabesque, Second Time. C. 1885–1890. Bronze. Ny Carlsberg Glyptotek, Copenhagen, photographer: Ole Haupt

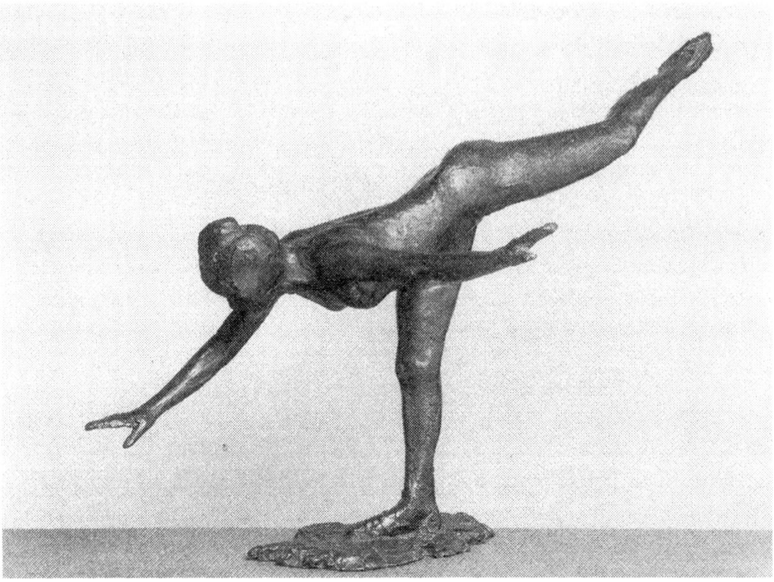

Edgar Degas. Grande Arabesque, Third Time. C. 1885–1890. Bronze. Ny Carlsberg Glyptotek, Copenhagen, photographer: Ole Haupt

Jean Sutherland Boggs identifies a similar sequence, roughly contemporaneous to the sculptures, in Degas's depiction of four bathers.[7] Boggs revealingly compares the sequence to a series of frames in a film: 'the camera circles the bather while she gathers the last drops of water in her sponge, and then comes in for a close-up as she shifts her weight, steadies herself with her left hand, and lifts her right arm to squeeze the sponge out on her shoulder' (Boggs 1988, p. 447). The sequence was never intended to be displayed as such – its unity is in the artist's mind and in his working practises. It is a slightly longer sequence than the arabesque sequence mentioned above. It captures the transitions from a stable posture, when the bather's legs are almost straight and she is fully bent over, to an unstable one, with the bending of knees and balancing and then finally we return to stability with the crouching position.

In his focus on the moment of action and the moment of being, as a dancer, as a body, as a person, Degas goes beyond the representation of movement and frequently draws and paints the subject not moving at all, in a conventional sense.

7. In order: Woman Bathing in a Shallow Tub, c.1885–6, Pastel, Hiroshima Museum of Art; Woman Bathing in a Shallow Tub, 1886, pastel, Hill-Stead Museum, Farmington; Woman Bathing in a Shallow Tub, 1885, charcoal and pastel, Metropolitan Museum of Art; Woman Bathing in a Shallow Tub, 1886, Pastel on heavy wove paper, Musée d'Orsay.

For example in his oil painting, *The Dance Lesson* (c.1879), [National Gallery of Art, Washington] there are a number of dancers but – startlingly – none is dancing. Just as he anticipates movement in his single figures, so here he shows us a scene before, or after the lesson itself. In so doing he invites us to look forward or back to what is about to or just has happened, but also is saying that just as important for his purpose are the stationary dancers standing or stretching. He is as interested in what they are doing and feeling in their bodies before or after practise as during it. Action and movement, he seems to be saying, are constant and present in the minute postural adjustments which occur during standing as much as in the more dynamic events of performance. Focus, he says, not just on the public displays of athleticism but on the experience of one's body at all times.

With Marey and Muybridge, the significance of each moment captured by the opening and closing of the camera lens is lost. The moment only counts in as much as it contributes to the construction of the sequence. The moment is subsumed by the sequence. Degas crops these sequences, thereby cutting movement and the moment from narrative. The removal of narrative is already achieved in the numerous practise scenes he depicts. Here, it is the repetition so essential to a dancer's training that suspends narrative.[8] Degas's nudes, his bathers in particular, are also involved in repetitive acts, such as wiping themselves. Repetition prevents the sequence from being closed. The moment can no longer be used in the construction of a bigger whole, as with Marey's decomposition of the phases of a jump, for example. Crucially, repetition allows Degas to explore part of a movement in and for itself, and the effort involved in carrying it out.

In a sculpture such as Paul Richer's 'French Boxing, Direct Kick' (1898–99), the split second that is captured clearly invites an imaginative reconstruction of a boxing match. Richer chooses to show the moment of impact, the most dramatic moment in terms of narrative. Degas chooses moments that are curiously suspended in between the moments that are of interest from a narrative point of view, or which occur before the action or movement has started, or that are difficult to locate within a diachronic sequence of movements, as is the drawing *Bather Sponging Her Knee*,[9] ca. 1883–4, Metropolitan Museum of Art, on which the pastel *After the Bath* is based (Lemoisne 717) (reproduced in Boggs 1988, p. 421).

Degas's paintings and sculptures of dancers aren't usually meant to invite us to imagine the dance, but the movements involved in dancing, or sometimes simply

8. He seems to have incorporated the idea of repetition from his drawings of the 1870's onwards (Ann Dumas, personal communication).

9. http://www.metmuseum.org/Collections/search-the-collections/90000045?rpp=20&pg=1&ft=Degas+Standing+bather&pos=7

in preparing for dancing. This is what we take him to mean when he says that, for him, dance is a pretext for rendering movement. The focus is on a moment of embodied experience, in movement or even in a static posture. Moments of being are to be found in repose as well as in dance, he is saying.

Degas's distinctive approach to movement is closer to that of philosopher Henri Bergson (1859–1941) than Marey or Muybridge's. The relations between Degas's artistic reconstructions of movement and Bergson's philosophy of movement remain unstudied, yet they provide rich contexts for understanding one another. Bergson's key philosophical texts on movement were published too late to have been an influence on Degas, who modelled wax and clay all his life and whose most innovative figures, his *Dancer Looking at the Sole of Her Right Foot* for example, are likely to date from the late 1880's; Bergson's *Matter and Memory* was published in 1896. Bergson's new conceptions about movement nevertheless emphasize a series of themes which fit Degas well. Bergson and Degas were both fascinated by the phenomenon of transition and with movement grasped in duration. Movement, until Bergson, was approached philosophically in spatial terms. It was decomposed into a series of positions in space corresponding to moments in time (the duration of the movement was plotted along a geometrical line). But this conception, Bergson showed, was problematic, because each moment is itself fixed in time and space. It is impossible, Bergson argued, to reconstruct movement by assembling a series of immobile moments. This was where Zeno went wrong and explains why his thinking about movement ends in paradox. It also explains why Marey and Muybridge ultimately also miss the essence of movement. Movement, Bergson emphasized, is what happens *in between* each position or moment. This was also part of what Degas intuited (see above, *After the Bath*, for example). In earlier two dimensional works, his unusual framing and cropping techniques interrupt movement in such a way as to capture it whilst still unfolding (you can see this in the feet descending the spiral staircase in *The Dance Class*).

3. Degas's development

Degas is well known for having worked on three subjects in particular, horses, dancers and bathers. This is what he depicted time and time again in his paintings, pastels and drawings. These are also the main subjects that he dealt with in his sculptural work. While it is true that he mostly worked on all three subjects in parallel, he made more horses earlier in his career and more bathers towards the end. The progression from one subject to another, at certain points in time at least, whilst not attributable to an overarching narrative about Degas's development, seems to have played an important part in allowing him to approach movement in different ways. Movement provides a thread for grasping one strand in Degas's complicated evolution as an artist. In very broad terms, Degas seems to have progressed from an exploration, in his early works, of what one might call movement-worlds to a more fine grained study not only of movement but of posture and of the human body itself in action and in repose. He progressively removed narrative and context and asked us to look directly, solely at the body. With each new step, Degas seems to have entered the body more deeply, showing that even in stationary positions we observe and feel the body and the myriad of small adjustments and movements we make.

Let us look more closely at this very schematically drawn progression. Many of the earlier works tend to represent multiple mobile figures interacting with one another. His depictions of dance classes or of jockeys, often carefully balance groups of figures that are in motion with others that are static. The oil paintings *Racehorses before the stands* (1866–68), also know as *Le défilé* [Orsay, Lemoisne 262] and *Dance class at the Opera* (1872) [Orsay, Lemoisne 298] are good examples. A comparison of these two works (others could have been added) suggests that the racecourse is a version of the dance floor. They are essentially the same stage, upon which Degas places his figures, imparting motion to some, whilst anchoring others firmly to the ground. One could think of these early racecourse and practise pictures as taking a Newtonian approach to movement in as much as they show systems of interacting moving figures, a sort of human version of a solar system. In a slightly later racecourse scene, considered to be one of Degas's major works, the oil painting *The Racecourse, Amateur Jockeys* (1876–1887) [Musée d'Orsay, Paris], the movement of the speeding jockey that has just entered the frame form the left (he is thematically related to the bronze *Jockey* (1881–1890) [Norton Simon Art Foundation, M.1977.02.48.S]) is mirrored by that of the speeding train in the hills behind him. Beyond the witty effect, noted by one critic, this visual echo serves to thematise speed itself. The train, shown minimally as a blurred dark line, is the representation of a pure vector of speed, and something like a signifier of the force to which the jockey racing across the middle ground of the canvas is also submitted. The train reminds us that both machine and human-being are being propelled along the same straight line by virtue of the same law of physics.

A key transition occurs round about the middle of the 1880's. The pastel *After the Bath* (1883–84), already mentioned above, is one of the works that marks this turning point. Jean Sutherland Boggs usefully points out (1988, p. 421) that it occupies a pivotal position between a series of earlier nude figures (pastelized monotypes), which were themselves related to a series of brothel scenes, and the famous (at the time infamous) series of larger format nudes that Degas was to work on for nearly a decade, from the mid 1880s onwards. These nudes, which mark a crucial development in terms of Degas's use of colour and line, take us a away from the worlds-in-miniature that were the racecourse or dance class to focus on single figures grasped through larger formats. In *After the Bath* (pastel and wash, c. 1883, Durand-Ruel collection), the model is seen from behind as she balances on her right leg, with the left bent at knee and hip as she dries or grooms her left thigh with a sponge or small cloth clasped in the left hand. The posture is unstable; she looks at the floor and the towel she stands on, her right hand grips a chair. It must have been unsettling for the model to hold for any time, but this is not apparent from the drawing. Instead we focus on the model's back and especially bottom. Perhaps a better term here is 'rump' for, in comparison with her slender legs and elegant breast, her posterior appears more prominent. She is one of the first of Degas's bathers to stand more or less upright (Boggs, ibid.) and Degas has made the most of her verticality, from the point of her movement. This, more than many of Degas' earlier drawings, brings you back to the sculptures. It is redolent of three dimensional representations (indeed, a series of sculptures explore similar postures). Her body, though in two dimensions, is showing the weight of – and in – her body, a weight that she is pushing up against as she balances.

Compared to the earlier racecourse and dance scenes, a different kind of movement emerges in these large nudes. The actions they carry out are almost all autotelic – they end in themselves and possess a complete, self-sufficient quality. The catalogue of the 1886 Impressionist exhibition in which a number of them were exhibited, refers to a "suite of female nudes, bathing, washing, drying themselves, wiping themselves, combing their hair or having their hair combed" (quoted in Shackelford & Rey 2011, pp. 129–130). His bathers, in particular, introduce us to a new kind of movement, sometimes referred to as active-touch, in which moving and touching have become inseparable and interdependent. Perhaps one could see the transition of the mid 1880's more generally as a reorganisation of Degas's artistic imaginary as he considered touch and the internal feeling of posture and movement. Rather than observing from the outside his work invites us to imagine the feelings of others from the inside. The highly original technique he developed for using pastels, in which he applied layer after layer of thickly encrusted colours is highly tactile and almost like a form of modelling. Later still, when making preparatory sketches, Degas is said to have discarded his paintbrush in order to lay down the tones of his composition with his thumb (Denis Rouart in Pingeot 1991, p. 22).

One of the new motifs that emerges at the time of these late bathers is the circular tub. It contains his bathers and provides a powerful visual symbol for the self-centred and self-sufficient world they inhabit. Beyond that, the tub may be seen as a symbol of the containing body itself, with which Degas seems to become increasingly preoccupied in his later years. Other motifs provide strong visual triggers for haptic experiences, such as the images of woman having their hair combed, which bring us deeper and deeper into the body. The evolution of Degas's reconstruction of movement may be seen as an involution. It reaches its culminating point in a work such as *Nude Woman Drying Her Foot* (c.1885–6) [Pastel, Musée d'Orsay, Paris. Lemoisne 874] in which the human body, as one critic aptly notes, has become almost snail-like (the female figures become increasingly distorted in Degas's late works).

4. Lessons from loss; proprioception and embodiment

It is a patient of Jonathan Cole's who best allows us to grasp the importance of an aspect of movement that is often overlooked yet is crucial for understanding Degas's project. Ian Waterman is one of a handful of people in the world to have lost, due to a virus, all sense of touch over the skin below the neck. But, more than this even, he has lost all movement and position sense too. This means that he has no awareness of where his arms, legs, hands or body are unless he looks at them (Cole 1995). Deprived of this proprioceptive feedback from his body and limbs he was completely unable to control any movement. Proprioception is so deep within us that we hardly think how we stand or walk or pick up a cup. But deprived of these, Ian found that what he used to do without thinking he could no longer do or even imagine how to do. Initially after his illness, which occurred when he was 19, his attempts at moving just led to unpredictable, uncontrolled lunges. Soon after the illness he needed full and complete nursing care since no movement was useful or appropriate.

After several weeks of despair he decided to try to move in a completely novel way, by concentrating on that movement, imagining that it was happening in his mind and by using visual supervision. Lying in bed he decided to try to control sitting up. He contracted his stomach muscles and found himself slowly sitting up. So euphoric was he at managing to sit that he lost concentration on that movement (or posture) and so the movement decomposed and he nearly fell out of bed. That single movement and moment was revelatory. He realised he could control movement, but also the sheer amount of mental concentration on movement he would need to do so. For the next 17 months he was an in-patient in a rehabilitation hospital, spending all day, every day, thinking about movement and its composition and his new requirements to move. He learnt to dress and feed himself, taking hours over each but determined to become independent. After 12 months he stood and two months later started his first unsteady but remarkable steps. No one with the same condition has learnt to walk unassisted.

Ian has lived with his extraordinary condition for more than 30 years now and all the time has to think about movement and his body's position and weight. No movements are spontaneous and all need mental concentration. He was so dependent on moment by moment concentration that if he sneezed when standing he would fall. He has to be aware the whole time of where his body is in space, and how vulnerable it is to other people knocking into him, to the wind, to slippery surfaces and to his own mental reserves to think about movement.

Degas's sampling of parts of movements, the attention he gave to issues of balance, the way in which he used modelling (see below for more on this) all confirm that his approach to movement was informed by an intuitive understanding of the sense that Ian has lost. Degas's originality lies, in part at least, in the fact that he investigated a terrain that was new not only to art but also to science, that of the inner perception of posture and movement, in particular through touch and proprioception. What comes across time and time again, is that he was less interested in the outer appearance of movement than its inner experience and feedback. It was in 1833 that Charles Bell first postulated the existence of a muscle sense on a par with other senses. Sir Charles Sherrington (1857–1952), who followed in Bell's footsteps, and was lecturing in physiology at St. Thomas's Hospital at more or less the same time as Degas was making his wax and clay models, elaborated Bell's intuition into a theory about the dependence of our consciousness of position and movement on a myriad of bodily sensations. It is precisely these sensations that Degas tracks across the skin surfaces of his models, with a relentless acuity and a new sense of realism. Bell illustrates his idea of a muscle sense with the example of a blind man leaning in the wind. Although he cannot see, he knows how far he is leaning. Like Bell's blind man leaning in the wind, Degas's figures seem to know the inclinations of their bodies, their postures, without having to look at them. Here too Degas rejoins Bergson, who notes that one gets a truer sense of movement when it is captured not, externally, by the eye, which has a tendency to segment, but from the inside by what Bergson calls 'muscular consciousness' in a similar way to Bell. Only then is each movement apprehended as an uninterrupted and undivided whole, as continuous (Bergson 2012, pp. 209–10).

Seen from the outside, movement consists in a change in place. But when you apprehend your own movements through an inner sense, they consist in changes in state or qualitative changes (Bergson 2012, pp. 217–19). The latter point of view is also Degas's. Degas was interested in the way in which a moving person apprehends his or her movements. He is interested in the first-person experience of mobility – indeed in multiple first-person experiences, since each person's way of being in the body and in movement is different. A trained ballerina has a very different relationship to movement than you and I, which is something that Degas's works convey.

5. Microscopies

The above narrative about Degas's interest in embodiment is confirmed if one is to consider his sculptural work. Degas's modelling is the means of an analysis of movement and of the body's relationship to motion and to weight and gravity which accords pride of place to proprioception. It is as if Degas had intuited that proprioception underpins locomotor movement and by extension our ability to imagine it. Let us look more closely at some of Degas's wax and clay models and try to tease out what it is about movement that he is trying to understand through them.

In the three works *Grande Arabesque, first time, second time* and *third time*, considered as a sequence, which they should be, Degas is perhaps making us aware not only of movement but of its velocity and the difficulties of movement at slow speeds. Each of these figures is also about the relationship between the head (where the figure is looking), feet and arms. In *Woman Arranging Her Hair*, what does Degas show us? A standing figure wringing out her hair. The hair is wet, matted and almost immeasurably heavy; their movements suggest a slow sensuousness. The standing figure is well built and well covered but, still, look at her hips and buttocks. They are tense and the gluteal muscles and back show the effort of leaning over. The figure tells us that standing is an exercise in physics, to quote Ian Waterman. In the bronzes one can see the effort of leaning and its effects on the trunk. The figures are quite poorly delineated in the face and legs, which are smooth, and even in their ample bodies. The focus is on the hair and its wringing, but mostly on the backs of the women; the statues make us see the hair as heavy not only by its mass but by the effect on the back muscles of the posture and movement.

In *The Tub*, Degas invites us to imagine not another movement but almost its complete absence, as the subject lies on her back. But there is still a tension with the left hip flexed and then internally rotated to have the foot over her body to the right. Without the right hand grasping it one feels the left leg would be unstable, with the left arm abducted at the shoulder to balance. Even in such an apparently static bronze, reflecting a static posture, Degas says, there is movement and tension; the body may be still but it is still poised and working to remain in position. The right foot is balanced on the rim of the bath but also curled over it, holding it. The face is not well delineated; the parts sculptured the most are the feet and hands, the body and legs; look at these, he is saying. It is a study in shape and in flexibility but also a study of how, within posture, even horizontally lying, even in a bath, Degas tells us there is tension and movement underneath. Even within stillness the body is not still. Even when we remove the outer appearance of movement, there is inner movement. If the figures drying their hair remind us of the work involved in standing, this bather tells us of the poise within a lying posture.

(Ian Waterman knows this too; sitting is a task for him, as is standing, which is more difficult than walking. The only time he can relax is when lying on a bed.)

A similar lesson about our inner sense of movement may be drawn from a comparison between Degas's horses and his human figures. Degas modelled horses throughout his career. Those that were found in his studio after his death show horses in a variety of postures: standing, passing, pulling a load, just rising off their front legs. All have refined attention to the head as well as legs and trunk. This shows how bodies differ in their expressivity. In man the need to balance on two legs creates difficulties since this is inherently an unstable position. The arms, trunk and head are used to balance with the muscles of the legs and trunk constantly adjusting to maintain our position. In humans, walking has been termed controlled falling forwards. For Ian standing, say in a queue, is torture as he has to balance upright and then move a small amount forward before stopping again. It is far easier to get into a rhythm for walking steadily at his own pace. Horses seem to have a different form of instability in movement. Their forward motion is less falling than propulsion with stability from the outstretched legs, without the need for retrenchment and rebalancing that we have, say, as we walk down a steep hill when each step brakes as well as balances us. Part of horses' freedom in movement, which we have lost with standing on hind legs, is a stability and abandon in movement which we can empathise with but not, alas, enjoy ourselves (see the bronze, *Horse Galloping on the Right Foot*, from the late 1880s). Dancers in their practised precision may appear abandoned to the moment and the music, but this usually depends on intense underlying control and practise. By constantly modelling dancers side by side with horses, Degas must have become aware of the differing needs for balance and movement, and their expression. In the BBC Horizon documentary *The Man Who Lost His Body* (1998), Ian told his story about picking up a swede. To grip something out from the body which is heavy, or even to put one's arm out, one would fall over without the compensatory leaning of the body and the weight the other way. Without that, you fall over, as Ian found. Degas, we would like to suggest, had to acquire a similar kind of understanding, albeit by different means – by modelling wax and clay.

Degas understood all this with some knowledge of science, perhaps, but he also had the physics of wax and clay figures to think about. The bathers drying their hair were a considerable engineering feat since that hair weighs a lot. Drawing is done at the end of a brush or charcoal; it is weightless (even if the resulting images convey the illusion of weight). Sculpture, in contrast, is under gravity's influence, just like the body is; Degas explored these similarities between body and sculpture again and again. Sculpture knows about the physics of movement and of posture, and is completely dependent on them. By moving between sculpture and drawing, between three dimensions and two dimensions, Degas moved between gravity and weightlessness. His genius was to use sculpture to inform and develop his drawings and paintings so as to convey, and invite us to imagine, the effort and weight of movement of his figures depicted on paper as he continually explored them in parallel through sculpture.

Nicolas Poussin's use of wax figures is sometimes cited as an antecedent to Degas's own modelling activity. As part of the preparation for a painting, Poussin modelled and placed wax figures in a box, which he illuminated through small apertures. This helped him to identify shadows, to render volume ('le modellé') and to stage his composition. But, as far as we know, Poussin's wax figures were not a means of experimenting with mass. The rendering of volume has been a central concern of pictorial art at least since the quattrocento onwards, and indeed has been equally important to architecture (Le Corbusier was concerned with what happened when light stuck different kinds of surfaces). But volume is not mass. Mass introduces a new, kinetic, dimension. The improvised external armatures that Degas used to prop up many of his sculptures (which art historian Bruno Gaudishon argues should be considered an integral part of his sculptures (Gaudishon 2010, p. 24)) tell us that mass and its distribution were key to his own experiments with modelling. Therein lies part of Degas's modernity. Many of Degas's sculptures were discovered unfinished, so their surfaces often haven't been smoothed over or worked to any extent (there are exceptions). But there is evidence to suggest that he may well have left them this way himself – what he enjoyed most of all was destroying the pieces he had made in order to start all over again. Degas, we would like to suggest, was interested in the properties of the raw wax and clay and of the inner and outer armatures which he cobbled together from bits and pieces found in his studio. His interests were arguably in their weight and tensile strength, which allowed him to make them stand and twist, to maintain the postures he sculpted, just as his models maintained them in life. Exploring the physics of his sculptures allowed him to explore the physics of being in posture and movement, just as Ian Waterman has too. His wax and clay figures were experiments in and at the limits of stability and balance. The difficulties inherent in standing which Ian was forced to consider and which we forget from our first childhood steps must have become apparent to Degas in modelling and, through that, informed his two dimensional weightless representations in his drawings.

Once you begin to look at mass, which he had to do with the sculptures, you need to think more about movement from the inside and about the proprioceptive loops involved in executing moves while balancing, and also the way in which proprioception projects movement into the spaces beyond the moving body, which with sculpture are the spaces occupied by the viewer. Walter Sickert tells a story about going to Degas's studio, rue Victor Massé (Pingeot 1991, p. 22). It was night time and Degas picked up a sculpture of a dancer, rotating it in front of a candle. Sickert recalls the *succession* of shadows projected by the light onto the sheet of paper that Degas used as an improvised screen. It is unclear to what extent this sequence constituted a sequence in Marey's sense, but what the exercise did make clear was that to perceive the movements that the piece represented requires mobility, here the mobility of the rotating sculpture which, in the gallery space, is replaced by the movement of the viewer around the sculpture. The work requires the viewer's own mobility to be actualised. The model moves as you move and register its movements in your consciousness.

Perhaps one could think of the particularity of our experience of sculpture by means of an analogy with active touch? If you put an object on your static hand, you can't explore it. You explore it by manipulating it, using movement of the fingers and the sensations of touch and proprioception to explore it. The vision particular to sculpture, which is in three dimensions, and from a number of locations, might be likened to a form of active touching, as one's eyes move across the sculptures contours. The two dimensional drawings that Degas based on models, particularly his nudes and bathers, carry over some of the modes of viewing particular to sculptures in three dimension. It is also in this sense that there is crossover between the different media used by Degas. The sculptures are more than substitutes for living models; they provide a model for a way of seeing.

In conclusion we suggest that Degas's art invites us to go beyond seeing a figure, to try and capture the inner sense of movement, whether dancing or bathing. Though his early work revealed a fascination with movement and action, in horses and dancers, which never left him, later he became as fascinated with what it felt like to be seated, or lying, or in a posture, in other words in the sense of being which emerges from poise and posture as well as movement and action. He removed narrative from his work and often removed an identifiable, individual person, being sometimes more interested in the body than the face. He anticipated the work of Maurice Merleau-Ponty philosophically and those experts in the body, whether modern choreographers or, for instance, Alexander or Feldenkrais practitioners. Look, said Degas, we are our bodies; see, feel, experience and be; through and in the body, whether in action or repose, for that is who and what we are.

References

Armstrong, C. (1991). *Odd Man Out: Readings of the Work and Reputation of Edgar Degas*. Chicago: University of Chicago Press.

Bergson, H. (2012). *Matière et mémoire*. Paris: PUF.

Boggs, J.S. (1988). *Degas*. New York: The Metropolitan Museum of Art.

Cole, J. (1995). *Pride and a Daily Marathon*. London: Duckworth.

Czestochowski, J.S., & Pingeot, A. (2002). *Degas Sculptures: Catalogue Raisonné of the Bronzes*. Memphis: Torch Press and International Arts.

Kendall, R., & DeVonyar, J. (2011). *Degas and the Ballet: Picturing Movement*. London: Royal Academy of Arts.

Jamot, P. (1924). *Degas*. Paris: Editions de la gazette des beaux-arts.

Kendall, R. (1996). *Degas: Beyond Impression*. New Heaven: Yale University Press

Marques, L. (2002). Mechanism and Classical Tradition in Degas's Bronzes. In J.S. Czestochowski, & A. Pingeot (Eds.), *Degas Sculptures: Catalogue Raisonné of the Bronzes* (pp. 109–115). Memphis: Torch Press and International Arts.

Pingeot, A. (1991). *Degas: Sculptures*. Paris: Reunion des musees nationaux.

Gaudichon, B. (2010). Et moi qui veux faire de la sculpture. In *Degas Sculpteur (Exhibition catalogue. Roubaix, La Piscine-Musée d'art et d'industrie André Dilligent, 8 Octobre 2010–16 January 2011)* (pp. 13–29). Paris : Gallimard.

Shackelford, G.T. M., & Rey X. (2011). *Degas and the nude (Exhibition catalogue. Museum of Fine Arts, Boston, October 9 2011. – February 5 2012, and Musée d'Orsay, Paris, March 12 – July 1, 2012)*. Boston: Museum of Fine Arts Boston.

Time lines

The temporal dimension of marking

David Rosand
Columbia University

The invitation to contribute to a volume on the motor dimension of imagination in the arts, gives me the opportunity to return to a theme I explored in my book *Drawing Acts* (Rosand 2002): namely, the phenomenology of drawing. The original subtitle that I proposed for the book was in fact "Studies in the Phenomenology of Drawing", but it was rejected by the publisher as somehow inappropriate, indeed off-putting, for the presumed primary audience, i.e. art historians. In the context of the present volume, however, my thoughts on drawing may find a more accommodating setting.

Returning to my theme, however, I realised that, beyond what I had already written, I might not have much more to say about the phenomenology of drawing. In light of that somewhat embarrassing realisation, I thought it might be useful for me – and, I hope, of some interest to the reader – were I in effect to comment on what I had written in the book. As the title of this chapter suggests, there was in fact a dimension of drawing that I had not taken fully into consideration: namely, time – the time it takes to draw a line and the time it takes to read or respond to that line.

Cy Twombly, an artist for whom painting and drawing seemed one, said that each line he made "was the actual experience" of making a line (Figure 1). "It does not illustrate," he said. "It is the sensation of its own realization." "It's more like I'm having an experience than making a picture." (quoted by Randy Kennedy in the obituary of the artist, *The New York Times*, July 5, 2011). From and through the picture we, as viewers, share that experience, that sensation of realisation. We rehearse the artist's gestures internally, follow their rhythms through space – which, inevitably, means through time. The issue I want to raise, then, is just how we might factor that temporal dimension into understanding our response to an image made by a moving hand.

Line is the central object of our study, that is, the trace of the movement of the hand – or the arm or, indeed, the full body – and line has been at the center of visual aesthetic inquiry since antiquity. The dominant ancient etiological myth

Figure 1. Twombly, Cy (1928–2011): Untitled, 1955. New York, Museum of Modern Art (MoMA). Pencil on paper, 24 3/8 × 361/8′ (62 × 91.7 cm). Gift of Jo Carole and Ronald S. Lauder. Acc. n.: 503.1992. © 2012. Digital image, The Museum of Modern Art, New York/ Scala, Florence

of painting locates its origins in drawing, specifically in contour. All early accounts, as summarised by Pliny the Elder, "agree that painting began with the outlining of a man's shadow" (this and subsequent are translations from Pliny 1968, *Historia naturalis,* XXXV.15). From that first primitive stage, of pure contour, art made steady mimetic progress toward tone and colour. The distinction between outline and modelling – between schematic simplicity and tonal or chromatic complexity, surface reality and representational illusion – was to become fundamental in Western thought, with ethical implications that could charge aesthetic commentary with particular urgency. In line was to be found the essential truth of representation, the basic structure of idea, to which colour could only add a superficial gloss of material nature, the appearance of a more contingent, less stable reality. Indeed, already in antiquity, in response to the full chromatic development of painting, there seems to have developed a sense of nostalgia for the primitive purity of linear expression. Thus, Aristotle could invoke graphic representation in arguing the priority of plot over character: "compare the parallel in painting where the most beautiful colors laid on without order will not give one the same pleasure as a simple black-and-white sketch of a portrait" (translation from Aristotle 1984,

II: 2321. *Poetics*, 1450a-1450b). Associated with the sure measure of mathematics, with the proportions of creation, line appeals to the mind. Colour, on a baser lever, appeals to the senses. This tradition, this appreciation of the purity of line, which runs from antiquity through the Middle Ages, serves especially in the Renaissance as the basis for a modern visual aesthetics based on drawing (*disegno*) and extends into the modern era. Drawing, in the words of Henri Matisse, "belongs to the realm of the Spirit and colour to that of Sensuality." (Letter to Henry Clifford (1948), in Matisse 1995: p. 183). I suspect that, from his own experience, the French master knew better; he surely knew the sensuality of the line.

We may return to Pliny the Elder and his studio history of art for the establishment of two fundamental aspects of line, qualities that were to prove essential to subsequent pictorial appreciation and analysis. The ancient encyclopaedist celebrated two lines in particular. One was the line of Apelles, a line so uniquely fine (*linea summae tenuitatis*) and inimitable that it could serve as a signature, the mark of the artist: from that single trace his admired rival, Protogenes, recognised the presence of Apelles (*Hist. nat.*, XXXV. 81–85). The other was the line of Parrhasios, a painter "unrivaled in the rendering of outline", which is "the highest subtlety attainable in painting", Pliny writes. "Merely to paint a figure in relief is no doubt a great achievement, but many have succeeded in that." Much more difficult, and where artist's are rarely successful, is "in finding an outline that can fully express the contours of the figure. For the contour should appear to fold back, and so enclose the object as to give assurance of the parts behind, thus clearly suggesting even what it conceals" (*Hist. nat.*, XXXV, 67–68).

These two lines embody basic polarities of picture-making: the mark on the surface and the illusion behind, graphic reality and representational fiction. And yet both are made by the tracing hand. The outline of a form is itself an abstraction in nature, but not in art. Painters recognise that the contours imagined surrounding solid bodies have no reality in nature. Leonardo da Vinci clearly distinguished the mathematical line from the drawn line: "The outlines which show the shapes of surfaces of dense bodies are called contours and… do not have substance." (Leonardo da Vinci 1956: ¶ 807, cc. 217v-218). But painters also recognise them as necessary graphic fictions, essential to representation. The substance of the contour is itself the drawn line, the very materiality of art. Its mimetic responsibility is realised in the act of being drawn, for the movement of the draughtsman's hand is simultaneously a tracing on the surface and a probing of a world beyond. And Leonardo's search for that non-existent contour is in effect a probing of the hand around an imagined form. Only by repeated tracing will he arrive at a graphic truth. And such repetition takes time, each probe of the draughtsman's hand representing a moment in the search.

In the very character of the bounding line of the drawing we recognise the object, not seen but projected, imagined. Whether the line is sharp and even or irregular and varied, whether it rhythmically expands and contracts, whether its edges are neat or fade into the surrounding surface, whether its texture is smooth or rough, its trace continuous or broken, firm or tentative, thick or thin: such variables will inevitably inform representation, determining the quality or character of the object rendered as well as its relation to the ambient ground, that is, to a virtual space. Changes in contour – a thinning of the ink, a lessening of the density of chalk or crayon – may record the velocity of the drawing gesture, which, in turn, is measured over time as well as space, adding yet a further dimension to our experience of the line. That velocity, moreover, may transfer to the depicted object, investing it with associated qualities, countering its own gravity and inertia. Or the kinaesthetics may be reversed. The draughtsman's hand may move with slow deliberateness, or it may return to repeat its motion, thickening the substance of a line, adding to its material as well as visual weight; the resulting line might then brake its directional momentum, becoming by its very thickness less a directed trace than a spreading mark, an object in its own right. Such an expansion of its own inner field modulates the directional impulse of the line, effectively diffusing linear energy laterally, over a broader spread of surface. When a contour becomes so heavy, when it thickens across its directional axis, becoming more a mark than a trace, blunting its own momentum, we may speak of a "pictorialisation" of the line – an extension into painting of the line of Parrhasios.

Paul Klee opens his *Pedagogical Sketchbook* by introducing the concept of line as an independent force, a momentum: "An active line on a walk, moving freely without goal. A walk for a walk's sake". However apparently casual, this energy is directed: "The mobility agent is a point, shifting its position forward". In his second lesson Klee immediately constrains that Euclidean freedom, deliberately limiting the active line in its movement by establishing fixed points, bringing linear impulse under control and transforming "point progression" into "planar effect". Its initiating vectorial impulse interrupted, Klee's line wilfully plots its irregular, unpredictable course. "Accompanied by complementary forms", it enters into varied relations with its surrounding field; "circumscribing itself" or engaging "secondary lines", it further complicates its relation to the ground, implicitly spatialising its path (Klee 1953, pp. 16–18).

Klee's demonstration, based on the axiomatic point-line-plane progression, participates in a long tradition of graphic speculation by artists fascinated by the transformative power of line – from Alberti, Piero della Francesca, and Leonardo to Wassily Kandinsky, Pablo Picasso … and, of course, Saul Steinberg. Artists do not speculate in the abstract, however. The line of their concern is a drawn line, traced by their own hand, and in the course of its making they can only become keenly aware of that pedestrian energy described in Klee's lesson. They know that linear momentum obeys no ready rule, that the trajectory of the line is open and that in such openness resides expressive potential. And they know that a diagonal line, freeing itself from the rectangular constraints of the field, almost automatically thrusts back beyond the picture plane into a notional space that it in effect creates. The draughtsman's gesture, recorded in its ink tracing, compels the viewer's own entry into a notional word beyond the paper's surface. No pedagogical abstraction, such a drawn line traces the gesture of the imagining hand, the reach of the draughtsman into an imagined world.

The draughtsman may begin a line with some goal in mind – whether to depict a particular object, jot down a compositional idea, or merely to break the surface tension of the paper. Once begun, however, the line itself may begin to assert a certain will of its own, to challenge the guiding control of the hand, suggesting, even urging its own agenda. Out of that tension there can arise the most creative conflict, as the drawing hand, which may have become complacent in its purpose, is forced to decision.

Leonardo's wandering pen finds in its own inscribing motion new purpose, independent of its originating scriptural purpose (Figure 2). What begins as a

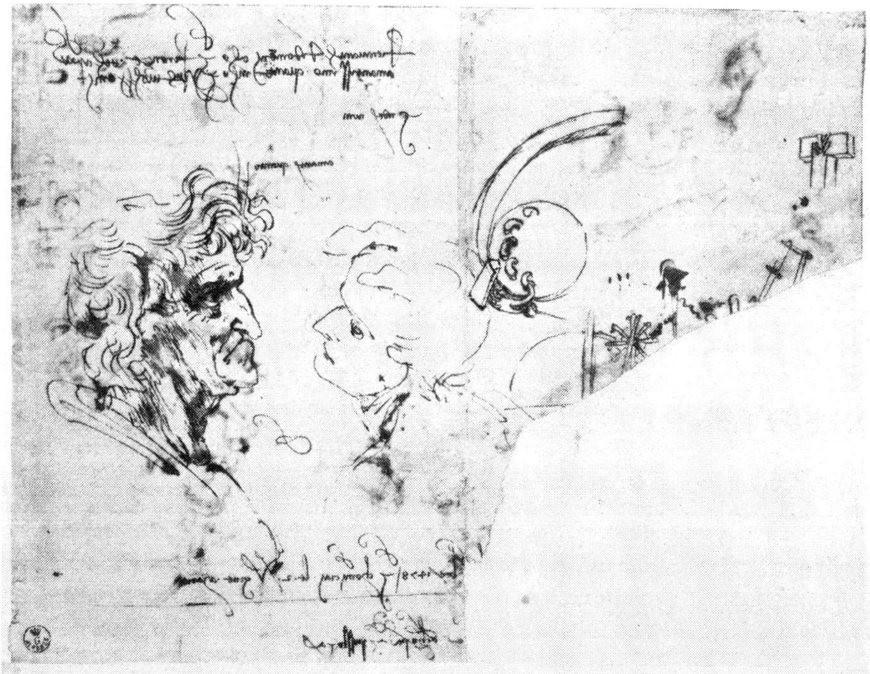

Figure 2. Leonardo da Vinci (1452–1519): Drawings of figures, probably studies for the Adoration of the Magi (facsimile). Florence, Gabinetto dei Disegni e delle Stampe degli Uffizi. © 2012. Photo Scala, Florence – courtesy of the Ministero Beni e Att. Culturali

calligraphic flourish in an exaggerated notarial handwriting liberates itself from verbal responsibility; it asserts its own graphic momentum. Literally taking off, repeating itself as an independent graphic exercise, the flourish leaves the word behind, and in so doing discovers and explores its new potential as independent grapheme. Above all, freed from scripted constraint, it more insistently asserts the spatial implications of drawing; it becomes a line curving through space. The pen declares its own will: an initial small curve continues on its elegant course, defining the surface over which it runs. Then it turns back upon itself, a movement natural to the alphabetic course of writing. But as soon as it crosses its own previous path – and without the governing verbal context of the letter/word – the line declares the challenge of pictorial art, its ambiguity. Does the line pass over or under? Either way, it has transcended the absolute flatness of the paper.[1] As soon as the line has crossed itself, forming a loop, it participates in what Paul Valéry has aptly described as "the *spatialization* of linear movement" (Valéry 1972, pp. 24–25). However it may seem a mere doodle for Leonardo, this calligraphic impulse nonetheless represents an epitome of the act of drawing – what Klee was describing as "an active line on a walk, moving freely, without goal", but whose path is nonetheless controlled by the habits of the trained hand. The movement of the line inevitably takes place in time. A walk in space takes time, and Valéry extends his comments to what he calls "the *chronolysis* of space" (ibid.).

Once begun, the line becomes more than a means toward an end. Insinuating itself into the drawing process, it insists upon its own role as protagonist, on establishing its own reciprocal relationship with its maker. Whatever initial intention may have inspired the making of a drawing, whatever external stimulus, the draughtsman inevitably finds his attention being commanded by his own line. Whatever its intended function in the structure of representation, the line becomes an active participant in the act of drawing, in the processes of its own making, even asserting its own creative independence. Whatever it may owe to the impulse of the drawing hand, it insists on a dialectic with its producer; once made, it in turn would seem to guide its maker. As Matisse recognised, "One must always search for the desire of the line, where it wishes to enter or where to die away." ("Matisse Speaks to His Students 1908: Notes by Sarah Stein," in Barr 1951, p. 551).

As viewers following that line, we become increasingly aware of that independence as we respond to the reality of the drawn line, to its substance, its body and personality, its idiosyncratic and vagrant qualities. In searching

1. For further analysis of Leonardo's drawing and its implications, see Rosand 2002, pp. 61–111 (Chapter 3: "The Handwriting of the self: Leonardo da Vinci").

for descriptive language adequate to our response, we invoke a full range of kinaesthetic experience. Mixing metaphoric allusion and psychological perception, tactile sensation and somatic awareness, we assign values and qualities, affect and character, to lines and marks.

The self-reflexivity of the drawn mark, alluding to its own making, quite naturally implicates the maker, returning us to an axiom of connoisseurship enacted in the line of Apelles: the presence in the drawing of the draughtsman. In the assertion of its autonomy, its innate resistance to the purpose of representation, the line recalls the process of becoming through the act of drawing, the gesture of the draughtsman.

Drawing something is a complex action; it involves subject and object, perception and representation, eye and mind, and, most obviously – yet too often the neglected components in critical discussion – hand and body. Nor is it merely a dialectical relationship between paired terms. Between perceiving eye and object perceived there intercedes drawing itself, as both gestural sequence (act) and evolving configuration (art). Once the first mark disrupts the blank paper, the draughtsman enters into a double dialectic: with the object before him (or the idea imagined) and with the emerging graphic construction itself. As the drawing develops, its demands upon the draughtsman begin to take precedence over those of the object (or idea) before (or within) him; the drawing asserts itself as the main object of concern, the primary other in the subject-object relation.

"There is a tremendous difference between seeing a thing without a pencil in your hand and seeing it while *drawing* it", as Valéry observed, "… the act of drawing a given object endows the eye with a posture of command which must be sustained by the will. In this case the *will* is necessary to *seeing*; and both the *end* and the *means* of this *willed seeing* is the drawing itself" (Valéry 1960, p. 36). Valéry, perhaps the most sensitive modern observer of the creative act, lays out the variables for defining a phenomenology of drawing, at the core of which is the role of the hand, of the body, in the artist's seeing the world.

Through the act of drawing the draughtsman reaches out, puts himself in active touch with the world, projects himself. To draw a line is to extend oneself into the world, to know it, and to recognise one's self. In a lecture "On the Nature of Vision," delivered in 1912, Oskar Kokoschka confessed: "Without intent I draw from the outside world the resemblance of things; but in this way I myself become part of the world's imaginings" (quoted in Hoffman 1947, p. 287).

The same object, necessarily, will be drawn differently by different draughtsmen. We may be tempted to say each "sees" a fruit differently (compare Figure 3 to Paul Cézanne's *Apples* 1891–94, pencil, 22 × 27.3 cm, present location

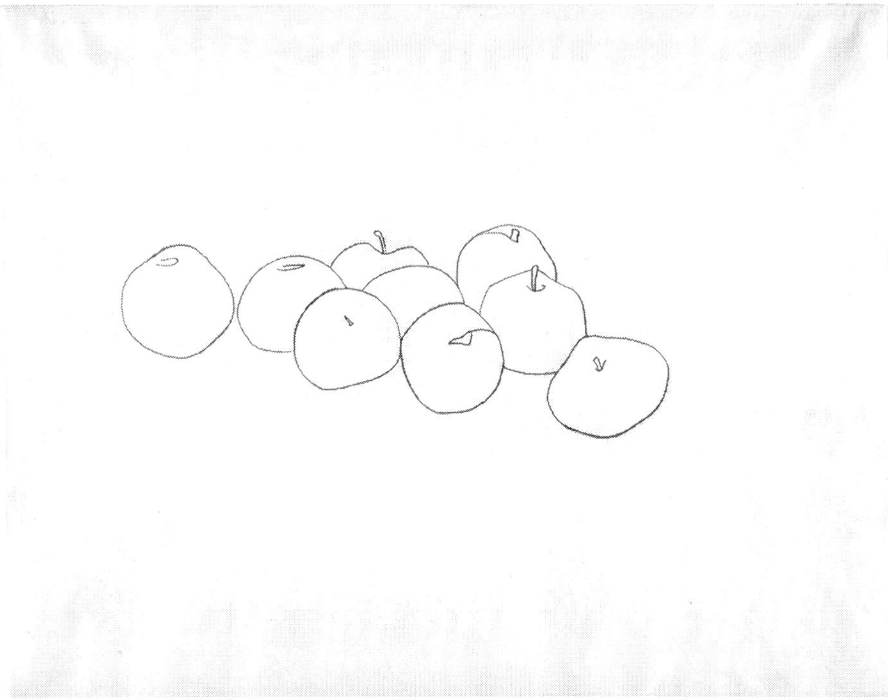

Figure 3. Kelly, Ellsworth (b. 1923): Apples 1949. New York, Museum of Modern Art (MoMA). Pencil, 17 1/8 × 22 1/8. Gift of John S. Newberry, by exchange. ©2012. Digital image, The Museum of Modern Art, New York/Scala, Florence

unknown).[2] Such a locution, however, risks metaphorising the verb, for we can hardly know what an other *sees*, only what he or she has represented. Through the drawing alone can we know the draughtsman, through whose vision, a fully somatic vision, we may believe we too see the world. Moreover, as Leonardo da Vinci consistently demonstrated, the draughtsman himself knows the world only by drawing it; the artist "sees" with hand – that is, hand with pencil – as well as eye. They work together as sensory extensors of the body in the world.

Different modes of drawing present us with different modes of knowing and understanding. The draughtsman who bounds an object with a firmer contour, which, like a horizon line, implies the far side of the globe, continues the legacy of Parrhasios, his line "clearly suggesting even what it conceals". Such a drawing depends upon and reveals a certain confidence: not only in the firmly drawn line and in its ability to perform that complex representational function, but a

2. Paul Cézanne's *Apples* 1891–94 can be found in Adrien Chappuis, *The Drawings of Paul Cézanne: a catalogue raisonné*. London: Thames and Hudson 1973, no. 1078.

confidence as well in the object represented, a faith, as it were, in the continuity of surface, in the existence of the far, unseen side. The unbroken continuity of the line declares that belief.

Conversely, the graphic shaping of an object through the accumulation of short, broken strokes that together suggest a boundary, not a contour but rather a liminal zone, reveals a different temperament. The tentative probing recorded in that collectivity of touches betrays a kind of groping, a scepticism in search of assurance; in the exploratory sequence of strokes we read the haptic ambition of the drawing hand, the repeated attempt to reach the object, to secure it for the grasp. Even as we are ready to interpret the phenomenon in purely visual terms – as a graphic rendering of the idea of passage toward and beyond the bounding line, as a rendering of successive vantage points of that disappearing edge – we come back to the gesture itself, as much the movement of the hand as of the eye. Interpretation involves us in the reconstitution of the act of drawing and, moreover, finds in that act the legitimate object of its own operation. In following that operation, we sense its temporal dimension, the time involved in reaching and feeling. The draughtsman's experience becomes ours.

"The painter 'takes his body with him." Evoking the words of Valéry, Merleau-Ponty continues:

> Indeed, we cannot imagine how a mind could paint. It is by lending his body to the world that the artist changes the world into paintings. To understand these transubstantiations we must go back to the working, actual body – not the body as a chunk of space or a bundle of functions but that body which is an intertwining of vision and movement. (Merleau-Ponty 1964, p. 162)

That observation is especially true of drawing, where the movements of the body, actual and imagined, are more directly recorded by the tracing hand. What we here call the imagined movements of the body, however, refer to and ultimately depend upon the body-image of the viewer, that is, upon our inner sense of our own body in the world – what Michael Polanyi called "the tacit dimension" (Polanyi 1966, esp. pp. 13–14)[3] – the body extending into the space around it and relating to other objects in that space.

The act of drawing, in particular, at once is and records precisely that extension. The apple rendered accommodates itself to the hand that brought it into being; seen at a distance, it is made proximate through drawing, accessible to touch, prehended. More obviously, and on a larger scale, the drawing of a figure relates to the bodily situation of the draughtsman. When the object of drawing is another

3. The concept of "tacit knowing" and the role of the body in such knowledge is elaborated more circumstantially in Polanyi (1962).

human being the entire body is involved. The model's pose is internalised by the draughtsman, measured against his own "body image" or "postural schema" – to recall the terms developed by Paul Schilder (cf. Schilder 1950).[4] The peculiar tensions of the pose, the balance of the body, its relative stability or instability, especially as gauged against the norm of the upright posture: these phenomena are instinctively felt, intuitively comprehended, rather than objectively analysed.

The analysis that occurs in the act of drawing, in the translation of perception to graphic mark, inflected contour or accentuated movement, is itself a response of the draughtsman's body. The thirty-second pose in life-drawing classes acknowledges just that phenomenon: with little time for sustained visual analysis, the student is forced to take in the model in an instant, to comprehend and internalize the pose kinaesthetically, to understand it in and through the very act of drawing it. And when the artist has so mastered the figure that he needs no model, that same internalisation of pose is projected on the paper. Realising such inner movements with pen on paper, the draughtsman's imagination is indeed somatic.

And that experience is true even for longer poses. However attentively the draughtsman's eye may scan the model, searching out contours and surfaces, the record of the drawing itself is, we might say, more an expression than a representation, more an internal than an external match – *pace* Gombrich's notion of "making and matching" (Gombrich 1960). With regard to "drawing from life", Valéry theorises "that the shapes our sight reveals to us as contours are produced by our consciousness of the concerned movement of our eyes as they register precise vision. This *registering* movement constitutes *line.*" His conclusion: "Seeing lines is copying them...." And as he further observes, "There is a tremendous difference between seeing a thing without a pencil in your hand and seeing it while *drawing* it."[5]

Drawing is (re-)enactment. So too is our response to drawing. Whether we are initially concerned with the mimetic function of the drawn line or with its calligraphic qualities as ornament, one aspect of its existence remains central: the line is a direct record of the draughtsman's gesture. On a fundamental level, it involves us, as viewers, in the kinaesthetics of the act of drawing: its qualities of direction, velocity, weight, its rhythm, pace, and inflection stand as permanent trace of the movement of the artist's hand – and of the body of which that hand is an extension.

4. Schilder's concept of body-image is further elaborated by Merleau-Ponty (1962); see also in the same volume "An Unpublished Text by Maurice Merleau-Ponty: A Prospectus of His Work", pp. 3–11, and "The Primacy of Perception and its Philosophical Consequences", pp. 12–42.

5. "Seeing and Copying," in Valéry 1960, p. 36. Valéry continues: "... the act of drawing a given object endows the eye with a posture of command which must be sustained by the will. In this case the *will* is necessary to *seeing*; and both the *end* and the *means* of this *willed seeing* is the drawing itself."

More than the hand may be directly involved. Depending on the size of the field, the artist may be working only with his fingers, or from the wrist, or elbow, or shoulder. The swing and range of the marking implement will vary: the larger the scale of operation, the more of the body involved. Thus, for example, the preliminary drawings (*sinopie*) done directly on the wall in monumental medieval and early Renaissance fresco painting required the full engagement of the artist's body: the very act of drawing on that scale involves a kind of imitation *avant le figure*, so to speak; drawing itself becomes a playing out of the figural action being rendered.[6] And the viewer surely responds more immediately and fully to a life-size figure represented by a series of graphic impulses, gestures of the creating body of the artist, than, say, to a thumbnail sketch.

The gesture of drawing is, in essence, a projection of the body, and, especially when viewing the drawing of the human figure, we are inevitably reminded of that. The conviction of such a representational image depends upon a kind of transference of energies felt. We might prefer to speak more conventionally of "imagination" or even of "mind", but the figures of an artist like Rembrandt are so intensely and fully realised in their summary graphic notation that our own response attests to what we may term the "mime" of drawing, the projection of self – or, rather, of the self-imagining of the body.

The drama is in the line. Meaning is generated in and by the act itself of drawing, for the act of drawing is already one of feeling, as Matisse confessed: "My line drawing is the purest and most direct translation of my emotion. The simplification of the medium allows that." (Matisse 1995, p. 130). Perhaps only dance offers a comparable art in which means and end, the how and what of significance, are so perfectly identified. Mallarmé, in responding to the figure of a dancer in motion, quite naturally spoke of "une écriture corporelle" (Mallarmé 1966, p. 304). Responding to drawings, we make our way, through line, to the originary impulse of the draughtsman. Interpretation involves a connecting act of *re*-creation, the self-projection of the viewer *re*-imagining the process of drawing.

Leonardo da Vinci, who was effectively the first to theorise the art of drawing and its affective dimension, recognised the active role of the viewer as, initially, a private dialectic between the artist himself, as first beholder, and his emerging work. That relationship ultimately extends beyond the studio, to us as viewers. The open structure of drawing, especially of the rapid sketch, invites our participation; indeed, it requires such active response for the completion or realisation of its significance. This is especially, and most obviously, true of our response to the rapid sketch. Recognising and exploiting the open quality of the sketch, Leonardo

6. For further discussion of *sinopie* as drawing and for further bibliography, see Rosand 2002, pp. 25–32.

welcomed its invitation to further imaginative exploration.[7] And it became axiomatic to the connoisseurs of the eighteenth century, who recognised that drawings that are "quickly executed and unfinished" invited the imagination to "supply the missing parts", to fill in the spaces between the lines. Each viewer thereby participated in the completion of the idea of the idea in his own particular way, "selon son Goût" (De Piles 1715, pp. 69–70).

Such engagement with suggestive graphic structure implicates the viewer in the creation of the drawing, as he or she is co-opted into furnishing the missing parts by act of the imagination. But drawing itself takes the initiative in this exchange; it sets the viewer on the right path ("dans un bon chemin"); it establishes the direction and momentum of interpretation. Only through such participation can the viewer become an active agent in the completion of the design.

Interacting with the linear configuration of the drawing, the imagination of the viewer expresses itself in a corresponding mode. Drawing, as I've been emphasizing, is the record of a physical act. Its invitation is, on a primary level, to the body of the viewer, whose own response will necessarily involve the somatic dimension. "Looking long enough", as Ernst Kris has written, "one tends to become aware of a kinesthetic reaction, however slight; it may be that one tries, at first imperceptibly and later consciously, to react with one's body, or it may be that the reaction remains unconscious". Following the linear patterns of a drawing, supplying continuity to the open gaps between points and lines, we engage the very energies and impulses that went into its making (Figure 4).[8]

"From looking at a whirl of lines", Kris continues, "from following them, we change imperceptibly from identification with the model into the state in which we 'imitate' the strokes and lines with which it was produced. To some extent we have changed roles. We started out as part of the world which the artist created; we end as co-creators: We identify ourselves with the artist" (Kris 1952, pp. 55–56).

The epistemological circle so nicely described by Kris is intuitively shared in the existential analysis of others – for example, by Jean-Paul Sartre, who speaks of the collection of lines being "animated by a certain attitude of my body, namely, by my body enacting a certain pantomime" (Sartre 1948, pp. 40–41). Draughtsman, drawing, and viewer complete a circuit of identity. The viewer enacts the drawing, mimicking it within his body. Through drawing the viewer meets the draughtsman. Criticism, which is response articulated, imitates creation in reverse.

7. For further discussion of Leonardo's discovery of the sketch, see Rosand 2002, pp. 50–54.

8. On Raphael's circling hand, see Rosand 2002, pp. 112–144 (Chapter 4: "Raphael and the Calligraphy of Classicisim").

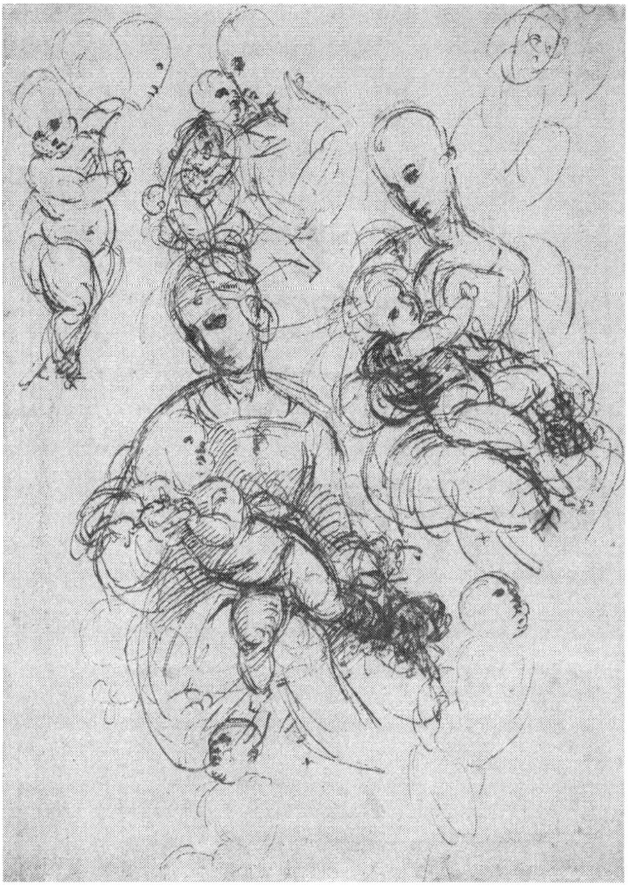

Figure 4. Raphael: Studies for a Virgin and Child in her arms, ca. 1506–1507, Pen and brown ink, over traces of red chalk, 25.3 × 18.3 cm ©The Trustees of the British Museum, London

Long before Klee's Euclidean description of a point as "the mobility agent … shifting its position forward", Leonardo had demonstrated his own working awareness of just this function of the line as a probe, but for him it was of necessity directed. Although he certainly appreciated its appeal as pure tracing or calligraphy, it was precisely the exploratory responsibility of a line that gave it purpose; its extension into the world made visible vectors of force and energies otherwise unperceivable to the eye. As the privileged organ of perception, the eye was a means of extension: "It carries men from east to west, it has discovered navigation … ", and, as he demonstrated, the lead of the eye is followed by the hand (Leonardo da Vinci 1956, ¶ 34, c. 15v.). Following it, the drawing hand will travel toward those distant horizons. In practice, however, the eye is urged on by the hand. Line makes the world imaginable.

"A line is made by the movement of a point." Leonardo begins one of his typical observations with this geometric axiom. But he then transposes the abstraction to the realm of lived reality: "the point may be compared to an instant of time, and the line may be likened to the length of a certain quantity of time" (Leonardo da Vinci 1939, ¶ 916). Time with a length: what Valéry summed up as the *chronolosis* of space. The moments of a line, the time of drawing – as Picasso put it, quite concretely: "The fatigue of one's hand as one draws is a perception of time." (Picasso 1972, p. 103). The implication is clear: it is through the body that we, both the artist and the viewer, perceive time.

How then are we to enfold that temporal dimension into criticism? How, indeed, can we begin to measure and evaluate the perception of time in the response to a drawing – or any work of visual art, for that matter? These are questions I never really confronted in *Drawing Acts*.

For example, in discussing Michelangelo's black chalk drawing of *The Risen Christ* (Figure 5), I was quite concerned with technique, with dispelling the

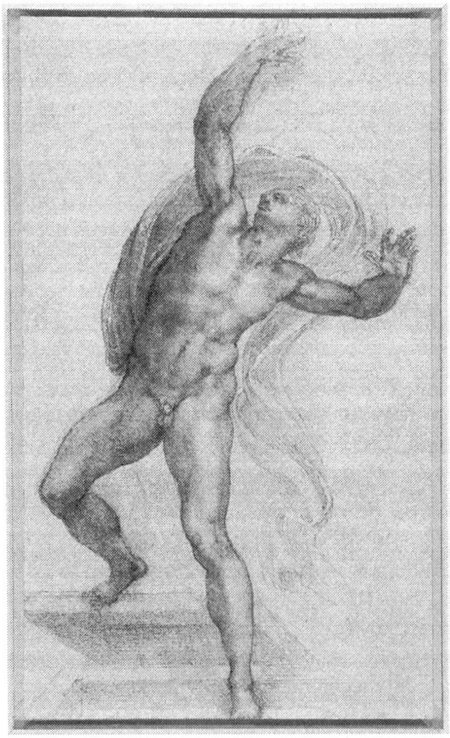

Figure 5. Michelangelo Buonoarroti (1475–1564): The Risen Christ, c.1532, black chalk, 37.3 × 22.1 cm. Royal Collection Trust / © Her Majesty Queen Elizabeth II 2012

erroneous notion that he had realised form through a process of stippling (Rosand 2002, pp. 182–219). Stippling involves the patient application of variously spaced marks or dots to produce tone. It is not a chalk technique; rather it is associated with shading in pen and ink and intaglio printmaking. It is essentially redundant in chalk drawing, where tonal modulation is the natural result of the interaction between the substance of the medium and the texture of the support, between the granules of chalk and the tooth of the paper. Michelangelo modelled his anatomical forms not by any laborious process of dotting, but rather by passing and re-passing his chalk over the surface in ever denser concentrations of hatching. Technique, I was arguing, mediates importantly between the artist and his creation. Moving over the paper, for the duration of its contact the drawing hand remains responsive to the feeling of its own movements. Evoking form from paper, each stroke affirms, even as it defines, the reality of that form. The intent is plastic: to give shape to the flatness of paper. The drawing hand is a forming hand. As Pierre-Jean Mariette, the greatest of the eighteenth-century connoisseurs, recognised in Michelangelo's highly finished drawings, "He caresses what he makes" ("Il caresse ce qu'il fait") (Mariette 1851–1860, I, p. 223). There is indeed a tactile and therefore somatic dimension to stroking the chalk that keeps the artist in constant, responsible and responsive touch with his emerging creation. In the physical engagement of such a graphic process time counts. Each stroke is a progress toward a mimetic end; it also represents a duration or, to quote Leonardo, a "space of time", a sustained period of contact with the drawing, of commitment to it. As Cézanne had groped for the body of the apple, stroke by stroke, so did Michelangelo seek out a body through drawing, although his stroking was less a search for boundary than for surface. For Michelangelo, the commitment to the drawing of a body inevitably meant a commitment to the body itself, especially when that body was the corpus of his Saviour.

Although the body in the work of Cy Twombly is strictly his own, his confession that each line he made was "the actual experience" of making a line, "the sensation of its own realization", seems quite relevant to a more general and deeper understanding of the temporal dimension of marking – an understanding I must confess I am still groping for.

References

Aristotle (1984). *The Complete Works of Aristotle: Revised Oxford Translation,* 2 vols. (ed. by J. Barnes). Princeton: Princeton University Press.

Barr, A.H., Jr. (1951). *Matisse: His Art and His Public.* New York: Museum of Modern Art.

Chappuis, A. (1973). *The Drawings of Paul Cézanne: a catalogue raisonné.* London: Thames & Hudson.

De Piles, R. (1715). *Abrégé de la vie des peintres, avec de réflexions sur leurs ouvrages, et un traité du peintre parfait; de la connoissance des desseins; de l'utilité des estampes* (1699) (2d ed.). Paris: J. Estienne.

Gombrich, E.H. (1960). *Art and Illusion: A Study in the Psychology of Pictorial Representation.* New York: Pantheon Books.

Hoffman, E. (1947). *Kokoschka: Life and Work.* London: Faber and Faber.

Klee, P. (1953 [1925]). *Pedagogical Sketchbook* (transl. by S. Maholy-Nagy). New York: F.A. Praeger.

Kris, E. (1952). *Psychoanalytic Explorations in Art.* New York: International Universities Press.

Leonardo da Vinci (1939). *The Literary Works of Leonardo da Vinci* (2 vols.) (ed. by J.-P. Richter). London and New York: Oxford University Press.

Leonardo da Vinci (1956). *Treatise on Painting [Codex Urbinas Latinus 1270]* (2 vols.) (ed. by A. Ph. McMahon). Princeton: Princeton University Press.

Mallarmé, St. (1966). *Oeuvres completes* (ed. by H. Mondor, & G. Jean-Aubry). Paris: Gallimard.

Mariette, P.-J. (1851–1860). *Abecedario de P.-J. Mariette et autres notes inédites de cet auteur sur les arts et les artistes* (ed. by Ph. de Chennevières, & A.de Montaiglon). Paris: L'Archives de l'art français.

Matisse, H. (1995). *Matisse on Art* (ed. by J. Flam). Berkeley/Los Angeles: University of California Press.

Merleau-Ponty, M. (1962). *Phenomenology of Perception* (transl. by C. Smith). London: Routlege & Kegan Paul.

Merleau-Ponty, M. (1964). Eye and Mind (transl. by C. Dallery). In J. H. Edie (Ed.), *The Primacy of Perception and Other Essays* (pp. 159–190). Evanston: Northwestern University Press.

Picasso, P. (1972). *Picasso on Art: A Selection of Views* (ed. by D. Ashton). New York: Viking Press.

Pliny (1968 [1896]). *The Elder Pliny's Chapters on the History of Art* (tranl. by. K. Jex-Blake, ed. by. E. Sellers, reprint with additional notes by H. Ludwig). Chicago: Argonaut.

Polanyi, M. (1962). *Personal Knowledge: Towards a Post-Critical Philosophy.* Chicago: University of Chicago Press.

Polanyi, M. (1966). *The Tacit Dimension.* Garden City, N.Y.: Doubleday.

Rosand, D. (2002). *Drawing Acts: Studies in Graphic Expression and Representation.* Cambridge/ New York: Cambridge University Press.

Sartre, J.-P. (1948). *The Psychology of Imagination* (transl. by B. Frechtman). New York: Philosophical Library.

Schilder, P. (1950 [1935]). *The Image and Appearance of the Human Body.* New York: International Universities Press.

Valéry, P. (1960). *Degas, Manet, Morisot* (transl. by D. Paul). New York: Pantheon Books.

Valéry, P. (1972). *Leonardo, Poe, Mallarmé* (transl. by M. Cowley & J.R. Lawler). Princeton: Princeton University Press.

Styles of observation and embodiment

Using drawing to understand Robert Morris' *Untitled 3 L-Beams* (1965)

Francis Halsall
National College of Art and Design, Dublin

To know anything in space (for instance, a line), I must draw it, and thus synthetically bring into being a determinate combination of the given manifold, so that the unity of this act is at the same time the unity of consciousness (as in the concept of a line); and it is through this unity of consciousness that an object (a determinate space) is first known.
Immanuel Kant, *Critique of Pure Reason*, B 138 (2007)

1. Introduction

My starting point for this chapter was Thierry de Duve's pencil drawing of Robert Morris' *Untitled 3 L-Beams*, a work of Minimalist sculpture from 1965 (Halsall et al. 2008, p. 91). De Duve produced the drawing from a well known photograph of an installation view of Morris' work at the Green Gallery in New York. In order to produce the drawing de Duve needed to apprehend the shapes of the sculpture (in its photographic representation) and re-present this apprehension according to the materials he had to hand, a technical schema and his own aptitude. In short there were four co-ordinates within which de Duve produced his drawing: (a) what he saw; (b) the pencil and paper he used; (c) the learnt techniques by which he drew; (d) his bodily actions.

My argument here is that drawings like this reveal another means by which to approach Morris' sculpture; that is, through drawing itself. My overall conclusion is twofold. First that, even though it is a 3-dimensional sculptural form, *Untitled 3 L-Beams* can be considered a form of drawing. Second that the perceptual ambiguity of *Untitled 3 L-Beams* creates a puzzle for the viewers and a challenge for them to attend to. In doing so it promotes a style of observation that one would adopt if drawing the sculpture. In short it puts the viewer into a position of someone who is drawing it.

There are 6 elements to my argument in reaching this dual conclusion. These are (and not in the order in which the discussion below follows):

a. That drawing is a process and a practice.
b. By arguing that drawing is a process I assert that it is not a medium. Instead it is a process that is not specific to a particular medium but rather one that can occur in different mediums. Hence,
c. drawing is a process grounded in particular activities, namely a type of observation and tactile action (and I will use examples to demonstrate this.) By means of describing this particularity I will use the word *style.* Thus, my claim is that drawing is a particular *style* of observation and action. Using *style* to describe processes of observation and action might seem odd at first, but my point in using it is to uncouple the specificity of the act of drawing from medium specificity.
d. The simple forms of *Untitled, 3 L-Beams* delineate forms in space and define them by means of an outline, which is to say that they are in the style of drawing. In short *Untitled, 3 L-Beams* is a 3-dimensional drawing.
e. The work positions the viewer in such a way that an interrogation into how the forms delineate forms in space is part of the meaning of the work.
f. *Untitled 3 L-Beams* puts the viewer into the position of someone who is drawing it; that is, of someone who must apprehend its forms and, in turn, reflect upon that apprehension.

2. Why I can't draw

I'm not very good at drawing and any efforts to do so are normally pretty clumsy. The main reason as to why I can't draw well is that I haven't learned to look in the appropriate style. David Hockney calls this particular style of looking to draw "eyeballing" which he says is,

> The way an artist sits down in front of a sitter and draws or paints a portrait by using his hand and eye alone and nothing else, looking at the figure and then trying to recreate the likeness on the paper or canvas. By doing this he 'gropes' for the form he sees before him. (Hockney 2006, p. 23)

Also, I can't seem to make my hands do what I'd like them to in order to make a satisfactory drawing. I don't have the technical facility to use the drawing materials effectively. In short, I don't have what Ernst Gombrich calls a "schema" for drawing.

A colleague once gave me a drawing lesson and I, apparently, made the classic mistake when trying to draw an object. In this case it was a beer glass. I first imagined the immediate experience of the glass as a conceptual object, which in this case was a transparent, open cylinder. I then attempted to rotate that cylinder in my mind's eye to bring it parallel with the picture surface in order to represent it through drawing lines. The reason that this does not work as a strategy for drawing is that it is the wrong style of looking. This style of looking takes first hand experience and attempts to mediate it conceptually according to a pre-existent shape (such as a cylinder) before attempting to re-present that shape according to the material of the drawing (pencil, paper and so on) and parallel to a picture plane.

The successful drawer, on the other hand, must attend to the specific experience of the object *as it is experienced*. They learn to attend to the gaps between things and treat the spaces between elements as something rather than nothing. They must then match their observations with a set of learned procedures and physical actions. The good drawer uses their arms and hands and thumbs and other parts of the body to relate the proportions of the viewed object to their own body. They must bracket (put out of action) a conceptual consideration of the object in favour of grasping its concrete particularity. The drawer must then translate this experience into the medium they have to hand according to the techniques they know.

I find such a style of "eyeballing" and close looking – what I am calling here the drawing style – actually very difficult to do. It is certainly the case that this is not how I experience the world on a day to day basis whereby my natural attitude to things is as something ready to hand to be used or understood. I rarely attend to door frames or tables as significant aesthetic experiences or perceptual conundrums. Even many works of art do not present themselves in such a way too. Recently, for example, I spent a considerable time looking at the Ghent Altarpiece or Adoration of the Mystic Lamb by van Eyck and marvelling at its complex iconography of saints, patrons, angels and so on. I was absorbed by the lustrous surfaces of oil paint. And puzzled by its weirdness. But I did not imagine myself drawing it. I was not in the drawing style of looking. There seemed to be too much going on, a surfeit of richness perhaps, to allow for this. My argument is that Minimalism helps achieve this very particular style of close looking. It does so, in part, by presenting a perceptually intriguing experience and also, in part, by keeping all other aesthetic elements to a minimum thereby drawing aesthetic attention to the conditions of looking itself. Morris' *Untitled, 3 L-Beams* provides a good example of this.

3. *Untitled, 3 L-Beams*

Morris' *Untitled, 3 L-Beams* is comprised of 3 identical L-shaped fibre-glass forms (243.8 × 243.8 × 61 cm) with a 90 degree angle in the middle. The forms are simple and they are painted white. Morris had planned to make nine forms although only three were built and this is the way the work is now exhibited (there are several versions).

Typical for works of Minimalism the forms are non-representational, have no surface ornament and no apparent expressive content. In 'ABC Art', her well known contemporary commentary on Minimalism from 1965, Barbara Rose observed:

> That these young artists [of which Morris was one] attempt to suppress or withdraw content from their works is undeniable. That they wish to make art that is as bland, neutral and as redundant as possible also seems clear. The content, then, if we are to take the work at face value, should be nothing more than the total of the series of assertions that it is this or that shape and takes up so much space and is painted such a colour and made of such a material.
>
> (Rose 2000, p. 214)

The effect of this simplicity is that in the absence of additional content the conditions under which the work is experienced is what it is about. This is the way that Morris talked about such work. He said: "I want to provide a situation where people can become more aware of themselves and their own experience rather than more aware of some version of my experience." (Newman & Bird 1999, p. 97).

In other words, Minimalism draws specific aesthetic attention to the conditions by which it is experienced. It does so by removing any elements that might be extraneous to an aesthetic experience. These are elements such as expressive, representational, iconographic, or decorative ones. In the absence of such features the primary meaning of the work lies in the manner by which it is experienced.

The *3 L-Beams* are identical but arranged differently to one another. Even though the objects have the same dimensions and shape, the work confuses this apparently easy interpretation so that their similarity is hard to grasp, at least initially, as Rose acknowledged:

> For the spectator this is often all very bewildering. In the face of so much nothing he is still experiencing something, and usually a rather unhappy something at that. I have often thought one had a sense of loss looking at these big, blank empty things, so anxious to cloak their art identity that they were masquerading as objects. Perhaps what one senses is that, as opposed to the florid baroque fullness of the *angst*-ridden older generation, the hollow barrenness of the void has a certain poignant if strangled expressiveness. (Rose 2000, p. 215)

There are three main reasons for this bewilderment. First scale; standing at eight feet by eight feet, they are simultaneously bigger than human dimensions, whilst being smaller than traditionally monumental sculptural (or architectural) forms. Those sculptural forms that are either on a human scale (like Auguste Rodin's work) or dwarf it though a monumental scale (Richard Serra) can be cognised through an association to our own bodies as we can imagine ourselves in relation to them. The scale of Morris' work on the other hand is neither one nor the other and is thus difficult to grasp.

Second the forms are arranged in a deliberately confusing way. They are re-iterated in three different positions and are rotated around three different axes which make the similarity between them difficult to perceive even if it is known conceptually. One knows of the similarity but cannot quite see it.

Third the work is often exhibited in a small and cramped exhibition space which hinders the easy apprehension of the forms in the round and at once. Unlike traditional sculpture which is plinth based and thus, generally speaking, is organised around a single axis and towards a single view-point, one cannot walk around the work in order to work out its forms easily. This exacerbates further the ambiguity of scale and arrangement.

The conditions of display often confound an easy experience and cognition of the work. As Rosalind Krauss argued it is precisely the position of the forms in space that creates the effect of confusion because they "suspend the axiomatic co-ordinates of an ideal space." (Krauss 1973, p. 50). Thus, the spatio-temporal positioning of the shapes has a direct consequence upon the experience of those shapes; and this is a dimension of the work's meaning. A comparison could be made, as de Duve does, with Rodin's work the *Three Shades*, the three figures that stand on the top of the *Gates of Hell*. This is, de Duve observed: "a work that is also composed of three identical sculptures arranged in such a way that they look and feel different; they manage to sustain that feeling, no matter how long you look at them and how well you know that they are actually identical." (De Duve 2008, p. 99) Similarly, *3 L-Beams* is three identical shapes arranged, in de Duve's words "to look and feel different", which address the viewer and positions them in a relationship that compels them to actively account for their similarity and difference. Fried captures this in his celebrated critique of Minimalism in claiming that such an address to a viewer should be thought of one that "extorts" its response.[1]

1. Thierry de Duve's discussion on the anthropomorphism in Fried's position is discussed at length by Susan Best who wrote: " 'Demands', 'addresses,' such terms are routinely used in art history to describe the accommodations a receptive viewer makes to the exigencies of different art practices. These terms, and our constant recourse to them, clearly indicate the ingrained and unavoidable nature of anthropomorphism. But Fried's term 'extorts' is in a slightly different register: there is both violence and unwillingness implicit in this term. Indeed, Fried's response to minimalist works, such as Tony Smith's *Die*, makes manifest an extreme form of anthropomorphism and a more profound entanglement of spectator and work." (Best 2006, pp. 127ff.)

De Duve returns to Immanuel Kant's account of aesthetic experience in the *Critique of Judgement* to frame his argument and states that:

> Morris' minimalist pieces need to be seen, perceived, and experienced in real time and space. They even emphasize the 'reality' or literalness of this time and space, presenting, as it were, time as duration and space as a function of gravity. (De Duve 2008, p. 90)

Kant is used by de Duve to argue that aesthetic experience is at the very heart of a satisfactory account of Morris' work. In doing so his argument runs counter to any argument which would read Minimalism alongside other tendencies in art after modernism (such as Conceptual Art) as anti-aesthetic.

There are two things at stake in this engagement in Kantian aesthetics. First there is the Kantian claim that we become conscious of the free play of our cognitive powers, which we experience when making an aesthetic judgement, through (pleasurable) sensation and not conceptually. This, crucially for my argument here, situates the experience as an aesthetic one occurring with a sensing body (and not merely a disembodied mind). Second, through Kant, de Duve demonstrates that it is through the power of imagination that the forms of Morris' work as they are sensuously experienced can be properly cognised and understood. As de Duve argues, imagination "schematizes and synthesises raw sense data; it unifies the manifold of empirical experience into a Gestalt, which it presents to the understanding." (De Duve 2008, p. 90).

It is my claim here that this is also what the drawer does whilst drawing; namely to schematize and synthesise raw – and perhaps bewildering – sense data and to unify the manifold of empirical experience into a Gestalt which is then presented through the material of the drawing.

4. Drawing is a process

I am arguing then, that drawing is a process. It is the translation of experience according to the material used in the process of drawing and the bodily procedures used by the drawer. However, before anything else, drawing is diagrammatic and non-mimetic. It is the construction of patterns and the making of marks. As Gombrich describes, the process of drawing does not sequentially proceed from observation to transcription. Instead the drawer works according to schemata. The artist, Gombrich argues, "begins not with his visual impression but with his idea or concept." (Gombrich 1960, p. 62) However even though they begin with a concept this is not the endpoint of the process. They must subsequently work from the originating concept towards reconciling it with experience. This is done according to a process of "making and matching" (Gombrich 1960, p. 29) whereby the image is made and matched to experience (this is the process which I assume I'm not so good at). In this account of image making schemata are, according to Gombrich: "the first approximate, loose category which is gradually tightened to fit the form it is to reproduce" (Gombrich 1960, p. 64). Thus, even though a drawer may take an idea as her or his starting point schemata both pre-exist, and are conceptually prior to, drawing, as Gombrich states, "you cannot create a faithful image out of nothing" (Gombrich 1960, p. 83). Further, the schemata of drawing will, in turn, frame the way which the drawer perceives and inhabits the world. For example in discussing John Constable's copying of the drawing book of Alexander Cozens (an eighteenth-century landscape painter) Gombrich observes: "we know by now what Cozens teaches Constable. Not indeed, what clouds look like, but a series of possibilities, of schemata, which should increase his awareness through visual classification." (Gombrich 1960, p. 151). He continues by further emphasising the relationship between schemata and perception:

> It matters little what filing system we adopt. But without some standards of comparison we cannot grasp reality. Having looked at Constable's creations we may also see clouds in a fresh way. If so we will owe this heightened awareness to the memory of the images created by art. (Gombrich 1960, p. 151–152)

There are limits to Gombrich's account that I do not want to dwell on here; in particular it is predicated on vision and representation and it leans towards an account of art grounded in pictorial illusion. However, what Gombrich's account does offer is an account of image making that is based on it being a physical activity rather than a disembodied or merely conceptual one; or a medium with specific qualities.

The schemata by which the drawer operates are the culturally situated parameters for the drawer's physical actions. In phenomenological terms there is an intentional horizon for the body's motor potentiality. The drawer makes and matches by observing and correcting their actions. There are two specific implications I want to take from this and carry forward into the remainder of my discussion. First, that the observation which frames making and matching need not be *visual* observation; one can observe through all the senses. Second, that the correction that accompanies observation, and hence artistic practice in general and drawing in particular, is a manual, embodied practice. As Richard Serra claims, "Drawing is a verb." (Hoptman 2002, p. 11). Drawing is something that is done; and done by a body.

5. Drawing and medium specificity

Once drawing has been identified as a process its status or definition as a medium is radically problematized. Even the now dominant expanded definitions of medium such as we find in Krauss might be too specific.

For example, Krauss has given an expanded definition of medium as the "technical support" for the work of art. The benefit of this is that it does not reduce medium to any specific material and physical attributes. Such a definition of medium as a technical support has the virtue of:

> acknowledging the recent obsolescence of most traditional aesthetic mediums (such as oil on canvas, fresco, and many sculptural materials, including cast bronze or welded metal), while it also welcomes the layered mechanisms of new technologies that make a simple, unitary identification of the work's physical support impossible (is the "support" of film the celluloid strip, the screen, the splices of the edited footage, the projector's beam of light, the circular reels?) If the traditional medium is supported by a physical substance (and practiced by a specialized guild), the term "technical support," in distinction, refers to contemporary commercial vehicles, such as cars or television, which contemporary artists exploit, in recognition of the contemporary obsolescence of the traditional mediums, as well as acknowledging their obligation to wrest from that support a new set of aesthetic conventions to which their works can then reflexively gesture, should they want to join those works to the canon of modernism. (Krauss 2006, pp. 55–62)

The idea that medium be understood as the technical support for a work of art means that its definition is grounded upon a set of practices rather than a particular set of material conditions. Thus painting, for example, is not definable through physical material like paint, canvas and brushes alone, but instead must be understood as the set of historical conditions that allow for the identification of a set of technical procedures (such as historical precedents and studio practices) to be acknowledged as painting. Such an argument is developed by Michael Fried who has discussed how the definition of painting as a medium is exemplified by Gustave Courbet *Painter's Studio* (1854–55). Courbet called this painting a "real allegory" of painting, meaning that it revealed the contemporary historical and technical conditions of the medium of painting. Fried develops this further by arguing that the painting is (along with Courbert's *The Wheat Sifters* (1853)) an "allegory of its own production" in which Courbet paints himself as "already immersed" in the medium of painting and "physically enclosed, one might say subsumed, within the painting he is making, wherever the ultimate limits of that painting are taken to lie." (Fried 1990, pp. 155–61).

However, whilst the particular instances of schemata of drawing will be historically and culturally framed there is, I argue, a more general activity of drawing that cannot be as specifically historically situated as painting might. As Emma

Dexter observes drawing is not weighed down by the baggage of history and no-one has ever declared the end of drawing or that drawing is dead as has been claimed of both painting and sculpture (Dexter 2005, p. 6).

Drawing is immediate in the full sense of the word, meaning the lack of an intervening and historically configured medium with its own protocols and expectations. Drawing is the creation of pattern and form. And if the most basic difference between form and non-form is a line, then the most basic form of a line is a drawn one. No matter what material it is drawn in. Drawing is a technologically simple activity in which only the drawn lines mediate between the artist and the viewer. And these lines may be drawn on and with potentially any material and still be recognised as drawing. One only need look at the diverse range of things called drawing from the last forty years to see how it is manifested in a wide variety of mediums such as: wire and string by Fred Sandback; projected light in Anthony McCall's *Solid Light Films*; and performance and film in Matthew Barney's increasingly elaborate *Drawing Restraint* projects.

Yet in claiming that drawing is not a medium one leaves it open to ambiguity and instability in terms of definition. For the purposes of my argument I will use the word *style* to address this ambiguity. Style is useful because it offers a way of identifying a coherence according to an organising principle; yet one that is not medium specific. The Baroque, for example, is a style that is manifest across a variety of mediums. Style is, in Meyer Schapiro's definition, "a system of forms", (Schapiro 1998, p. 143) and for Gombrich: "Style is any distinctive, and therefore recognizable, way in which an act is performed or an artefact made or ought to be performed and made." (Gombrich 1998, p. 150).

I speculated above that drawing might be conceived of as a practice or perhaps certain processes (of looking and acting) which have a certain style. The reason for suggesting this was to uncouple drawing from any material or medium specificity. The consequence of this uncoupling is that drawing is no longer conceived as a medium; this was because even in expanded definitions of medium such as Krauss term of "technical support" it would need to be too broad to have a meaningful critical or descriptive purchase.

Throughout his artistic career Morris has repeatedly engaged in interrogating medium specificity. In *Notes on Sculpture* he explores how sculpture provides the opportunity for this interrogation:

> The primary problematic concerns with which advanced painting has been occupied for about half a century have been structural. The structural element has been gradually revealed to be located within the nature of the literal qualities of the support. It has been a long dialogue with a limit. Sculpture, on the other hand, never having been involved with illusionism, could not possibly have based the efforts of the last fifty years upon the rather pious, if somewhat contradictory, act of giving up this illusionism and approaching the object. (Morris 1995, p. 3)

Sculpture in general, and Minimalist sculpture in particular, for Morris, provides the conditions by which to destabilise medium specificity because it directly addresses the spectator as an embodied subject:

> Not only the production of objects, but the perception of them as well involves bodily participation in movement in three dimensions. It might be said that the construction of rectilinear objects involves a split between mental and physical activity and a simultaneous underlining of the contrast; on the one hand, the obviousness of the prior plan, and on the other, the extreme reasonableness of the material used to manifest the structure. (Morris 1995, p. 89)

On the one hand this address to the viewer undermines the modernist tenet of the autonomy of the work of art and hence the specificity of its form and medium. If the forms of the art are forms of the viewer's experience then they have lost their medium specificity and are instead relative to the contingent conditions of the observer's subjectivity. Such an argument formed the basis of Fried's critique of the "theatricality" of Minimalism in his famous essay, "Art and Objecthood" (Fried 1992, pp. 822 ff.).

On the other hand this mobilization of the perceiving subject to complete the work (as Marcel Duchamp had argued for in "The Creative Act" text (Duchamp 1967)) as it is being perceived places a sensuous and, crucially *embodied* human subject at the very heart of the experience of art. It is the centrality of the embodied human subject in the completion of the work which opens up the possibility of the conflation of sculpture and drawing that the two elements of my conclusion (where it's claimed that Morris' work is a drawing; and that it positions the viewer into a drawing mode of observation) are based on.

Sculpture shares with drawing the condition of being a sufficiently open medium as to render the question of the conditions of its medium specificity an unanswerable one. Yet, although Morris argues that sculpture is always literal (physical) and three dimensional, I want to argue that it can be enacted in different styles; and that drawing is one such style. And that this is possible because drawing also follows from a certain style of observations to a tactile process with its own, also particular, style.

What *Untitled 3 L-Beams* reveals is that both experiencing sculpture and drawing are embodied, tactile processes that take place in particular times and spaces. They are processes that have a particular *style* because they require a particular type of observation: namely the drawing style of close observation. As Morris acknowledged: "Since Rodin, all modern sculpture has pre-supposed drawing. Especially since the 1960s, nearly all three-dimensional work has proceeded from drawing." (Morris 1995, p. 199).

6. Showing drawing as an embodied practice: Morris' *Blind Time Drawings*

In his series of *Blind Time Drawings* Morris shows how drawing is first and foremost an embodied, tactile process (and is hence comparable to the embodied, tactile process of experiencing sculptural forms.).

Blind Time Drawings are a sequence of drawing Morris made between 1973 and 2000. Morris would give himself a set of instructions, in which, he states, the "body addresses the sheet of paper under various constraints" (Morris 2008, p. 204) for the drawing and in a single session perform them with his eyes closed. He would then estimate the time the task had taken. The instructions and time estimate would then be copied out beneath the drawing.[2] For example:

> With eyes closed, graphite on the hands and estimating a lapsed time of three minutes, both hands attempt to descend the page with identical touching motions in an effort to keep to an even vertical column of touches. Time estimation error: + 8 seconds. (Morris 2008, p. 15)

Morris claimed to have been motivated by a desire to find a "basis for drawing" (Morris 2008, p. 204) and what they seem to reveal are the structures of process and the structures of perception by showing their limits and the places where they break down. These works point toward the physical limits of Gombrich's schemata. Or, in phenomenological terms, they gesture at the horizon of motor intentionality within which the act of drawing is positioned.

In short, what these drawings show is that drawing is on the one hand clearly not about illusionism and on the other that it is a somatic (bodily) process which has a particular style.

The process of drawing whilst blind is consistent with the set of artistic practices that emerged in the wake of modernism which signal a move away from the aesthetic prioritization of the optical elements in art that had characterised modernism. This move was, in part, a move away from Greenberg's prioritization of what Caroline Jones has called "eyesight alone" (Jones 2005) as a privileged mode of engaging with painting. Artists such as Johns, Rauschenberg and Morris who reacted against Greenberg's Modernism did so by explicitly returning to the body to disrupt the hygiene of pure visuality and did so by re-mobilising Duchamp's distrust of vision and what he called "retinal art". In part this also occurred

2. With one exception, in 1976 in the *Blind Time II* sequence when Morris worked with A.A. a woman blind from birth who he met through the American Association for the Blind.

through a reading of Jackson Pollock as a performative, that is *bodily*, painter found in accounts by Allan Kaprow and Morris who sees in Pollock's paintings an: "interaction of body and materials as they exist in a three-dimensional world" (Morris 1995, p. 78).

In the *Blind Time Drawings* this provided Morris with a means by which to move away from the modernist (Greenberg) pre-occupation with the two-dimensional picture plane that presents itself to vision toward a three-dimensional object that presents itself to the multi-sensory experience of an embodied subject.

The *Blind Time Drawings* demonstrate this clear bracketing out of vision in the field of artistic production by showing that drawing is an embodied and tactile process. In his response to them the philosopher Donald Davidson agreed with Morris that they are illustrations of "forms of human behaviour". Morris also claimed:

> I believe there are "forms" to be found within the activity of making as much as within the end products. These are forms of behaviour aimed at testing the limits of possibilities involved in that particular interaction between ones actions and the materials of the environment. This amounts to the submerged side of the iceberg. (Morris 1995, p. 73)

7. Conclusion

In Descartes *Optics* he claims that sight is analogous to a blind man's stick that is a way of "feeling" our way through space and around objects:

> For just as our blind man can sense the bodies which are around him, not only through the action of these bodies when they move against his stick, but also through that of his hand, when they are only resisting it, so we must affirm that objects of sight can be felt, not only by means of the action which, being in them, tends toward the eyes, but also by means of that which, being in the eyes, tends towards them [...] (Descartes 2001, p. 68)

This feeling is what the drawer attempts to make concrete as Emma Dexter says: "Drawing is not a window on the world but a device for understanding our place in the universe." (Dexter 2005, p. 5). The drawer is a subject struggling to capture their object and its essence. They struggle with the material by which they draw, with the means by which they know how to draw, with their apprehension of what it is they want to draw and with the possibilities that their bodies allow them.

Untitled 3-L Beams coerces its viewers into a similar struggle to drawing. *3 L-Beams* situates the perceiving subject in relation to its shapes. It thus draws that viewer into the *style* of phenomenological observation that one adopts when drawing.

As Davidson claims:

> Morris has depicted, then, the essential element on which the concept of an autonomous object (and world) depends: an intersubjective measure of error and success, of truth and falsity. He has put his viewers in a position to triangulate with him the location of his creative acts. (Davidson 1993, p. 614)

He does so presenting by a piece of work that addresses an embodied subject. In *Notes on Sculpture* written in 1966 just one year after *3 L-Beams* Morris explained his aspirations for such work: "the better new work takes relationships out of the work and makes them a function of space, light and the viewer's field of vision. The object is but one of the terms in the newer aesthetic" (Morris 1995, pp. 11–21). Or, as De Duve argues: "when the spectator turns around the object and grasps it in its differences, he is attending to his own differentiation, a becoming-other which is not the sudden astonishment in front of an alienating mirror, but a passive process resulting from his own actions." (de Duve 1983, pp. 234–60).

It is my argument here that if, as Thierry de Duve argues, "one of the functions of contemporary art is to construct models of the contemporary subject" (de Duve 1983, pp. 234–60) then *Untitled 3-L Beams* constructs the subject as *one who is observing it before drawing it*; that is, *as one who is drawing*. The best illustrations of this are any of the subsequent drawings made of its odd, taciturn forms. However, even though the work positions its viewers as drawers – that is as observing in the drawing style – not all of those drawers will be good ones. They would still need to use their bodies to achieve a concrete outcome in whatever medium they have to hand, and with varying degrees of success.

References

Best, S. (2006). Minimalism, subjectivity, and aesthetics: rethinking the anti-aesthetic tradition in late-modern art. *Journal of Visual Art Practice, 5*(3), 127–142.

Davidson, D. (1993). The Third Man. *Critical Inquiry, 19*(4), 607–616.

de Duve, T. (2008). Kant's "Free- Play" in the Light of Minimal Art. In F. Halsall, J. Jansen, & T. O'Connor (Eds.), *Rediscovering Aesthetics* (pp. 87–101). Stanford: Stanford University Press.

de Duve, T. (1983). Performance Here and Now: Minimal Art, a Plea for a new Genre of Theatre (transl. by D. Guilbaut), *Open Letter,* 5–6, 234–60.

Descartes, R. (2001). *Discourse on method, Optics, Geometry, and Meteorology* (transl. by P. Olscamp). Indianapolis, Indiana: Hackett Publishing.

Dexter, E. (2005). Introduction. In E. Dexter (Ed.), *Vitamin D: New Perspectives in Drawing* (pp. 5–11). London: Phaidon.

Duchamp, M. (1967). The Creative Act (Read by the author). A paper presented to the Convention of the American Federation of the Arts at Houston, Texas, 1957), *Aspen Magazine*, 5 & 6 (33 1/3 rpm record).

Fried, M. (1990). *Courbet's Realism*. Chicago: University of Chicago Press.

Fried, M. (1992). Art and Objecthood. In C. Harrison, & and P. Wood (Eds.), *Art in Theory 1900–1990* (pp. 822–833).Oxford: Blackwell.

Gombrich, E. (1960). *Art and Illusion*. London: Phaidon.

Gombrich, E. (1998). Style. In D. Preziosi (Ed.), *The Art of Art History* (pp. 150–163). Oxford: Oxford University Press.

Halsall, F., Jansen, J., & O'Connor, T. (Eds.). (2008). *Rediscovering Aesthetics*. Stanford: Stanford University Press.

Hockney, D. (2006). *Secret Knowledge*. London: Thames and Hudson.

Hoptman, L. (2002). *Drawing Now: Eight Propositions*. New York: The Museum of Modern Art.

Jones, C. (2005). *Eyesight Alone: Clement Greenberg's Modernism and the Bureaucratization of the Senses*. Chicago: University of Chicago Press.

Kant, I. (2007). *Critique of Pure Reason* (transl. by N. Kemp Smith). London/New York: Palgrave Macmillan.

Krauss, R. (1973). Sense and Sensibility: Reflections on Post 60s Sculpture, *Artforum*, 50, 149–156.

Krauss, R. (2006). Two Moments from the Post-Medium Condition. *October, 116*, 55–62.

Newman, M., & Bird J. (Eds.). (1999). *Rewriting Conceptual Art*, London: Reaktion.

Morris, R. (1995). *Continuous Project Altered Daily*. Cambridge, MA: MIT Press.

Morris, R. (2008). *Blind Time Drawings* (ed. by J.-P. Criqui). London: Steidl.

Rose, B. (2000). ABC Art. In J. Meyer (Ed.), *Minimalism* (pp. 214–217). London: Phaidon.

Schapiro, M. (1998). Style. In D. Preziosi (Ed.), *The Art of Art History* (pp. 143–149). Oxford: Oxford University Press.

Cy Twombly

Gesture, space, and writing

Rajiv Kaushik
Department of Philosophy, Brock University

Over the course of his career, Edwin (Cy) Twombly developed an ability to address himself to the expressive potential of the mark, smudge, line, or dot – the smallest expressive units of paintings. He continually revealed that these rudimentary elements of the image bear in themselves a compelling force that his own creative impulses follow. If Twombly's entire oeuvre appears dedicated to discovering what these rudimentary elements of the work of art contain, it is not to arrive at their final definition but to show a painter's endless efforts to confer into existence their own internal fragility, openness, and indeterminacy. As Marjorie Welish writes in *Signifying Art*, the Twombly image is, "searching for a pictorial solution whose outcome is unknown", and "[s]uspended between coming and going". The painter's "small, disconnected touches", she continues, "carry the sense of being forever hypothetical, doomed to partake in an open-ended discourse on painting where marks will continue to accrue without ever arriving at a definition of painting" (2000, p. 35).

I want to explore the basic elements of Twombly's work as open-ended discourse on painting, revealing that whatever can be said of the painting remains indefinite and on going. If this unfinished and indeterminate discourse on painting, in which talk about Twombly's work can proliferate endlessly, is parasitic on the basic expressive potential of the markings on a canvas, it first behooves us to reflect on how the markings operate for the painter to produce this proliferation. These markings, I want to say, are sites in which the body is opened up into the space around it in a very real way in order to show an incarnate site that is neutral with respect to phantasy and existence. They are each instances in which the difference between the two, between the interior and the exterior, is no longer. In this context, I would like to explore in the final section of this chapter how we might understand Twombly's so-called language paintings. These works, I will argue, show us the very origins of language from out of the interplay between the body and its space.

Because the basic markings of Twombly's works are, as Welish suggests in the above, unfinished, we must first understand that they are not the result of a formalism. Thus they must be distinguished from the gestures we find in abstract expressionist work. Yve-Alain Bois points out in an *Art Forum* conversation with Rosalind Krauss and others that Twombly's place alongside his contemporaries in the New York School is not an easy one:

> When you look at Twombly's early development, before the graffiti pieces, you see a step-by-step imitation of different Abstract Expressionists. He tries to emulate them but cannot; he realizes that for him it's a fraud. So he gradually moves to a position of paradox and dismissal. He then thinks: How can I debase, smear, erase that thing? (Bois 1994, p. 10)

Twombly, according to Bois here, cannot come to a position of a pure formalism because he covers over the shape of things rather than abstracts them. In this covering, Bois could point out, Twombly first moves from his scrupulous taxonomy of markings to a felt physical presence. By the early 1960's blobs and smears of pigment – red, browns, pinks, and black, sometimes introduced straight from the tube – are laid out on the canvas almost undifferentiated in form. It is suggested that this reintroduction of matter, from which Twombly had previously abstained, occurs at this point because he had explored enough the primitive potential of the drawn line so that he was now ready to add pigment and colour to his characteristic inventory of demarcations. Take for instance *The Ides of March* (1962). To understand Twombly in the context of erasure and debasement – and Bois is using these terms in the sense that Georges Bataille means them in which there is a negation irreducible to a being or to a positive determination but rather effects us from itself – is to place the painter in the context of a persistent negativity that makes representational and self-transparent consciousness impossible. It is to place Twombly in the context of a negativity as such, without reference to any determination outside of it. Here erasure differs from abstraction in the sense that it gives a role to the negative that is independent of things, whereas abstraction implies that the negative can be obtained from out of things. Bois is suggesting, then, that the fundamental indeterminacy in Twombly's images betray an original negation and erasure that imposes itself, overlays, and forever stands outside of things. He is suggesting, in other words, that insofar as Twombly's works refuse to refer to anything outside themselves they cover over things and disclose the positive role of negation – they consign them to a role outside of the artwork and disclose another process apart from the representation of things. What we have in the Twombly image, in this case, is the painter succumbing to that which remains outside of possible representation, fundamentally negating, erasing and smearing out determinate things in the service of indeterminacy itself.

But is it true that Twombly is *erasing* things in this sense that he conveys a negation that is originally separate from things? He would famously point out in a 1957 interview that,

> Most painting defines the image. It is at this point that I break with the more general process of painting. Each line is now the actual experience with its own innate history. It does not illustrate, it is the sensation of its own realization. The imagery is one of private indulgences, rather than an abstract totality of visual perception. (Norden 2003, n.p.)

In the first two sections of this chapter I want to focus on what I find key to a reading of Twombly in this remark of his: the basic markings of the Twombly are not only acts of erasure but self-referring or self-intimate acts so that if "the thing is debased", as Alain-Bois says, we also see this very process – the continual deformation of the thing; the sensation of this process is rendered such that we can witness a body opened up and in response to the very process of marking up the canvas. In this case, the negativity to which the painter succumbs does not impose itself immediately but it does so by degrees. Erasure, the Twombly image reveals, is a process, event, or a happening that spans and takes place in time. But neither is it derived from things, like abstraction. Erasure is a process that, found in the basic element of the artwork, occurs prior to any possible representation of things, and Twombly's images are able to convey a body as it gives itself over to this potentiality contained in the basic markings of a canvas.

I will argue that, as a result, the Twombly image may be seen not in the context of a negative dialectic but in the context of what Maurice Merleau-Ponty calls a hyper-dialectic that makes evident the place from out of which interiority and exteriority diverge from one another. Hyper-dialectic refers, then, to a region of human consciousness that is indifferent to interiority and exteriority, the cognitive and the non-cognitive, activity and passivity, and even the human and the animal. This reading in particular, I think, will be helpful later to understanding the many paintings or drawings of Twombly that are described by Roland Barthes as "work[s] of language" (Barthes 1985, p. 158). These images, as well as containing scrawls, make use of words, both legible and illegible. According to Barthes, such works are the most "subversive" of Twombly's images because they "traverse the aesthetic stereotype" (ibid). They call into question the very activity of writing words down, with the same inscribing hand that draws and paints, and thus they force us to question the idea of a linguistic system independent from the body that paints and draws. The scope of Twombly's images goes beyond even artwork as a practice, and towards its penchant to classify in terms of a language.

Consider for instance his *Quattro Stagioni: Autumno* (1993–95). This work and other works like it will be my focus at the end of this chapter. Here the appearance of the word "AUTUMNO" scrawled onto the canvas, as well as the title appearing alongside it, resists ectopizing the body as if it is something outside the play of signification. That is, it snatches the body away from its ordinary place of instrumental value, outside of signification, and puts it back into the very process of a symbolic play. The title is not produced in the context of a self-referential mode of language independent of the work of art, but rather is produced in the context of the self-referential aspect of the basic markings of the work. Thus Twombly's language paintings help us think through what it means for signification to emerge from out of, and screen off, the space of sensible bodies.

1. Rendering the process of mark-making

Barthes writes in "Cy Twombly: Works on Paper" that Twombly, "shows the gesture" so that "[w]e are not asked to see, to conceive, to savor the *product*, but to review, to identify, and, so to speak, to "enjoy" the movement which has ended up *here*" (ibid. 164). In showing the gesture, Barthes suggests, a viewer is not captivated by an autonomous artwork that depicts a world apart from its creator. In the Twombly image each marking is self-referential in the sense that, rather than referring to the external world of things, it refers to nothing outside of its own origination. To "show the gesture," then, is to shift fundamentally from simulacra to self-referentiality in which each time the brushwork reveals the event of its own production and the otherwise hidden movement of the artist's bodily intentions. The mark is just what ended up *here*, as Barthes says, because it immediately directs back into itself and towards the singular gesture that remains identical to itself in the phase of its own movement. In effect, Twombly is able to capture in each marking that which alone has animated it, an intrinsic and motivating force with respect to its own being. In revealing the gesture that created it, in other words, each marking of a Twombly image comes into contact only with itself, its own origination, and is never linked any other set of external and contingent associations.

When looked at from a viewer's standpoint, however, we do not just see discreet "heres", and Barthes also suggests that the Twombly canvas shows us mark-*making*, a process that unfolds through a certain span of time. If Barthes insists that Twombly's gesture is just what has shown up *here*, in this instance and in this image alone, he is also just as insistent that this gesture exists and persists only because it is in some sense spatio-temporalized. The gesture in the Twombly image is here, singular and in the phase of its own movement alone, but only because it is opened and spread out into a spatial world to which it has addressed itself. There is a communion between what would otherwise be assumed as two mutually exclusive and foreign terms, so that the space that circumambulates the body is not just its "outside" but the field of its possible expression. One must notice, in other words, that in being self-intimate the basic markings of the Twombly image are the expression of a hand *in movement* or *in transit*, which has just now *taken place*. Every line of the Twombly presupposes a secret activity that is working out an original being-in the environment as though for the first time. It is perhaps even impossible to separate the created product from the painter's posture, his stance in relation to the image, his gait, etc. The environment that was previously invisible has now, however indirectly, been rendered in visible terms.

It is said that we can "read Twombly's work through the metaphor of the body" (Bird 2007, p. 498) and thus there is a difficulty in moving from representations of the body in specific works to the body itself as an inscribed surface. I would add, and for reasons that should become clearer in the following section, that if we give priority to the expressive capabilities of the mark that is before any possibility of representation, then *the metonymic is prior to the metaphorical*. That is, in reducing to the original indeterminacy of the scrawl, Twombly's images cannot first give metaphorical reference to the body but are rather vestigial objects that bear in themselves the traces and markings of a specific body as it has moved through its own space in a certain way. Only on this basis does one then read the metaphorical references to the body in Twombly's images.

Hence in his writings on Twombly Barthes gives priority to the alchemical notion of the *materia prima*. The *materia prima* refers to the brute moment of materiality prior to creation. It is that from out of which creation happens, and refers to the initial moments in which the body finds itself in the midst of the materiality and needs to create from out of it. It thus refers to a moment of creation in which things are chosen and other things are rejected, the filial moment in which creation begins to crawl out of a morass. This sort of emphasis on the materiality of Twombly's art that precedes and succeeds any secondary representation gives ultimate importance to corporeal presence transmitted via instrument (e.g. brush or pencil) and matter (e.g. paint or graphite) into a surface so that we should see the direction, weight, rapidity of motions, and finally all the motor-reflex operations that contribute to the nature of a mark-making process. It is possible to say that the Twombly image is the very act of composing caught in its midst, not a fully formed composition but the process of composing itself coming into appearance. One can even wonder if "composition" is "a useful term to describe [the] process of making, unmaking and remaking' evident in Twombly's images" (ibid., 501).

2. The body's intentions opened up into mark-making

Now we are able to shift registers. We can see the mark's realisation of itself, prior to the intentions of the artist, and we can witness what is like for the painter to be guided by this prior realisation. Now there is painter's own sensation of what it is like to mark up a page or canvas, where this process of mark-making implicates a subjugation to a set of external forces not the artist's own. As Bird writes, Twombly's images give us a metaphorics of the body in which the body is understood in the midst of the interplay between what Jacques Lacan called the imaginary symbolic as opposed to the real that frustrates meaning and refuses to lend itself to symbolization (ibid., p. 499). "There are many *petits morts* in the works by Twombly", Bird thus writes, referring to the brief time (as in an orgasm) in which Lacan says the symbolic/real opposition is no longer, "a line, smear or trace expires, suddenly, in the midst of frenetic activity…" (ibid.). But, again, I would emphasize here that the Twombly piece refuses to accept that this overcoming is just metaphorical simulation of the symbolic in the real. There really are a series of *petit morts* in Twombly's works, I would say, and this is because Twombly's pieces are metonymic insofar as they reveal an original continuity between the symbolic and the real, prior to their separation, by means of his radical reduction to the mark that the painter has inscribed onto the surface. It is otherwise difficult to see the overcoming of the break between symbolic and real by referring only to the symbolic that occurs within the painting and then reading it out from there. In any case, I think, we can witness the concrete site of a reconciliation between symbolic and real at work in the image itself.

Take, just as an instance, the image from the *Bacchus* series of 2005, *Untitled VII*. Here we see active lines, rendered without any fixed representational or even compositional goal. They are just a set of scrawlings looped, with various densities and weights at the tops of the loops or at the bottoms. These variations are apparently not the result of any advanced deliberations but, if they are deliberated over, one can surmise that it is in relation to, and from out of, what has just now occurred on the canvas – the behaviour of the paint, the surface onto which it is conferred, the workings of gravity. Gesturing is inevitably opened up to something outside of itself – it is at a distance or even *ek-static* – so that in a very literal sense it passes into what is un-conscious, e.g. when the paint is inevitably forced downward to the bottom of the painting by gravity. If we describe the paint as a blood-like red that drips, expires, terminates, and thus calls to mind several *petits morts*, we must see that this is due to the more primal register of the material in which the basic markings call into question the specific animating body that inscribed them, which is then subjected to a set of un-reflexive aspects. In his last provocative thoughts on the recurrent theme of Dionysian bacchanale in

Twombly's images, Bird does point to this very complex of "the interplay between the intentional and accidental accumulation of marks across their surfaces" (ibid., p. 503). There is, he writes, "the scribble as both a trace of the body's rhythm and as the origination of an intentional marking of surface..." (ibid.), which is then subject to "the downward pressure of gravitational force returning the *materia prima* to the earth from whence it came..." (ibid., p. 504). Though he does not quite say it explicitly, it is the accidental aspect of the gravitational force that serves as a "reminder...that at the culmination of every Dionysiac ritual there has to be a reckoning" (ibid.). These accidental and unwilled aspects of the artwork, in other words, disclose that each and every event of creation inevitably falls back into the very materiality from whence it originally came. It is first on the basis of this return and upsurge of the material, the accidental and un-volitional, into the activity of creating the work of art, that colour can only subsequently be read metaphorically, as "both mimetic – the red of wine and blood – and symbolic – the Dionysian bacchanale" (ibid., p. 503).

Another aspect of Twombly's work appears here in the Bacchus image that I would like to explore further in the following section: there is not yet any concrete distinction between the symbolic and the accidental, or between the bacchanale and the un-willed behaviour of the material, until Twombly assigned the name 'Bacchus' to the image. The name, functioning to deepen the problem of the symbolic/real by showing us both the moment the symbolic becomes distinguished from the real, the imaginary from the material, forces us to wonder how the sign comes to be from out of the accidental aspects of the material. This is what I want to focus on below.

3. Language/writing – gesture

It is one thing to suggest that Twombly announces a gesturing body that is open, and homologous to, and within, the play of the symbolics of the unconscious itself, and thus that he questions and even undermines the rupture between the symbolic and the real, but it is quite another to make this claim where language is involved. Language is not normally thought to be about the body at all, and it is often thought to disclose an autonomous and self-sufficient symbolic play apart from the real. Yet, in Barthes' essays on Twombly he asks us to see the artist's writing in the light of his own poetics in which there is interaction between language, text and the mark-making of images. Barthes points out in this context that Twombly's writing is primarily a graphism, so that, though "it presents itself as writing," nevertheless "the letters formed no longer participate in any graphic code..." Twombly's 'writings,' in other words, do not function in the way legible text normally does, in order to fix meaning to the otherwise indeterminate image. His writing is instead really a "graphic texture," which is not simply this writing or that, nor even the Being of writing," but rather the elements of writing that are not necessary to and even in excess of it (1985, p. 162). Here, in Twombly's graphism Barthes says we witness,

> certain opaque, non-signifying elements – or rather, elements of a different signification – catch our attention…the nervous turn of the letters, the spurt of the ink, the tensile quality of the strokes, all those accidents which are not necessary to the functioning of the graphic code and are consequently, already, surpluses. (ibid., p. 169)

It is in the context of these other, outside elements of the graphic text that Barthes calls Twombly's "*gauche* (left-handed)" such that they "refer to the circle of the excluded, the marginal…" (ibid., p. 163).

Barthes makes a similar claim about Twombly's titles when he describes them as not referring to anything but something excluded: "In Twombly's titles, we must not look for any induction of analogy", he says. "If the canvas is called *The Italians*, do not look for the Italians anywhere except, precisely, in their name" (ibid.). Barthes points out that if this "pictorial nominalism" does not operate by the terms of analogy (representation, likeness, mimesis), it nevertheless has another mode of operation called the "performative" (ibid.) One way to treat this modality of language is to insist, as Krauss does in her reading of Barthes' essay, that the sense of a linguistic sign is thereby "suspended" (1994, p. 74 and p. 118) in favour of a specific act or performance in order to ultimately accomplish something pre-linguistic, pre-verbal and pre-symbolic "through the act of dirtying, smearing, scarring, jabbing" (1993, p. 259). In Twombly's graffiti pieces the activity of marking something up is "violent", "an invasion of a space that is not the marker's own" that "takes illegitimate advantage of the surface of inscription" (ibid., p. 118). Furthermore, she writes, this resultant mark "is the trace of an event, torn away from the presence of the marker" (ibid). This tear between the mark and the marker, for Krauss, shows the impossibility of a continuity between the two terms because, though the "graffiti's graphic lash strikes in the present", nevertheless "it registers itself as past, a mark whose violence dismembers the very idea of the image in the mirror", or the very idea that the painter is reflected in his or her creation (ibid.).

One has to question Krauss' treatment of graffiti in order to see why Twombly's performative use of language in his pictorial nominalism is not quite a matter of suspending the sign's sense and emphasizing a pre-symbolic erasure of it. The very point of graffiti, it could be said, calls into question the marked up surface as illegitimate for the marker. The marker means to indicate that the surface is legitimately his or her own, and thus the marked up surface is the result of an act of usurpation, a reclamation of a surface that is seen as properly one's own. Seen from the point of view of an unsuspecting viewer, surely this act appears illegitimate. It gives the feeling to its viewer of arbitrariness, possibly applied to any random surface, turning up especially on billboards, sides of buildings, walls, etc. But this randomness to its viewer, from the point of view of the artist, is in fact its very point. I would go so far as to argue that the strategy of apparent randomness only aids in the image's usurpation. The placement and glyphic character of the graffiti, its use of the surface on which it applies, gives it a lack of defined space, and this lack is used for the marker's own ends. A reclaimed surface is a political act that reorients space to the marker's own ends; it forces the viewer to confront the possibility of another condition other than her own. I would say that, since there is no illegitimate use of surface for the graffiti artist, from this point of view there is also no separation between marker and marked up surface like the one Krauss describes as violent and illegitimate. In fact, the very surface on which the graffiti is applied conveys its meaning. Twombly may be a graffiti artist in the same way Stéphane Mallarmé, with whom he was obsessed, reclaimed the white of the page as a surface that conveys the meaning of the black ink applied to its surface. The point is that language is opened up and it means something tactile, something available to touch. The performative act of language, such as the one in a Twombly images, does not erase sense but rather it is itself sense, and thus it implies that the sense of language can be at an intersection between itself and the world in which it is enacted.

It is furthermore impossible to consistently read Twombly's performative language in the way Krauss suggests when we consider recurrent images like *Orpheus 1979*, from a 1979 series in which he makes relatively clear recurrent iconographic and iconological references to Greek and Roman figures. Though still child-like, the names of these figures are clearly legible and have a referent. One theory has it that names such as Orpheus or Pindar are to be understood in the light of mythology, in which Twombly was deeply interested, and so we are not really meant to follow their lives or stories but to shift from the register of definition and into the realm of metaphor and connotation. But I refuse this route if I am to attempt to consistently read the basic expressive quality of his markings as the primal aspect of Twombly's work, existing neither merely in the symbolic or metaphorical nor merely in the real.

Although Krauss' treatment of performative language in Twombly's paintings is not meant to explain images such as *Orpheus 1979*, once we take into account the doubts raised to her reading we see that we do not need to adopt yet another explanation for such an image. If there is good reason to doubt that graffiti suspends signification in such a way as to question the impossibility of a continuous relation between the marker and the mark, Twombly's performative language may not reveal a break between signification and act. We could rather say that, at the same time that his images are enactments, they are also the site of signification and intellect. Bird himself comes close to saying this when he writes that, "the gestural aspect of writing as an identifiable linguistic sign emerges painfully, but also sensuously, from the chaos of scribble" (Bird 2007, p. 489). Here we could have a material semiosis: though it is a cognitive activity, language is now seen to derive from out of the sensible, which is therefore not the erasure or eclipse of a sign-system (in an above reference, for instance, Barthes himself uses the phrase "a different signification"). Notice, for instance, how the name "Virgil" in *Virgil 1973* seems to *come to be written* from out of a process in which there is scribbling, writing, scratching out, and then again re-writing. Everything is at work here all at once for Twombly: there is what Barthes calls the non-signifying elements of a graphic texture (the non-volitional tendencies of inscribing), a graphic code (the word 'VIRGIL' is legible), as well as a pictorial nominalism (the image is subsequently, in a reflective moment, named for what is inscribed in it). The idea is that Twombly shows a commonality between painting drawing and sculpting, and even how they coincide in the same artist. The co-origination between painting or drawing and language or text undermines the difference between discourse and figure.

So long as one appeals to an erasure that prohibits reference to a sensible world apart from language and denies meaning to the sensible apart from the meaning imparted by signification, the solution to the problem of reference cannot occupy the conceptual space in which it is posed. That is, it refuses to explain the problem of reference, how it is possible that words refer to the sensible world. The strategy here is not to deny the existence of the extra-linguistic, but rather to assert that all reference to things is mediated by the signifiers through which such reference is made. On this view there is no way to exit signification. But, nevertheless, the question still arises as to the nature of this mediation, and this question is understood as one about a fundamental discontinuity and heterogeneity. A canvas such as *Virgil 1973*, however, asks us to reconsider the symbolic play of signification as indistinct from the gestures of the hand. I want to say that Merleau-Ponty offers us a way to think through the Twombly canvas, and in particular his language paintings. Merleau-Ponty, too, sees that understanding language as originally an autonomous system is deeply problematic. The mediation that links the two terms, language and unconscious, is discontinuity or erasure, but the very attempt at *mediation* is an attempt to link the two. The challenge, for Merleau-Ponty, is to conceive an unconscious that intersects language and world becomes the challenge of what he calls in *The Visible and the Invisible* a "good dialectic" or a "hyper-dialectic", which could only be a "dialectic which criticizes itself and surpasses itself" (1968, p. 94). It is interesting to note that for Merleau-Ponty this hyper or good dialectic can be contrasted with "bad faith and bad dialectic" and is instead simply the return to *Syge*, the abyss" (ibid., p. 159).

Merleau-Ponty uses term "hyper-dialectic" to indicate that he is looking for a relation between terms before the thought of their relation and before a philosophy that begins by proceeding dialectically. The term invites us to think of the relations of matter and form differently than do materialism, spiritualism and criticism. It invites us to conceive these relations of matter and form in such a way that they do not originally oppose but rather inhere in one another. His ultimate goal is to get us to think of relations of matter and form as different in a non-substantial way such that meaning can come to live in a fragment of matter. Hyper-dialectic, then, refers not to a third and transcending moment of the relation between opposing terms but to the incarnated site of their self-mediation. This form of dialectic implies that the process of coming into appearance is grounded in the specific things themselves, bound to the concrete content, instead of being dictated from above by a supervenient logic that imposes its own requirements onto that which it seeks to explain. The term rediscovers the process of change in time such that differences are continually emergent. Here we may consider oppositions instead as broken up or as divergences, and thus as originally outside of or absent from themselves in order to become themselves. Hyper-dialectic thus finally discovers that this form of mediation in the incarnated site is made possible not by a uni-dimensional structure sustaining things from underneath them, but by a sensible logic that makes possible both the reflection and the thing upon which reflection reflects.

Thus, I would argue, the recourse to hyper-dialectic, insofar as it implies the discovery of an enjambment between self-reflexion at the heights of its self-torsion and the sensible world, allows us to grasp Twombly's language paintings in a new light instead of the negative dialectic suggested earlier by Yves Alain-Bois in reference to erasure and debasement. Rather than giving us a moment of erasure and frustration, I want to say, Twombly's language paintings reveal the incarnate place of the origins of language. This place is not negativity as such. But, in view of this sensible, it also just as true that language does not originate purely from out of the intentional and volitional. Though there is in Twombly's "childhood calligraphy" an "unsentimentalized beginning" that gives clarity anew to an original "affective expression", there is also the process of restoration and recovery at work in Twombly's images that requires cultivation and mastery" (Welish 2000: 62). There is a "virtuoso technique" that at the same time indicates its openness to its origins, an openness and origination from out what is other to it. For example, when describing an image such as *Leda and the Swan* (1962), Linda Lindstrom remarks on Twombly's virtuoso technique in his movements: "next come single arcs", she writes, "still made by the original swinging movement of the arm, but now in one direction only, the tool being lifted at the end of the first stroke instead of being returned to the starting position" (Lindstrom 1957, p.18).

If hyper-dialectic applies to Twombly's graffiti pieces, it is because his inscribed words are the result of a reflection on language carried to the extreme, so that language itself may be recovered in the process of its own formation – seen once again from the point of view of its origination in the context of "a hard-won and deliberate process of enunciation" (Bird 2007, p. 501). Once an identifiable and written linguistic sign is seen to emerge from out of the gesture, all the characteristics of Twombly's otherwise non-linguistic gestures apply to it. It, too, is founded by the expressive potential of the mark, and can be seen as such once the draughtsman-writer allows himself to feel what it is like to be given over to this expressive potential that precedes him. Already Twombly has discovered in these markings a way in which the body is opened up affectively to what is other than it. They announce unpredictability by letting the gesturing body follow what is un-willed and beyond volition. The disclosure of thinking and writing from out of the un-thought and non-verbal, from out of nothing more than the sensible, is the result of a reflection carried out so exhaustively that it finds the birth of its own origins in a sensibility that would have otherwise remained hidden to it. This is what Twombly himself described as the marking's private indulgences.

References

Barthes, R. (1985). *The Responsibility of Forms* (transl. by R. Howard). New York: Hill and Wang.

Bois, Y.-A., Buchloh, B., Foster, H., Hollier, D., Krauss, R., & Molesworth, H. (1994). The Politics of the Signifier II: A Conversation on the *Informe* and the Abject, *October*, 67 (Winter), 3–21.

Bird, J. (2007). Indeterminacy and (Dis)order in the work of Cy Twombly. *Oxford Art Journal*, *30*(3), 484–504.

Krauss, R. (1993). *The Optical Unconscious*. Cambridge MA/London: The MIT Press.

Krauss, R. (1994). Cy Was Here: Cy's Up, *ArtForum International*, *33*(1), 118.

Lindstrom, M. (1957). *Children's Art*. Berkley: University of California Press.

Merleau-Ponty, M. (1968). *The Visible and the Invisible*. Evanston: Northwestern University Press.

Norden, L. (2003). What Painting Can Contain. In L. Norden (Ed.), *Cy Twombly: A Gathering of Time, Six Paintings and a Sculpture (exhibition catalogue* (n.p.). New York: Gagosian Gallery.

Welish, M. (2000). *Signifying Art: Essays on Art After 1960*. Cambridge: Cambridge University Press

Pre-motor and motor activities in early medieval handwriting

Jan W. M. van Zwieten & Koos Jaap van Zwieten
University of Hasselt

1. Introduction – the Beatrice saga

At age nine, Dante Alighieri first caught a glimpse of Beatrice Portinari, also nine, who would symbolize for him perfect female beauty and spiritual goodness in the coming decades. Portinari however did not seem to return his feelings, which Dante described (±1292) in terms of the inner movements of organs. In those days, the understanding of how our organs function as a mechanism was rather elementary. It is worthwhile to read Dante's own description of this love at first sight, which he wrote down between the ages of twenty seven and thirty, but "emotions and the ability to love do not disappear along aging" (Määttä 2011, p. 15). In boys, the age of about nine years marks the onset of quantitative development of the structures in the brain (basal ganglia) that are involved in affective states (Giedd 2008, p. 338). These structures can nowadays be visualized when active (Bartels & Zeki 2004, p. 1160).

She appeared dressed in noblest color, restrained and pure, in crimson, tied and adorned in the style that then suited her very tender age. At that moment I say truly that the vital spirit, that which lives in the most secret chamber of the heart began to tremble so violently that I felt it fiercely in the least pulsation, and, trembling, it uttered these words: Behold a god more powerful than I, who, coming, will rule over me. At that moment the animal spirit, that which lives in the high chamber to which all the spirits of the senses carry their perceptions, began to wonder deeply at it, and, speaking especially to the spirit of sight, spoke these words: Now your blessedness appears. At that moment the natural spirit, that which lives in the part where our food is delivered, began to weep, and weeping said these words: Oh misery, since I will often be troubled from now on! From then on I say that Amor governed my soul… (Dante 1292, p. 1).

Although in this commentary "Dante shows a thorough knowledge of the scholastic method of reasoning" (Greenfield 1981, p. 73), it may be interesting to concentrate on his precise explanations on the internal organs and their presumed motions – better known as somatisations. "Somatizations may be considered untransformed sensory impressions and emotional experiences" (Fischbein 2011, p. 209). No wonder that today too, vague and diffuse e.g. gastro-intestinal symptoms are well-known in medical records (Guedes et al. 2008, p. 138).

"Most individuals indicate that they desire a complementary partner instead of a similar one", Dijkstra and Barelds conclude (2008, p. 600). This is how Dante describes his feelings, especially when he pictures Beatrice as someone who removes all evil intentions from him. Recently, various studies appeared concerning various styles of flirting and their backgrounds. Within five dimensions of flirting, the physical and sincere dimensions appear to be second and third in rank, as they "correlate with rapid relational escalation of important relationships with more emotional connection and greater physical chemistry." (Hall et al. 2010, p. 365). Spitzer (2011, p. 858) confirms that the "sincere dimension" is marked by interest in emotions. Further, Dante's high esteem for Beatrice (although he later married Gemma Donati) seems to confirm what was found in the participants in a recent study by Swami and Allum (2012, p. 89), namely that the participants also rate former partners as more attractive than themselves.

2. Movements of inner organs

When we concentrate on the description of Dante's inner movements today, these can now be easily explained in terms of activity of the autonomic nervous system, especially the sympathetic division of it, which generally causes arousal of all body functions, including our internal organs. In a much comprehensive article, Potts (2008, p. 21) sufficiently explains this autonomic nervous system response in romantic love, while Codispoti et al. (2006, p. 217) investigated a.o. autonomic heart rate responses in viewing emotionally arousing pictures. Such present-day explanations can be useful to better understand Dante's descriptions. The "greater physical chemistry" (Hall et al. 2010, p. 365) may also have been literally present. Emanuele (2011, p. 265) could identify "a positive association between the intensity of early romantic feelings and serum levels of nerve growth factor (NGF)". Moreover, Govoni et al. (2011, p. 266) speculate that nerve growth factor may be modulated to influence specific stages of heart function. In other words, the "neurochemistry of love" is an intriguing area of study. Meanwhile, Parkinson (2006, p. 3) warns for the neediness correlated to NGF in passionate love. Both heart activity modulation and a lifelong fascination for Beatrice marked Dante indeed. Beside unraveling the autonomic processes that come into action when there is love at first sight, the traditional descriptive explanation of emotion as a result of impression may still be useful (Whiting 2009, p. 290). A specific medical background is not required to understand this.

3. Handwriting and neuromotor characteristics

Apart from this "centrally oriented" approach of the description of emotions, namely starting from points of view of internal medicine and neuroscience, we now hypothesize that visible traces of emotional states may also be found in the enormous wealth of various historical handwritten texts – as long as the current characteristics of quill pen writing, and the processes of writing by hand are taken into account. It is evident that a skilled mastering of the precise positions and movements of hand and fingers is a prerequisite for successful handwriting.

Although nowadays the teaching of handwriting has been criticized (Trubek 2009, p. 2), current behavioural studies still make use of handwritten letters' characteristics like strokes, roundedness, etcetera. In consequence, Fisher et al. (2010, p. 57) studying brain activation during rejected love, noticed typical pre-motor activity patterns, as suggested by irregular writing patterns as well, due to basal ganglia dysfunction (Mergl et al. 2004, p. 387). The basal ganglia and other deep brain areas are also known as the "emotional circuits" of the brain.

> The subjective ease with which we carry out simple action plans…(like) making a downstroke while writing – masks the enormously complex integrative apparatus needed to achieve and maintain coordination among the thousands of sensors, neurons, and skeleto-motor units that contribute to any act's planning and execution. (Bullock & Grossberg 1988, p. 49)

A typical "downstroke" asks for flexion of the both interphalangeal joints of the finger. This requires the coordination of the extrinsic, but especially the intrinsic hand- and finger-muscles (Napier 1966, p. 15). Rounded letterforms ask for well-coordinated interphalangeal joint motion.

Further, it should be noted that both interphalangeal joints move simultaneously in all "free" i.e. unresisted hand- and finger-movements and during precision-handling, like the picking up of small objects (van Zwieten et al. 2008, p. 171). In consequence, appropriate finger positions in handwriting normally also show such comparable simultaneous ("coupled" or "coordinated") slightly curved interphalangeal flexion, no matter which arm and hand muscles are active. The "automatically" coordinated unresisted finger motions have their functional-anatomical and kinematical basis in a tendon-like extensor apparatus that is known as the extensor assembly of the finger (Bunnell 1942, p. 10;

van Zwieten et al. 2002, p. 354). It is noteworthy that especially such hand- and finger-positioning during writing with a feather quill is advised in a woodcarving by the humanist Mercator, who rightly characterizes it as "Bona gubernatio" which means: a good steering (of the pen) (Mercator 1540, p. 10). He further comments: "Bona comprehensio calami" which means: a good grasp of the reed (the shaft).

With respect to the feedback of the finely tuned hand- and finger-motions, by sensory as well as by motor representation, recent publications have thrown a new light on this highly complex subject. Barton et al. (2010, p. 3873) used text stimuli and functional and structural imaging of their subjects, while Tsapkini and Rapp (2010, p. 200) succeeded in localizing orthography-specific functions within the left fusiform gyrus of the cerebral cortex. Tavares et al. (2011, p. 102) demonstrated activity in *both* fusiform gyri, when offering emotional contents. From this, it is clear that deep brain areas like emotional circuits may influence handwriting.

4. Traces of emotion in a handwritten text

In view of the aforementioned search for traces of emotion in historical handwriting, we checked a short handwritten 11th century Flemish poem for typical characteristics in the light of hypothesized finger- and hand movements (Kobayashi 2003, p. 3; Zanone et al. 2005, p. 2) that were possibly influenced by some presumed pre-motor (emotional circuit-driven) activity during another example of unrequited love (Mergl et al. 2004, p. 387). Our analysis concerned the compact types of Early Gothic/Carolingian minuscule (Morgan 2006, p. 129) in:

"Hebban olla uoga__ nestas _agunnan hinase hi _nda thu uu__ unbiadan __e nu"

This text reads as follows: Hebban olla vogala nestas hagunnan (All the birds have begun their nests) hinase hic enda thu (except me and you) uuat unbiadan uue nu (what are we waiting for) (Weel 2005, p. 5). "It looks Flemish!" authoritative Oxford-bred scholar Sir Kenneth Sisam seems to have exclaimed, when first noticing this phrase 80 years ago at the end-leaf of "Mss. Bodley 340" (Kwakkel 2005, p. 30). Especially in the last decade, extensive research has been performed concerning the language, history, identity, nationality and/or gender of the scribe who wrote this typical, poetic phrase (de Grauwe 2004, p. 52; van Oostrom 2006, p. 98).

In analysing historical texts, written with a feather quill, some know-how on quill pens and on how to trim a nib may be helpful (Morgan 2006, p. 36). Conventionally one wrote some probatio pennę ("pen test") first. In our analysis, we did not take into account qualities of quill-sharpening or ink fluency because the scribbling itself pretends to serve as a test of this.

5. Historical backgrounds of the text

When in 1066 William Duke of Normandy conquered England, it had an enormous impact. Even from the 1173 Earl of Leicester's army a satirical song-cum-dance remains (until today), ascribed to Flemish and Norman noblemen alike: "Hop(pe) Willy'ken, hop(pe) Willy'ken, Ingland is thyne and myne, &c." (Friedman 1959, p. 1). In the slipstream of William's army, clergymen followed, some of which may have been Flemish indeed. One such (late 11th century) scribe at Rochester St. Andrew's wrote down this possibly oldest known Flemish (i.e. Old Low Franconian) verse plus its Latin translation. At present, many see this verse as South-West Flemish (also in view of the scribe's possible origin) (de Grauwe 2004, p. 53). Their analyses, however, are mainly devoted to the linguistics of the text (Louwen 2009, p. 63). Meanwhile, the handwritten phrase lends itself very well to a search after emotional traces, as "it looks most like a love poem, or at any rate the beginning of one" (Meijer 1978, p. 2). Many linguists therefore presume an emotional state having been present in the mind of the scribe, writing on the occasion of a (possibly anecdotic) unrequited love (van Oostrom 2006, p. 102). Handwritten manuscripts expressing disappointment, or emotions in general, look far more irregular, however. Today's scientific analyses on this very topic usually make use of a person's writing performance registration in real-time, i.e. by means of video cameras, writing tablets, cyber-gloves etcetera (Kobayashi 2003, p. 2). Of course, analyses of texts handwritten ages ago do ask for different techniques, like the so-called "digital paleography" (Brink et al. 2012, p. 167). At present however, searching for *emotional* traces too, by such techniques, is not possible. We therefore first screen our short text, referring to some comparable (historical) handwritings, whether or not emotionally influenced, by character size and then by regularity.

6. Preliminary screening of character size and regularity

The handwritten letter to the Galatians, dated 56–57 (Rolland 2001, p. 124), is the letter where St. Paul refers to his own writing in large letters – most likely on a wax tablet, however (Mitternacht 2007, p. 58). His original Greek "Idete pelikois humin grammasin egrapsa te eme cheiri" is translated as "Ye see how large a letter I have written unto you with mine own hand" (Holy Bible, Galatians 6, 11), but also reads as "See what big letters I make as I write to you now with my own hand!" (New Testament in Today's English Version 1971, p. 462). Emotionally influenced persuasion may have lead St. Paul to switch temporarily to a large handwriting, called "macrographia" only if the writing *stays* abnormally large (Beversdorf et al. 2001, p. 99). Although far-reaching diagnostics on St. Paul's health condition have been made, the possibility "that it is hyperbole [...] is more probable" (Landsborough 1987, p. 660).

Some one and a half millennium later, we find a testimony on how to produce properly sized handwritten characters, using italics in particular, in the manual by Mercator (1540) that we already referred to. The author patiently explains, by writing examples and instructions, how to position and move each individual finger during the writing process. Further, special emphasis is laid on the contact of the lower arm with the writing desk. Too large an area of contact increases the force needed for writing, evoking fatigue and unpleasant sensations and causing "peccantes" i.e. writing mistakes (Mercator 1540, Chapters 2 and 3). This careful description makes perfectly clear that the ease and legibility of writing as well as the comfort of all psychomotor elements concerned, are acknowledged as interdependent.

A very recent report convincingly illustrates the diminished size of handwritten characters, also known as "micrographia", in the case of a transient mental depression related to an eating disorder (Sekar et al. 2010, p. 763). In this case history of an adolescent girl, just before her psychomotor disorder became apparent, "the shape of [her] letters did not alter much but the size was reduced to almost one third of the size of the individual alphabets of her previous handwriting". The authors postulate that "the symptoms of micrographia [...] could [...] be aspects of the communication difficulty observed in this patient" (Sekar et al. 2010, p. 765). The authors also report that the girl was later successfully treated.

Yang and Kao (2003, pp. 7–8) give a scientifically justified state of the art, as well as an overview, of 35 graphological parameters that are related to personality traits, to be found in the regularity of individual characteristics of today's handwriting. Apart from their two parameters related to handwriting pressure, most of them may be applied to our Flemish text. Also because these authors focus on personality styles in *bi*cultural contexts, their (negative as well as positive) correlations can be used for our text in view of the scribe's bicultural identity Flemish – English. Although negatively correlated in Yang and Kao (2003, p. 9), in our text we note in particular: open "a" and "o" openings (tolerance to be a good listener), absence of left slant (attuned to needs of subordinates), pointed "m" and "n" tops – i.e. "prickly" characters (quick thinking and curiosity). Positively correlated (Yang & Kao 2003, p. 9) was: the wide word spacing in the text, meaning: affectionate relationship between the workers.

After this preliminary screening, based on character size and regularities as seen in (historical) examples of handwriting styles, we summarise that in our 11th century Flemish text no clear traces of emotional involvement, depression, or psychomotor dysfunction were observed. Instead, personality traits currently appreciated as positive, could be traced in the manuscript.

7. Further analyses, results and conclusions

1. To analyse handwritten forms, letters or characters, highly refined methods are available today, some of which are based on more or less automatic recognition of patterns by a. o. grid representations (Zhang & Lu 2004, p. 13). Several of these methods depend on matching techniques. Lu et al. (2011, p. 883) compared speed and accuracy of various methods. These authors expect that application of high-dimensional index technologies may improve their results in the near future. Falk et al. (2011, p. e104) developed elegant user-friendly computer-based handwriting assessment set-ups to quantify the handwriting proficiency in children.

In our further analysis we compared – by means of careful and repeated visual checks – each character of the handwritten 11th century text (Weel 2005, p. 5) with its standard model form as taught by instructional textbooks on historical calligraphy fonts, especially that of Morgan (2006, p. 129).

As typical features we (again) acknowledged: fluency, regular or irregular downstrokes and upstrokes, and presence or absence of rounded letterforms. Parallel to this, we determined letter frequencies. Such a rather traditional application of letter frequencies (Di Mascio 1959, p. 586) is nowadays also used to analyse phrases (MacKenzie & Soukoreff 2003, p. 755). Further, individual characters were also clustered according to difficulty of writing technique.

2. To test whether or not traces of emotion are found in this 11th century manuscript on presumed unrequited love, its (somewhere "prickly") characters were compared to standard types. In comparison to the compact standard Carolingian minuscules, each character of the manuscript displays fluent, regular downstrokes and upstrokes.

3. For teaching purposes, the following 8 groups of increasing difficulty are currently used: ceo, irnmu, lbh, dqp, fs, at, g, and xyz. Most characters of the text are in the first 4 groups (Table 1).

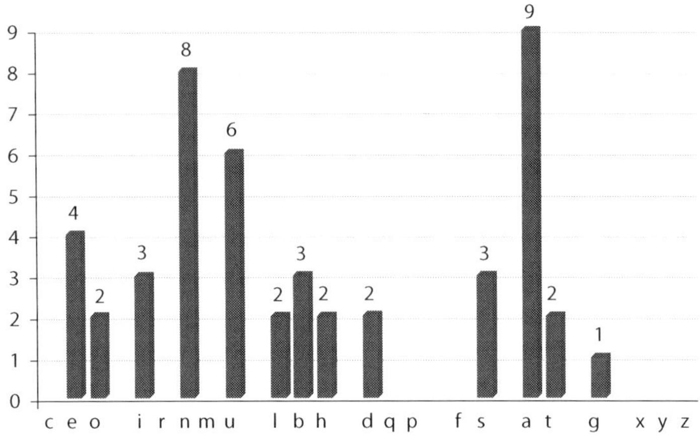

Table 1. Letter frequencies as found in the manuscript, clustered within eight groups of three letters which are ranked according to the increasing difficulty of handwriting (see text)

4. Varying in frequency, the text shows 13 individually different characters i.e. half our alphabet (Table 2). Although Carolingian texts do not use characters "k, j, v and w", the manuscript still may be seen as (half) a pangram like today's: "The quick brown fox jumps over the lazy dog" (Falk et al. 2011, p. e104).

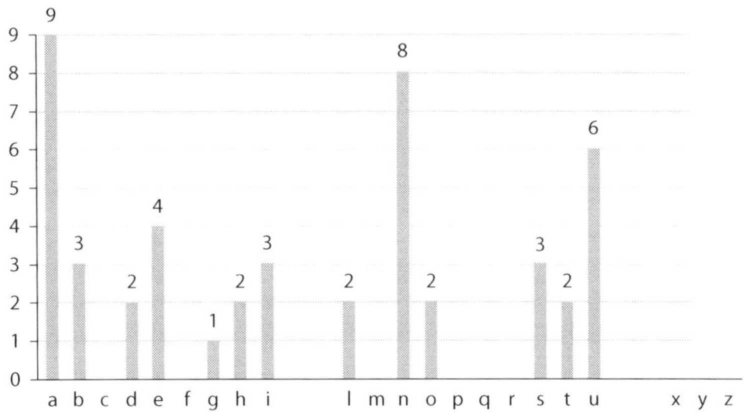

Table 2. Letter frequencies found in the manuscript, as divided over the modern alphabet

5. As the handwriting itself does not display typical "inner movements", it may represent a first Flemish hemi-pangram rather than being an emotional outcry of a romantic unrequited love.

8. Discussion

After the clear results from our analysis, it may be useful to discuss three aspects that possibly need some more explanation. Firstly a short comment on Dante's description of his "spirits". Caciola (2000, p. 280) gives this comprehensive view on the medieval concept of "three spirits":

> Medical theorists subdivided the human spirit into three different categories according to function and placement within the body. The "vital spirit" regulated the vital signs from the heart, maintaining heartbeat, pulse, and respiration. In fact, the vital spirit was the basic principle of life itself; and the heart was the physiological seat of life [...]. After leaving the heart, the vital spirit could be transformed into either the "natural spirit," which was based in the liver and controlled a variety of involuntary activities, including digestion and sexual response; or could be purified into the "animal spirit" as it ascended to the head through a sort of fine sieve at the base of the brain known as the retus mirabilis. Named for the soul, anima, the animal spirit resided in the brain, regulating the nervous system and intellectual responses to sensory stimuli. (Caciola 2000, p. 280)

It becomes clear from this, that Dante perfectly interpreted and described his feelings according to the current medieval concepts. In other words, within the scholastic tradition, his description was right. Besides, the description by Dante of one (the vital) spirit uttering words to another (the animal) spirit, which then starts to speak, and so on, nicely accords with the original meaning of the designation "sympathetic" nervous system (van Zwieten 2005, p. 33). This original concept namely included a certain notion of some presumed mechanism by which one organ could communicate with another organ, so that they were able to "sympathize" with each other. In other words, if one organ suffered, the other organ would suffer too (sym-pathein is translated: suffering together). This concept more or less agreed with the verse "And whether one member suffer, all the members suffer with it" (Holy Bible, 1 Corinthians 12, 26a). This explanation made sense also, because the whole nervous system was considered to be composed of a network of fine hollow pipes, through which spirits could "pneumatically" send their messages. Even in the age of psychodynamic theory, as propagated by Sigmund Freud, the nervous system was still conceived in terms of "hydraulic force" (Daugman 2001, p. 28). But as said above, nowadays sympathetic activity is synonymous to arousal ("stress", "adrenalin") preceding some kind of physical action. Moreover, Brussels-based anatomist Andreas Vesalius himself had also depicted the aforementioned "retus mirabilis" in his famous 1538 Tabulae Anatomicae Sex. There he commented: "Plexus reticularis ad cerebri basim, Rete mirabile in quo vitale spiritus ad animalë prępáratur" which means: "Fine network at the base of the brain, wonder-net in which the vital spirit is prepared to (become) the animal spirit" (van Zwieten 2005, p. 30). This arterial plexus later turned out to be the "circle of Willis" which is responsible for much of the brain's arterial blood supply.

A second, completely different aspect concerns the process of quill-sharpening that is inevitably inherent to the short Flemish 11th century manuscript which was subject of the present study. This "pen test" was actually first noticed and described by Sisam's Ph.D.-student Mr. N.R. Ker (Kwakkel 2005, p. 30). The "scribbles in [...] Latin and Dutch on the end-leaf of Bodl. 340, (340.169v)" (Kwakkel 2005, p. 30) are namely preceded at several places by the words "probatio pennę si bona sit", which means: "testing the pen if it is good". Such tests, apparently written by the very same hand, indicate that the feather quill point had just been (re)sharpened indeed before actually continuing to write the manuscript. Archaic as it seems to be now, pen-sharpening was current practice until halfway the 19th century. Therefore, it is not surprising to find these frequent activities not only depicted, but also described by many painters and writers of the Dutch and Flemish school. As a vivid example of the allusions to the (re)trimming of a feather quill, the next lines may serve, taken from "Founding Father of Flemish Literature" Hendrik Conscience's famous 1849 novel De Loteling (The Conscript) (Conscience 1884, pp. 2–11). As a matter of fact, these lines come right at the start of a love story.

> Jan and Trina (Trien) – they did not know it – loved each other with the unspoken and timid feeling that makes the heart beat at the slightest sign, that gives blushes to the forehead at the slightest word, that changes life into a long dream, a blue sky full of glittering stars of happiness and immeasurably deep as if the human heart should stay forever as during the first sigh of love. [...] In one hand she [Trina] held two large sheets of writing paper, in the other a pen with a newly sharpened quill and a bottle of ink, given to her by the verger. [...]
>
> "Look, so it always begins: – very honored parents, all trembling I take the pen in hand, in order to ... – I don 't remember it anymore!" [...]
>
> The girl started working. After a while, salty sweat drops glistened already on her forehead, she held her breath, her face was glowing. A long sigh almost escaped from her breast, and, as if she felt relieved of a heavy burden, she said with joy: "Phew! That b is the hardest character of them all ! But now it still stands there, with its long head!" The two other women stood and gazed with astonishment on a character, at least as large as the member of the finger. [...]
>
> *(After her younger brother accidently spills the pot of ink over the letter, she decides:)*
>
> "I was still planning to rewrite the letter, the first time it was not good, the letters were too large and the writing was too crooked. Now I will do better, I have got the courage. But first let me rush to the village to run after paper and ink and to let sharpen my pen again ... " (Conscience 1884, pp. 2–11)

The technique and manual dexterity of how to sharpen a quill formed a crucial part in the training of primary school teachers, as de Booy (1977, p. 219) reports. From about 1850 however, the use of feather quills gradually disappeared, because of the general introduction of steel pens. With regard to letter frequencies in the grades of increasing difficulty we saw that most characters in the analysed 11th century manuscript (in grades of increasing difficulty) are from relatively easy, to moderately difficult (Table 1.). Thus it makes sense, as told by Conscience, that the writing of the character "b" (that we found within middle groups of increasing difficulty) as Trina endeavored, might be regarded as rather difficult indeed.

For a third and last aspect in this discussion it is necessary to return to the most evident result from our analyses, namely that within the handwritten poetic phrase, no traces of whatever emotion could be found that possibly might have led to deviant hand- and finger movements. Be it so, it may still be possible that emotional factors did exist, around the very era of writing. From Friedman's (1959, p. 673) original review it becomes clear that in the late 11th century the English population perceived their Norman "visitors" plus their companions (clergymen) not as friendly tourists, but as invaders and conquerors instead. The mockeries and provocations, as sung and danced by (the opponents of) the 1173 Earl of Leicester's army – be it one century later – might have been the hostile and grim result. Thus Weel (2005, p. 7) rightly argues that while scribbling, the scribe possibly tried to find some mental rest for this overall unhappy situation. Now recent reports demonstrate that this so-called "expressive writing" may help persons to overcome negative emotions like anxiety and grief (Baikie & Wilhelm 2005, p. 343; Furnes & Dysvik 2011, p. 17). Also when such persons were university students, Piolat and Bannour (2010, p. 2) obtained comparable results in their study after the effects of expressive writing concerning the positive and negative events on anxiety levels. Further, in a clinical setting, people with serious illnesses may experience the benefits of writing poetry as an adjunctive treatment (Rickett et al. 2011, p. 268).

And here the poetic character of the short manuscript comes back again. Now we are entering a different world. As rightly noted by Weel (2005, p. 6), this end-leaf of Bodleian 340 also contains a wealth of other try-outs in Latin: texts of hymns, songs of praise and so on. Some of these are more or less related to the eschatologically much dreaded year of 1000 ("1 K") that still echoed in the late 11th century. But more important in this respect is the upper left quadrant of the end-leaf, displaying a dozen of musical notes in the Gregorian Chant notation, to be more precisely: Scandicus subtripunctis, Virga, Porrectus and Climacus respectively. (The terminology of these different neumes is based on Harrison (1920, pp. 9–10). Neumes are groups of one to four notes, all of which fall on the same syllable of the text.) The musical notation also makes sense in view of the other texts of hymns and songs of praise on this end-leaf, originally written down in the Benedictine monastery of St. Andrews at Rochester where the manuscript came from. (Plain) chant is deeply rooted in the Benedectine tradition indeed.

Impressive research e.g. by Mannaerts (2009, p. 11) and in particular by Krispijn (2002, p. 469) who independently succeeded to reconstruct melodies from historical texts of thousand years ago, and even much older, now suggests that the words of our analysed manuscript too might have been accompanied by some (unknown) melody. Although rather speculative, the singing of such a song could have helped to overcome the aforementioned unhappy feelings. Because of the conclusion by Clift et al. (2010, p. 20) in their study on choral singing and psychological wellbeing, that women endorse the wellbeing effects of singing more strongly than men, the suggestion that scribe or poet might have been female (a musically talented novice like Maria in The Sound of Music) as van Oostrom says (2006, p. 106), seems right too. The novice's wish to share her original verse (as usual in community singing) with other e.g. non-Flemish novices might also explain the "simultaneous" Latin translation, handwritten right above the Flemish phrase, meanwhile perfectly following the Flemish metrical pattern in a most ingenious way. Once more, the community-oriented character of this text has become evident.

9. Summary

A curiosity-driven search for traces of emotion (or inner movement) presumed in the historical record consisting of early medieval texts and manuscripts, first focuses on Dante's precise and scholarly report of his own emotions evoked by love at first sight as a pre-teen. After explanations on bodily experiences and their neurochemical and physiological backgrounds, the focus then shifts to motions of hands and fingers influenced by emotions, as apparent from the possibly irregular handwriting, to be found in an 11th century Flemish manuscript. A screening for traces of emotions, known from other historical manuscripts, was done first. Analysing this handwritten short poem by comparison to standard orthography and with the help of letter frequencies did not reveal irregularities that were caused by emotion. The phrase, meant to be a pen test, should therefore rather be considered as half a pangram. Taking into account the historical circumstances in which the text was written, some emotional factors could nevertheless have been present. By the presence of Gregorian chant notation elsewhere in the manuscript, we hypothesize that the poem was originally accompanied by a melody, so that it could be sung as well, most likely within some choral setting. The emotional benefits of such choral singing in general are finally considered.

Acknowledgements

We would like to thank Nathalie Theunissen and Stefanie Van Mierloo, MSc Students of Medicine, as well as Jirka Cops and Yörg Dillen, BSc Students of Biomedical Sciences, for their kind interest during the preparation of this study. Hippus Handshoemouse® and Musica Sacra Tongeren are thanked for their long-standing endorsement. This study was initiated on the occasion of a 2006 project kick-off meeting on *The Chant of the Secular Clergy in the Low Countries: Music and Liturgy at the Collegiate Church in Tongeren*. It was performed under the auspices of the "Cultuurraad Tongeren". Several elements had been discussed in the annual *Summer Course of Dutch Language and Culture* of the University of Hasselt Belgium.

References

Dante, A. (ca. 1292). *La vita nova (The New Life), Section 1,II: The first meeting with Beatrice* (transl. by A.S. Kline). Available at: http://www.poetryintranslation.com/PITBR/Italian/TheNewLifeI.htm#_Toc88709644 (Accessed on October 18th 2012).

Baikie, K.A., & Wilhelm, K. (2005). Emotional and physical health benefits of expressive writing. *Advances in Psychiatric Treatment, 11*, 338–346.

Bartels, A., & Zeki, S. (2004). The neural correlates of maternal and romantic love. *NeuroImage, 21*, 1155–1166.

Barton, J.J.S., Sekunova, A., Sheldon, C., Johnston, S., Iaria, G., & Scheel, M. (2010). Reading words, seeing style: The neuropsychology of word, font and handwriting perception. *Neuropsychologia, 48*, 3868–3877.

Beversdorf, D.Q., Anderson, J.M., Manning, S.E., Anderson, S.L., Nordgren, R.E., Felopulos, G.J., & Bauman, M.L. (2001). Macrographia in high-functioning adults, *Journal of Autism and Developmental Disorders, 31*(1), 97–101.

Brink, A.A., Smit, J., Bulacu, M.L., & Schomaker, L.R.B. (2012). Writer identification using directional ink-trace width measurements. *Pattern Recognition, 45*, 162–171.

Bullock, D., & Grossberg, S. (1988). Neural dynamics of planned arm movements: emergent invariants and speed-accuracy properties during trajectory formation. *Psychological Review, 95*(1), 49–90.

Bunnell, J.S. (1942). Surgery of the intrinsic muscles of the hand other than those producing opposition of the thumb. *Journal of Bone and Joint Surgery, 24*, 1–31.

Caciola, N. (2000). Mystics, Demoniacs, and the Physiology of Spirit Possession in Medieval Europe. *Comparative Studies in Society and History, 42*(2), 268–306.

Clift, S., Hancox, G., Morrison, I., Hess, B., Kreutz, G., & Stewart, D. (2010). Choral singing and psychological wellbeing: Quantitative and qualitative findings from English choirs in a cross-national survey. *Journal of Applied Arts and Health, 1*(1), 19–34.

Codispoti, M., Ferrari, V., & Bradley, M.M. (2006). Repetitive picture processing: Autonomic and cortical correlates. *Brain Research, 1068*, 213–220.

Conscience, H. (1884). *De Loteling*. In *Volledige Werken*. Brussel: A.N. Lebègue & Co.

Daugman, J.G. (2001). Brain Metaphor and Brain Theory. In W.P. Bechtel, P. Mandik, J. Mundale, & R.S. Stufflebeam (Eds.), *Philosophy and the Neurosciences: A Reader* (pp. 23–36). Malden Mass./Oxford: Blackwell.

de Booy, E.P. (1977). Het 'basisonderwijs' in de zeventiende en achttiende eeuw – De Stichtse dorpsscholen. *BMGN – Low Countries Historical Review*, 92, 208–222.

de Grauwe, L. (2004). Zijn olla vogala Vlaams, of zit de Nederlandse filologie met een koekoeksei in (haar) nest(en). *Tijdschrift voor Nederlandse Taal- en Literatuurwetenschap, 120*(1): 44–56.

Dijkstra, P., & Barelds, D.P.H. (2008). Do people know what they want: a similar or complementary partner? *Evolutionary Psychology, 6*(4), 595–602.

Di Mascio, A. (1959). Learning characteristics of nonsense syllables: a function of letter frequency. *Psychological Reports, 5*, 585–591.

Emanuele, E. (2011). NGF and romantic love. *Archives Italiennes de Biologie, 149*, 265–268.

Falk, T.H., Tam, C., Schellnus, H., & Chau, T. (2011). On the development of a computer-based handwriting assessment tool to objectively quantify handwriting proficiency in children. *Computer Methods and Programs in Biomedicine, 104*, e102–e111.

Fischbein, J. (2011). Psychosomatics: A current overview. *International Journal of Psychoanalysis, 92*, 197–219.

Fisher, H.E., Brown, L.L., Aron, A., Strong, G., & Mashek, D. (2010). Reward, addiction, and emotion regulation systems associated with rejection in love. *Journal of Neurophysiology, 104*, 51–60.

Friedman, A.B. (1959). Medieval Popular Satire in Matthew Paris. *Modern Language Notes, 74*(8), 673–678.

Furnes, B., & Dysvik, E. (2011). Results from a systematic writing program in grief process: part 2. *Patient Preference and Adherence, 5*, 15–21.

Giedd, J.N. (2008). The teen brain: insights from neuroimaging. *Journal of Adolescent Health, 42*, 335–343.

Govoni, S., Pascale, A., Amadio, M., Calvillo, L., D'Elia, E., Cereda, C., Fantucci, P., Ceroni, M., & Vanoli, E. (2011). NGF and heart: Is there a role in heart disease? *Pharmacological Research, 63*, 266–277.

Greenfield, C.C. (1981). *Humanist and Scholastic Poetics, 1250–1500*. East Brunswick NJ/London: Associated University Presses.

Guedes, C.R., Nogueira, M.I., & de Camargo, K.R. (2008). Vague and diffuse symptoms in biomedicine: a review of the literature. *Ciência & Saúde Coletiva, 13*(1), 135–144.

Hall, J.A., Carter, S., Cody, M.J., & Albright, J.M. (2010). Individual differences in the communication of romantic interest: Development of the flirting styles inventory. *Communication Quarterly, 58*(4), 365–393.

Harrison, J.O.P. (1920). *How to sing Plain Chant*. Ditchling, Sussex: S. Dominic's Press.

Holy Bible, King James Version, 1 Corinthians 12, 26a. Cambridge Edition.

Holy Bible, King James Version, Galatians 6, 11. Cambridge Edition.

Kobayashi, K. (2003). Finger and wrist coordination during handwriting movements. *The International Journal of Forensic Document Examiners, 6* (1), 1–6.

Krispijn, T.J.H. (2002). Music in cuneiform script. Contributions to Old Oriental musicology 2. In E. Hickmann, A.D. Kilmer, & R. Eichmann (Eds.), *Orient-Archälogie 10, Studies in Music Archaeology III* (pp. 465–479). Rahden: Verlag Marie Leidorf.

Kwakkel, E. (2005). Hebban olla vogala in historisch perspectief. *Tijdschrift voor Nederlandse Taal- en Literatuurwetenschap, 121*(1), 1–24.

Landsborough, D. (1987). St Paul and temporal lobe epilepsy. *Journal of Neurology, Neurosurgery, and Psychiatry, 50*, 659–664.

Louwen, K. (2009). Zur Lesart und Hybridität der Altniederländischen Federprobe. *Amsterdamer Beiträge zur älteren Germanistik, 65*, 61–86.

Lu, W., Wu, J., Wei, B., & Zhuang, Y. (2011). Efficient shape matching for Chinese calligraphic character retrieval. *Journal of Zhejiang University – Science C (Computers & Electronics), 12*(11), 873–884.

MacKenzie, I.S., & Soukoreff, R.W. (2003). Phrase sets for evaluating text entry techniques. In G. Cockton, & P. Korhonen (Eds.), *Extended Abstracts CHI 2003*. (pp. 754–755). New York: ACM Press.

Mannaerts, P. (2009). Observations on the performance of plainchant in the Low Countries (10th–18th centuries). *Trans: Transcultural Music Review, 9*, 1–23.

Määttä, K. (2011). The fascination of love never fades – how do the elderly describe their experiences of falling in love? *International Review of Social Sciences and Humanities, 2*(1), 14–25.

Mercator, G. (1540). *Literarum latinarum, quas Italicas, cursoriasque vocant, scribendarum ratio* (Reason for the writing of Latin letters which the Italians call cursive). Leuven: Rutger Rescius.

Mergl, R., Juckel, G., Rihl, J., Henkel, V., Karner, M., Tigges, P., Schröter, A., & Hegerl, U. (2004). Kinematical analysis of handwriting movements in depressed patients. *Acta Psychiatrica Scandinavica, 109*, 383–391.

Meijer, R.P. (1978). *Literature of the Low Countries. A short history of Dutch literature in the Netherlands and Belgium*. The Hague/Boston: Martinus Nijhoff.

Mitternacht, D. (2007). A structure of persuasion in Galatians: Epistolary and rhetorical appeal in an aural setting. *Acta Theologica, 28*(2) Supplementum 9, 53–98.

Morgan, M. (Ed.). (2006). *Lettres enluminées – Carnet pratique de calligraphie ornamentale* (Édition française par C. Dandres-Franck & H. Pouchot). Rennes: Edilarge SA – Editions Ouest-France.

Napier, J.R. (1966). Functional anatomy of the fingers. In R.G. Pulvertaft (Ed.), *The Hand* (pp. 9–17). London: Butterworths.

New Testament in Today's English Version, Good News for Modern Man, 3rd *Edition* (1971). *Galatians 6, 11*. New York: American Bible Society.

Parkinson, P. (2006). Is there a neurochemical basis for falling in love? *The Science Creative Quarterly*, September 13 2006. (cf. http://www.scq.ubc.ca/is-there-a-neurochemical-basis-for-falling-in-love/, accessed October 2012).

Piolat, A., & Bannour, R. (2010). Effects of expressive writing concerning positive and negative events on anxiety levels of university students, *Psychologie française, 55*, 1–23.

Potts, G. (2008). Your brain on love: the three stages to euphoria. *Oakland Journal, 15*, 16–27.

Rickett, C., Greive, C., & Gordon, J. (2011). Something To Hang My Life On: The Health Benefits Of Writing Poetry For People With Serious Illnesses. *Australasian Psychiatry, 19*, 265–268.

Rolland, Ph. (2001). *L'origine et la date des évangiles* (Nouvelle édition électronique). Paris: Saint-Paul, Site de la Congrégation du Clergé.

Sekar, M.K., Arcelus, J., & Palmer, R.L. (2010). Micrographia and Hypophonia in Anorexia Nervosa. *International Journal of Eating Disorders, 43*, 762–765.

Spitzer, M. (2011). Die Wissenschaft vom Flirten. *Nervenheilkunde, 30*, 855–862.

Swami, V., & Allum, L. (2012). Perceptions of the physical attractiveness of the self, current romantic partners, and former partners. *Scandinavian Journal of Psychology, 53*, 89–95.

Tavares, P., Barnard, Ph. J., & Lawrence, A.D. (2011). Emotional complexity and the neural representation of emotion in motion. *Social Cognitive and Affective Neuroscience, 6*(1), 98–108.

Trubek, A. (2009). Handwriting is history. *Miller-McCune magazine,* available at: http://www.miller-mccune.com/culture-society/handwriting-is-history-6540/(accessed 17 December 2009).

Tsapkini, K., & Rapp, B. (2010). The orthography-specific functions of the left fusiform gyrus: Evidence of modality and category specificity. *Cortex, 46,* 185–205.

van Oostrom, F. (2006). Poëzie als pennenproef. In F. Van Oostrom (Ed.), *Stemmen op schrift* (pp. 93–107). Amsterdam: Bert Bakker.

van Zwieten, K.-J., Lippens, P.L., Geusens, P., Kowalski, M., Sholukha, V.A., & Zinkovsky, A.V. (2002). Clinical application of finger mathematical modelling. *Acta of Bioengineering and Biomechanics, 4*(1), 354.

van Zwieten, K.-J. (2005). Wetenschap en waarneming. *Gamma, 12*(4), 30–33.

van Zwieten, K.-J., Lippens, P.L., Gelan, J., Adriaensens, P., Schmidt, K.P., Thywissen, C., & Duyvendak, W. (2008). Coordination of interphalangeal flexion in the human finger. *Journal of Hand Surgery (European Volume), 33*(1), 170–171.

Weel, G.J.I. (2005). *Probationes pennae rond "Hebban olla uogala...".* available at: http://www.gerardweel.nl/probatio/index.php (accessed 19 May 2005).

Whiting, D. (2009). The feeling theory of emotion and the object-directed emotions. *European Journal of Philosophy, 19*(2), 281–303.

Yang, T., & Kao, H.S.K. (2003). Chinese leadership styles assessed by English handwriting, National Central University, Taiwan, available at: http://hr.mgt.ncu.edu.tw/conferences/09th_/1-1.pdf (accessed 11 November 2003).

Zanone, P.-G., Athenes, S., Sallagoïty, I., & Albaret, J.-M. (2005). Switching among graphic patterns is governed by coordination dynamics of handwriting. In A. Marcelli & C. De Stefano (Eds.), *Proceedings of the* 12th *Biennial Conference of the International Graphonomics Society (IGS2005), 26–29 June 2005, Salerno, Italy* (pp. 255–260). Civitella, Italy: Editrice Zona.

Zhang, D., & Lu, G. (2004). Review of shape representation and description techniques. *Pattern Recognition, 37,* 1–19.

The neurophenomenology of gesture in the art of Henri Michaux

Jay Hetrick
Universiteit van Amsterdam

In this chapter, I argue that the work of the Belgian poet and artist Henri Michaux contributes to discussions concerning the methods of neurophenomenology. First, I describe the development of Michaux's artistic practice from his earliest experiments with pictorial writing systems, to his more gestural *art informel* paintings, and to his infamous mescaline drawings. He describes this last stage of his work as expressing the "pre-gestural", a term used to refer to the affective and kinaesthetic inner movements that we might locate along the central nervous system, from the synaptic movements within the brain to those that stimulate a quivering hand. Second, I show how Oliver Sacks' neuroscientific research on migraine aura corroborates Michaux's claim that this domain of the pre-gestural reveals something fundamental about the human brain. In accord with Francisco Varela's vision for a neurophenomenology that takes equal account of first- and third-person investigations, Michaux's and Sacks' findings mutually reinforce each other and, together, help construct a neurophenomenology of gesture.

1. From gesture to the pre-gestural

In 1972, the French art historian Margit Rowell developed a concept of gesture in order to analyse the type of "action paintings" that were produced on both sides of the Atlantic in the mid-20th century, namely, those described under the rubrics of abstract expressionism and *art informel*. She argues that, for this type of art, gesture should be clearly distinguished from the brushstroke, which is merely its trace:

> Gesture is an irrational movement of the hand. It should not be confused with the stroke, which is a pictorial technique that refers to aesthetic considerations (for example, filling a space, modulating a surface), and which, because of its reflexive nature, is voluntary. Additionally, a stroke can only exist in space (it needs specific pictorial material to exist) and it expresses no existential connection to the space of Being.... By contrast, gesture is immaterial, abstract, and emanates

> from the inner movements of psychic life. It does not take into account pictorial space, but only the need to express itself. And, as an incidental seizure regarding a movement that is primarily immaterial, in relation to the stroke, we can say that it is disembodied. When the stroke stops, the gesture continues moving. The stroke is a technique of communication, the gesture is a dialogue within the self.
> (Rowell 1972, p. 67, my translation)

Subtracted from the existential terminology that informs and indeed fundamentally supports her analysis – which in this sense follows the typical art historical framework for understanding such gestural abstraction – the very separation of the concept of gesture from the formal marks, strokes, splatters, spots, and drips of these works allows us to in fact challenge this normative art history. But if we agree to this operation, what ultimately remains of gesture? In other words, how can we understand it as a type of "seizure" regarding the "inner movements of psychic life" as opposed to the more formal and material aspects of the brushstroke we see traced upon a canvas? In order to attempt an answer to these questions, I will look at the case of Henri Michaux, one of the main figures of Rowell's study along with Georges Mathieu, Pierre Alechinsky, Asger Jorn, Wols, and Jackson Pollock.

Of all these artists, Rowell claims that Michaux "attained a more profound level of experience" in his work through an "irreducible coincidence of thought and body" (Rowell 1972, p. 109). By this, she means that he went further than any of these other artists in reaching a "middle way" between the production of conscious, voluntary, and ultimately mechanical works and the kind of spontaneous automatism that most of them abhorred about Surrealism. The Buddhist connotations of the term middle way refers to the fact that, within this tradition, East Asian calligraphy was often evoked as an exemplary model for the creative process. By relying on the idea that the practices of "Oriental" painting are more "meditative" than their Western counterparts, Rowell argues that Michaux attained through his work "a self that knows no mind/body dualism", which serves as "a starting point for a new form of creation". This ground of creation is the informal and the insignificant, which themselves appear in a work only when "the pure motor activity of life is united with thought" (Rowell 1972, pp. 109–110). This is the context in which we should understand her otherwise obscure claim that "more than any other artist, with the exception of Pollock, Michaux has sublimated his story in nature" (Rowell 1972, p. 112). Regardless, even if we were to go along with this slightly Romantic line of thought, in the last analysis it undermines her own quite useful conception of gesture. If Michaux's work goes beyond the dualism of mind and body – whatever that means, and however we might asses that possibility – thereby proving itself to be one of the most successful examples of *art informel*, how can Rowell understand the gestural in his work, since her very concept of gesture is based upon its absolute difference from the material brushstroke? Although Michaux, like many of the artists in this tradition, was indeed interested in East Asian calligraphy and thought, perhaps by revisiting the trajectory of his work, including his own self-reflective writings about it, we might arrive at a more sober solution to this problem.

Michaux's shift from poetry to the visual arts, albeit gradual, was motivated by his lifelong search for an adequate means to express speed and movement. The literary critic and filmmaker, Jean Epstein, wrote in 1921 that "spatial speed, mental speed, multiplication of apparent diameters, extension of self-observation, the importance given to inner life, cerebral life and the resulting fatigue are the most important conditions of modern artistic production" (Epstein 1921, p. 96, my translation). And it is clear, both implicitly and explicitly, from Michaux's very first essays published in the surrealist journal *Le disque vert* in the early 1920s that he shared this sentiment with Epstein. Furthermore, one could argue that this desire to express the various speeds of movements within the human body became the key motivating factor that shaped the entire trajectory of his poetic and artistic output. This is how we can make sense of his early experiments with creating new hieroglyphic alphabets, which were his first attempts to produce signs that go beyond closed systems of linguistic signification in order to communicate directly certain affects that traverse the lived body. The search for an alternative and unmediated form of expression led him to study, like so many of his contemporaries, pre-historic cave paintings, which seemed to offer the promise of shifting attention away from what graphic signs mean towards a more performative understanding of the act of writing or drawing itself.

The French archaeologist André Leroi-Gourhan argued that in the visual cultures of the paleolithic and neolithic periods, mark-making was as much a corporeal practice as it was a symbolic one. Artists and philosophers, from Joan Miró to André Masson, from Georges Bataille to Maurice Merleau-Ponty, read and published accounts of this phenomenon in avant-garde journals like *Cahiers d'art* and *Documents* in the mid-20th century. For Michaux, the gestural energy of these cave paintings suggested the possibility of attaining a form of expression rooted in the raw kinetic and kinaesthetic body. These pictographic signs appealed to him because they were not only visual and gestural but also visceral and powerful, that is, somehow closer to the texture, rhythm, and intensity that fundamentally informs all expression. They were a model that might serve to help Michaux move beyond the more mediated type of writing systems with which he was becoming increasingly frustrated, writing systems that were altogether inadequate in expressing the affective sensations and movements of the body. It should be noted that, like the other proponents of so-called "new primitivism" like Antonin Artaud and Jean Dubuffet, Michaux was neither interested in fetishizing the exotic nature of these cave paintings nor in mimicking them in order to reach a kind of authentic spontaneity in the wake of the failures of Surrealism. Rather, these paintings simply illustrated to him the *possibility* that a writing system could be much closer to the gestural intimacy of bodily movements than the French language. This whole artistic process was – as he admits in a reflection on a work from 1927 entitled *Alphabet* – an attempt to "decondition" himself, to rid himself of his linguistic and cultural habits. The rest of his career as a visual artist can be seen as a slow apprenticeship in the lessons of these cave paintings, a critical and self-aware apprenticeship fueled by the visceral imperative to express movement and speed beyond naive spontaneity.

This apprenticeship can be clearly seen in a new series of *Alphabets* Michaux created in 1944, in which he clearly repeats not only the formal characteristics of Neolithic battle scenes depicting strange animals and spear-throwers; he confines their gestural movements within a type of taxonomic gridding that he most certainly appropriated from books – like Leroi-Gourhan's *Préhistoire de l'art occidental* – which attempted to archive these figures. The pseudo-archival structure of these alphabets suggests that Michaux was directly copying the formal layout of certain illustrations from this type of archeological book. It also evokes the gridded pages of children's exercise workbooks, suggesting again his posture of apprenticeship towards these archeological books. However, in Michaux's next major visual work, entitled *Movements*, this apprenticeship in taxonomy is gradually loosened in favor of allowing the force of the gestures to break free from confinement. In this coherently conceived artist's book, published in 1951, the rather tentative experiment with sign-producing gestures of both *Alphabet* works is now pursued in a more rigorous and confident way. It is book composed of sixty-four reproductions selected from over twelve hundred paintings in Indian ink. While still retaining a connection to the pre-historic paintings, both formally and structurally, *Movements* also vaguely bring to mind certain works of East Asian calligraphy. Indeed, it is known that Michaux owned manuals on Chinese ideograms and actually spent a great deal of time in his youth trying to learn the fundamentals of their calligraphic forms. Furthermore, by choosing the number sixty-four, he seems to be evoking the sixty-four hexagrams of the *I Ching*, the ancient Chinese divination manual that uses a combination of long and short brush strokes in order to predict movements and changes in the universe. One important aspect of this series is that, as we turn each page, the figures seem to slowly evolve from relatively small and timid strokes that are still contained within an implicit grid towards larger and wilder strokes that shatter the taxonomic structure of *Alphabets,* as if we are watching the secession of individual film frames or are flipping through one of those picture books Walter Benjamin described as prefiguring the cinema. Furthermore, in line with his interest in East Asian aesthetics – and invoking Sergei Eisenstein's identification of scroll paintings as proto-cinematic art forms – Michaux would later claim that "a scroll, a *kakemono*, would have shown it better than a book, provided that it could be unrolled, or a book of one single page folded over and over again" (Michaux 1976, n.p.).

These *Movements* mark an important stage in Michaux's progression as a visual artist since they link the earlier, meticulously controlled, forms of plastic writing to the later *art informel* paintings in which Indian ink is thrown straight onto the paper, spreading out into big blots, rather than being applied directly with a paintbrush as it still is here. Another important aspect of this artist's book is that it contains both a poem inserted in the central pages and a postface that briefly describes the work. Together they articulate – in addition to the task of communicating something beyond the confines of words – Michaux's motivation for producing the original twelve hundred pages as an "envie cinétique" (Michaux 2001, p. 440). But this kinetic desire, or desire for kinesis, is further explained not in terms of the physical or gestural movements of the brush, but the kinesthetic and sensual pleasures of the act of painting itself. Rather than attempting to transmit symbolic knowledge, even the coded or esoteric knowledge of *Alphabets*, *Movements* should be understood as a series of indexical traces of this impulse to move. We can now come back to Rowell, who makes a distinction between the gesture as an immaterial and irrational movement that we might locate along the central nervous system – from the synaptic movements within the brain to those of the quivering hand – and the material stroke that is simply an abbreviated and incidental trace of this inner movement. Indeed, the poem indicates that Michaux's desire for kinesis involves a reciprocal movement between the performative act of creating *taches*, the free marks or stains that are the formal characteristics of *tachisme* – the branch of *art informel* of which he is considered to be a part – and the more immaterial or psychic movements that traversed his entire being:

taches
taches to obscure
to reject
to uninhabit
to destabilise
to be reborn
to erase
to pin down
to spill memory
to depart
(Michaux 2001, p. 439, my translation)

The act of creating this type of free mark on the paper was seen by him as a kind of exorcism through which he was, again, deconditioning himself, not in order to create a beautiful work of art but in order to unleash the latent movements within himself and to form a kind of circuit between them and the material world. Incidentally, it should be noted that one of Michaux's earliest essays was a rant against André Breton's conception of the "absolute marvelous" in which Michaux characterized automatic drawing as the "incontinence of gestures" (Michaux 1998, pp. 60–61). His method should therefore not be seen as another incarnation of spontaneous automatism, but rather as a more deliberate and balanced practice that takes inspiration from East Asian calligraphy. In the last few lines of the poem, he describes these *taches* as

> signs of the ten thousand ways of keeping one's balance in this
> moving world that scoffs at adaptation
> signs above all to retrieve one's being from the trap of the language
> of others …
> a direct writing for unwinding
> from the compact spool of forms
> to unchoke, to revoke
> to clear the billboard mind of our times from its cluttering of images
> lacking aura, at least let's cast our effluvia to the winds
> (Michaux 2001, p. 440, my translation)

While the free marks and blotches testify to the fact that gestural movement has taken place, they are merely truncated figures which, although they supplant given or stable forms, ultimately belie the "quite extraordinary mobility" of which Michaux himself claims to be the "counterpart and the motor". Furthermore, the artist, who inhabits a paradoxical space at the center of this movement, himself remains "unmoving and slothful", highlighting the importance of inner movements over and above outward expressions (Michaux 2001, p. 598, my translation). As he continues in the postface:

> Their movement became my movement. The more there were of them, the more I existed. Creating them, I became quite other. I invaded my body – my centers of action and repose – which is often a bit remote from my head. I held it now, tingling, electric. Like a rider on a galloping horse which together make one. I was possessed by movements, on edge with these forms which came to me rhythmically. (Michaux 2001, p. 598, my translation)

The *Movements* project taught Michaux that the creation of this type of informal art – without abandoning oneself to an entranced spontaneity but instead riding the "middle way", as Rowell puts it, between conscious and unconscious practice – reveals a movement much larger than either the implied movements of individual figures or the kinaesthetic movements that traversed his mind and body. These *Movements* actually involve an alternating circuit *between* himself and the work, between gestures and strokes in Rowell's terminology, or in his own words, between the pre-gestural and the *tache*. In one of the most beautiful and revealing stanzas of the poem included in the book, Michaux finally discusses what he means by gestures:

> gestures
> gestures of unknown life
> of impulsive life
> that we are happy to squander
> of jerky, spasmodic, and upright life
> of wretched or whatever kind of life
> of life
> gestures of confrontation and retreat
> and of escape from strangulation
> gestures that exceed
> exceed
> and especially exceed
> gestures we feel but cannot identify
> (pre-gestures in themselves, much larger than the visible
> and practical gestures that will follow)
>
> (Michaux 2001, p. 439, my translation)

These "much larger" pre-gestures – characterized by a "SPEED!" and excess that must be contrasted with the timid strokes we see on the canvas – are, according to Michaux, "movements of dislocation and inner exasperation more than marching movements … inward foldings … in place of other movements which cannot be shown but inhabit the mind". (Michaux 2001, p. 438, my translation).

This articulation of the pre-gesture was an insight that stayed with Michaux and informed his art-making from this point onward. For example, when he reflected on the *Movements* project three years later, in a prose-poem entitled "Signs", he still speaks of

> interior gestures, for which we don't have limbs but desires for limbs, stretching, impulsive movements and all this with living ligaments that are never thick, never big with flesh nor enclosed in skin.... What an experience it will be when the time is ripe at last and, having got into the habit of thinking in signs, we are able to exchange secrets with a few natural strokes like a handful of twigs.
>
> (Michaux 2001, p. 431, my translation).

And even in poem written at the end of his life – which is interspersed with figures reminiscent of those depicted in *Movements* and *Alphabets*, and which even ends with a symbol that evokes the *I Ching* – Michaux explains that, in such figures,

> line is not an abbreviation of volume or surface, but an abbreviation of hundreds of gestures and attitudes and impressions and emotions…. A dynamic abbreviation made up of spears, not forms.
>
> What I wanted to represent was the gesture *within* the human, taking off from the inside, releasing, ripping free; the *eruption* of this intense, sudden, ardent concentration from which the stroke will proceed, rather than the stroke's arrival at its destination. (Michaux 2006, n.p., translation modified)

This concept of the pre-gestural deeply qualifies the context and motivation behind Michaux's artistic output and, crucially, marks the difference from his contemporaries. It also provides a key for understanding the more refined works for which Michaux is known: the Indian ink paintings of the mid-50s, which secured his place within *art informel,* as well as the so-called mescaline and post-mescaline drawings that dominated his creative output for nearly fifteen years.

Michaux's large Indian ink paintings from 1954 onwards, instead of utilizing cautious and controlled micro-movements of the wrist, vastly open up the painterly field both by his use of a larger canvas as well as by his more physical throwing and dripping ink directly on the canvas. Reluctantly taking the advice of a friend – that while "charming" the movements should be made bigger – Michaux was initially excited and almost overwhelmed by the liberatory potential of expanding the scope of the paintings. He said that "the fullness of gesture necessitated by the characters that were supposed to come out bigger had changed the spirit of the drawings. Instead of characters, instead of notations of an undefinable 'something,' they became propulsion, participation, released torrent. Through amplitude I was able to connect with my own speed" (Michaux 2000, p. 7). That is, these new paintings seemed to come much closer to fulfilling his expressed desire for *kinesis.* And this internal success was mirrored in the fact that Michaux began to exhibit in the company of Wols, Jean Fautrier, Jean Dubuffet and Jackson Pollock. The connection with Wols and Dubuffet is not surprising since Michaux had already been a part of their circle for at least ten years. But it is difficult today to comprehend the affinity between Michaux and Pollock that so many Parisian artists and critics – including Michel Tapié, Geneviève Bonnefoi, Jean-Louis Schefer, Claude Georges, and Jean Degottex – repeatedly insisted on articulating. It is glaringly obvious that while Michaux's large Indian inks had indeed transgressed the rather restricted boundaries of his earlier work, they remain quite timid and delicate compared with Pollock's huge and explosive canvases. Margit Rowell suggests that the resemblance these artists and critics saw between Michaux and Pollock is more than a formal equivalence and has to do with the fact that each, in his own way, invested gesture with the capacity to undo socialization, culturalization and to return to the different speeds and movements that pulse through body and mind.

For both, she argues, "gesture is a motivation, a tendency," "the manifestation of a primal state of being" that connects the artist to "the original source of all … creation" (Rowell 1972, p. 49, my translation).

The problem with such an easy and unconvincing conflation of Michaux and Pollock, aside from Rowell's existential rhetoric, is that it obscures one of the most important aspects of Michaux's work, the idea of the pre-gestural. While Pollock had no problems pushing the limits of outward gestural spontaneity using industrial materials and the full force of his body, Michaux had understood the Romantic trappings of surrealism. His continued use of Indian ink and canvases that never exceeded one meter in length should be interpreted as an expression of extreme caution against falling completely on the side of the external brushstroke at the expense of loosing his conscious connection to the delicate pre-gestural movements that coursed through his interior. This is corroborated by the Irish artist Francis Bacon, who owned one of Michaux's large Indian ink paintings, and who stated in an interview that "Michaux is a very, very intelligent and conscious man … who has made the best *taches* or free marks that have been made. I think he is much better in this way, in making conscious free marks, than Jackson Pollock" (Bacon 1987, p. 17). This is also evident when we read Michaux's own remarks about these larger paintings which stress not the visible qualities of the strokes but rather the kinaesthetic experience of making them, an experience that can only be had if one remains vigilant and self-aware, resisting the urge to succumb to a wild gestural frenzy which ends only in catharsis and exhaustion. In fact, Michaux was ultimately sceptical of these paintings, even though they did allow for a liberatory moment beyond *Movements*. He reflected back, exclaiming that "I hate them … they disgust me … so I fight them, whip them, should like to be done with them". More than anything, the blots, marks, and smears of these works should be interpreted as the expression of Michaux's frustration with the impossibility of "allying them with everything that moves in the unnamable crowd of beings and non-beings … insatiable desires or knots of force, which are destined never to take form". He ends this rant saying: "If I'm a *tachiste*, I'm one who can't stand *taches*" (Michaux, quoted in Spira 1999, n.p.).

These *taches* ultimately remain too unwieldy to adequately express Michaux's inner speeds and movements, which was the main motivation behind the production of both his visual art as well as his writing, a motivation made evident by the very titles of some of his poems, such as "Inside-space", "The Distant Interior", and "Life within the Folds". If we look closely at the trajectory of his career, it becomes clear that it is only with his infamous mescaline period from the mid-50s to the mid-60s that his quest to find an adequate medium to express the pre-gestural finally looses its compulsive urgency. He referred to these mescaline drawings as kinematic "attempts to draw the flow of time" rather than physical *taches* that exist only in space as a kind of after-image or after-thought. They are works of typically black ink on paper which very rarely depict glimpses of colour emerging from the movement of "countless lines, no longer static or immortal, but active, agitated, scurrying around, animated by a life all their own, zigzagging like mad across surfaces as if they had been cinematographically projected onto them" (Michaux 2000, p. 64). The drawings are indeed psychedelic – in the literal sense of "mind manifesting" – and they are kinetic, vibrating, endlessly seething and bubbling. Michaux admitted that he was not completely satisfied with these drawings since cinema "blessed with motion, seemed to have far more success when it came to expressing" the vibrational movements that connect us directly with the "cinematic" mechanisms of the brain (Michaux 2000, p. 66). But with these drawings, his almost compulsive search to express the pre-gestural was over and the last two decades of his artistic output can be seen as a recapitulation and refinement of the various techniques he had already experimented with. Michaux had finally discovered a way to transcribe directly what Margit Rowell calls the "immaterial and abstract … inner movements of psychic life", movements that we might locate along the central nervous system. Indeed, she describes his mescaline drawings as having "the homogeneity of a cellular tissue, consisting of undifferentiated small vibrations repeated to infinity … movements that are interwoven at a fundamental level (that is, within the body), in a kind of network like the nervous system" (Rowell 1972, p. 111). The abstract and dense swarms of seismographic scribbles, the very quality and quantity of the lines which repetitiously fill entire sheets of paper, are indeed reminiscent of early medical sketches of Golgi-stained neural pathways.[1] But more than simple *illustrations* that evoke images of the nervous system, Michaux believed that these mescaline drawings

1. Michaux had always been intrigued by the invention of scientific apparatuses that measured and recorded very small phenomena. For example, around the time of *Movements*, he declared that "one day in the not so distant future, you will find a device for measuring brain power, the force of this power station [*centrale*] to which we owe what we are. I hope to learn from this *cérébromètre* that which is really mine" (Michaux 2001, p. 292, my translation). It has been suggested that using such scientific vocabulary is therefore appropriate in describing his mescaline drawings: "The hand works like a seismograph, registering the smallest and most imperceptible nerve currents. Multiplication and division to infinity, sharp acuity into the innumerable swarm, repetition and symmetry lead to a form of vertigo, which outweighs the infinity and number. Each perception divides itself into an infinity of sensations which are divided in towards an indefinite abyss. Entering its microscopic dimension, matter reveals itself as and endless and groundless, like a maelstrom of sensations. But the sum of all these petite perceptions, usually unnoticed and that blends into an indistinct mass, offered here by Michaux, clearly and distinctly, in a state of total exacerbation of vision" (de Mèredieu 1994, p. 211, my translation).

render visually and directly the type of vibratory waves that might appear on the "bristling" encephalogram of a subject under the influence.

2. Michaux's mescaline work as a model for neurophenomenology

In some remarkable words that suggest a kind of neurophenomenology *avant la lettre*, Michaux asks: "Is it absurd to think that cerebral waves, which are on the whole slow, become perceptible in certain states of violent nervous hyper-excitation, especially of the visual cortex? New experiments are required in this field as well as more thorough studies of encephalograms of patients in a state of mescaline intoxication" (Michaux 1963, p. 7). While this ultimately remains open-ended speculation, it is the closest Michaux gets to articulating and expressing what he calls the pre-gestural. But before we dismiss outright this comment as the groping words of a naive poet, it should be noted that Michaux attended medical school for a year before dropping out to sail the world and to attempt putting his creative impulses into motion. His interest in the natural sciences was always in the background of his thinking and informed all of his work in one way or another. His particular initiation into the mescaline experience – which evokes the infamous *Club des Hashischins* – was provided by a series of monitored medical studies that included several other artists and writers, under the supervision of the psychiatrist Julian de Ajuriaguerra.[2] And Michaux's four books on the drug experience are pseudo-scientific treatises filled with references and footnotes that cite the latest neuroscientific literature. It is the scientific attitude of these books that lead Eric Duvivier, after reading *Knowledge through the Abyss*, to approach Michaux in order to make a film about mescaline. Therefore, the context in which we should attempt to fully understand this phase of Michaux's *oeuvre* is not only poetic and artistic, but also a context that utilises, interrogates, and responds to properly neuroscientific problems. I would like to suggest that the frame for understanding this *scientific* context began to be systematised only after Michaux's mescaline period. Of course, scientific research into hallucinogenic substances began in the mid-19th century – mostly with the

2. The *Club des Hashischins* was a Parisian group of artists and writers, including Charles Baudelaire, Théophile Gautier, Gérard de Nerval, and Eugène Delacroix, who explored the effects of hashish under the direction of the psychiatrist Jacques-Joseph Moreau. Similar to Moreau's account of these experiments, Dr. Ajuriaguerra wrote a book to document Michaux's controlled experiments with mescaline entitled *Contribution à la connaissance des psychoses toxiques: Expériences et découvertes du poète Henri Michaux*, which was published by Sandoz Laboratories, Basel in 1964.

intention of studying potential treatments for mental illness – and intensified in the 1950s and 1960s after the synthesis of lysergic acid diethylamide. Michaux was interested in the much more ambitious question of how these substances might bring to light certain fundamental mechanisms of the human brain, an aspect of his work that has been glossed over as utterly naive. But in 1970, immediately following Michaux's intense decade of mescaline use, Oliver Sacks published his first book entitled *Migraine*. Incredibly, this book discusses – in more "legitimate" scientific detail from the pen of a respected neurologist – precisely what Michaux was attempting to articulate through his mescaline writings and drawings. Sacks argues that migraine experience, pushed to its limit, is accompanied by hallucinations that seem to be analogous to drug-induced hallucinations. Reciprocally, Michaux notes that his mescaline trips were usually accompanied by some form or degree of migraine and scotoma (retinal blind spots), and that these two phenomena continued for decades after he stopped experimenting with the drug.

Sacks' book is a neurological and psychiatric study of the different manifestations of migraine, including the more extreme experiences of visual hallucinations as well as affective distortions of space, time, and body-image. Most interesting for the present discussion are the chapters in which Sacks discusses the so-called migraine "aura", a term originally used to describe the sensory hallucinations that sometimes precede epileptic seizures, but which has been increasingly used to depict analogous symptoms that inaugurate a certain class of intense migraine. Sacks meticulously relates these experiences not only to the hallucinations that can be experienced at the onset of an epileptic attack but also to acute states of psychosis, whether drug-induced or schizophrenic. His bold conclusion – which draws on the work of Ilya Prigogine and suggests that the model of self-organizing systems should be applied to the study of neural growth and functioning – is that certain "hallucinatory constants" give us a direct and privileged understanding of neuronal organization and the fundamental workings of the human brain. The specific hallucinations and disorders experienced in migraine aura include visual, tactile, and other sensory hallucinations, the most complex of which "take the form of synaesthesia and other sensory interactions, and dream-like sequences involving sensory images of every modality" (Sacks 1992, p. 199). There can also be muscular spasms suggestive of an epileptic seizure as well as alterations of affect and mood. Disturbances to higher-order brain functions include difficulties in the perception and use of the body, the entire range of speech and language disorders, states of double consciousness associated with feelings of *déjà vu,* other dislocations of time-perception, and elaborate dreamy, nightmarish, or trance-like states. Finally, amongst the higher-order disturbances are complex disorders of perception, the various types of which Sacks rather poetically labels – in a way that immediately evokes some of Michaux's descriptions of the mescaline trip – "lilliputian", "mosaic", and "cinematic" (Sacks 1992, p. 73–74).[3] And again reminding us of Michaux's experience, Sacks further explains that these latter cinematic visions "flicker" at more or less the same "scintillation-rate as migrainous scotomata (6 to 12 per second.)" (Sacks 1992, p. 75). But instead of attempting a reductive analysis of Michaux's mescaline drawings and writings *vis-à-vis* these neuroscientific findings, I would simply suggest that Sacks' research helps to legitimate Michaux's seemingly naive claim that science would one day be faced with the task of taking seriously and properly analysing the mescaline-induced visionary world, which he vehemently believed "*reveals* more than it creates" (Michaux 1974, p. 22):

> I believe that I am showing a basic phenomenon which was bound to be discovered one day … a primeval and general phenomenon which underlies even the most placid consciousness, the most strictly controlled and headstrong intelligence, and which, perhaps vaguely felt, but not seen, passes by unperceived behind other perceptions which are of greater interest. (Michaux 1976, n.p.)

Ultimately, his mescaline drawings should be understood as "pre-gestural" in the sense that they attempt to directly express inner neural movements and vibrations onto the canvas rather than trace the gross outer movements of twitching muscles of the arm or hand.

Sacks begins the last chapter of his book with a review of several first-person accounts of the various sensory disturbances that occur in the migraine aura by mid-nineteenth century scientists and physicians. The most thorough of these accounts have been written by John Herschel and Hubert Airy, who – through the analysis of their own experiences as well as those of others – independently came to the same conclusion as Michaux, namely, that hallucinations point to universal and fundamental structures of either the workings of the mind, in the case of Herschel, or of the brain, in the case of Airy. Herschel explains that, while perceptual representations and imagination are personal, what he calls the abstract "geometrical spectra" of migraine hallucinations seem to arise *de novo* from some impersonal and unconscious "geometrizing" part of the mind that works as a kind of "kaleidoscopic power" inherent to its organization and functioning, which remains "distinct from that of our own personality" (Herschel 1858, quoted in Sacks 1992, p. 274). Similarly, Airy noted that the brilliant geometrical patterns

3. Michaux explains that, "When the action of mescaline is at its height, it produces blinding images, or images ringed with lightning, trenches of fire, as well as, in the distance, lilliputian men whose motions are more like those of the pistons of an engine than human gestures" (Michaux 2002, p. 58).

of migraine aura are invariant and therefore constitute a "photograph" of some, equally invariant, structure in the brain (Airy, quoted in Sacks 1992, p. 274). These geometrical hallucinations are typical in advanced stages of the migraine aura, normally occurring only after one has progressed through the experience of phosphenes, or "seeing stars", and scotoma. Differing descriptions of such geometrical hallucinations bear striking resemblance to each other and usually consist of a multitude of polygonal shapes, each of which contains tiny replicas of itself, giving rise to a kind of self-transforming fractal mosaic or, in terminology of the nineteenth century, an arabesque. One envisions, for example,

> a form of visual tumult or delirium, in which latticed, faceted and tessellated motifs predominate – images reminiscent of mosaics, honeycombs, Turkish carpets … or moiré patterns.… These figments and elementary images tend to be brilliantly luminous, colored … highly unstable, and prone to sudden kaleidoscopic transformations. (Airy, quoted in Sacks 1992, p. 276)

John Herschel was perhaps the first scientist to make the connection between migraine hallucinations and those of a drug-induced vision, when he provides a fascinating description of complex geometrical patterns under "the blessed influenced" of chloroform, namely, "a kind of dazzle in the eyes, immediately followed by the appearance of a very beautiful and perfectly regular and symmetrical 'Turks-cap' pattern, formed by the mutual intersection of a great number of circles outside of, and tangent to, a central one" (Herschel, quoted in Sacks 1992, p. 277). But it is only with Heinrich Klüver's extensive research on mescaline hallucination that Sacks really begins to understand the extent of what he comes to label "hallucinatory constants". Klüver was a physiological psychologist who made several contributions to neuroanatomy and wrote two short but influential works on mescaline, *Mescal: The "Divine" Plant and Its Psychological Effects* (1928) and *Mechanisms of Hallucinations* (1942) (both included in Klüver 1966). Proceeding from his own first-person experience, as well as accounts of mescaline intoxication which proved to be strikingly similar despite very different cultural contexts, Klüver extracts certain universals of hallucinatory experience, which he calls "form constants". He shows that similar form constants may appear in a variety of conditions including – in addition to migraine aura – hypnagogic hallucinations, insulin hypoglycemia, fever deliria, cerebral ischemia, some epilepsies, exposure to rotating or flickering visual stimuli, and sensory deprivation. Explicitly building upon Klüver's schema, Richard Cytowic has recently added natural and induced synaesthesia to this list of pathological conditions that may produce form constants within a subject's peripersonal space (Cytowic & Eagleman 2009, pp. 56–60). With so many aetiologies producing more or less the same phenomena, Klüver argues that there must be a universal mechanism at work in the sensory cortex. More or less in line with the positions of Herschel and Airy, Klüver argues that form constants must correspond to constants of cortical structure or organization and, more specifically, that they reveal something fundamental about the functioning of the sensory cortex and the nature of sensory perception. Remarkably, this somewhat speculative view has recently been empirically corroborated by a group of computational neuroscientists (Bressloff et al. 2002).

The main form constants Klüver names are gratings, cobwebs, tunnels, and spirals. But he also discusses at length two other fundamental characteristics of advanced-stage hallucinations that in fact undo form altogether. Both concern psychological affect and the crossing of sensory modalities. The first is the simultaneous seeing and feeling of movement: "slow, majestic movements along differently shaped curves simultaneously with 'mad' movements. Feeling there is motion *per se*". (Klüver, quoted in Sacks 1992, 281). The second is what he calls "haptic hallucinations" that are synaesthetic and kinaesthetic amalgams involving both the visual and tactile spheres:

> a luminous spiral forms itself through the active movement of stripe. This quickly rotating spiral is moving back and forth in the visual field. At the same time … one of my legs assumes spiral form.… The luminous spiral and the haptic spiral blend psychologically … one has the impression of somatic and optic unity. (Klüver, quoted in Sacks 1992, 281)

Taken together, Sacks argues, these are not merely *visual* phenomena nor even sensory *form* constants, but "hallucinatory constants" that should be described "most generally, as forms of organization, presumably physiological, which can become apparent to any spatially-extended sense" (Sacks 1992, p. 282). Relying upon more recent neurological studies of drug-induced hallucination, Sacks further argues that

> Klüver's use of the term "form constants," with its purely spatial connotations, gives a misleading impression of stability and invariance in time. This is not a stable, equilibrium sate, but a highly unstable, far-from-equilibrium state, which is continually reorganizing itself. There is incessant movement at this stage of hallucinosis, not only concentric, rotational, and pulsating – some form of oscillation is almost invariable – but with sudden fluctuations as well, sudden replacements of one pattern or one image by another, which Herschel, a century ago, had called "kaleidoscopic". (Sacks 1992, p. 284)[4]

4. The most detailed analysis Sacks relies upon is Ronald Siegel, "Hallucinations" in *Scientific American* 237 (4) (October 1977), pp. 132–140. Sacks claims that, while Klüver's approach is more anecdotal and qualitative, Siegel's is experimental and quantitative. Furthermore, Siegel uses his data to extend the number of Klüver's form constants to nine and adds "constants of movement", which include concentric, rotational, and pulsating movements.

Sacks' term "hallucinatory constants" is therefore meant to correct and extend Klüver's pioneering research on form constants by adding the category of movement. But as Klüver's own analyses suggest, the hallucination of movement should be understood both as the perception of the movement of kaleidoscopic forms as well as the sensation of movement within the body (affective kinaesthesia) and the movement between sensory modalities themselves (synaesthesia). He believes that this understanding of hallucinatory constants provides a clearer and more complete picture of the dynamism and complex organization of both hallucinations and their physiological origin in the brain.

In the last few pages of *Migraine,* Sacks constructs a theory for the neurological mechanisms of such hallucinatory constants. He traces a lineage of research from the early nineteenth century which seems to support Michaux's claim that geometric patterns perceived in a strong hallucinatory experience are the result of the wavelike diffusion and interference of nerve impulses in the brain. He shows that, while this proposition began as a kind of metaphor for explaining how nerve transmission spreads through a particular region of the brain – "like the ripples in a pond into which a stone is thrown" (William Gowers 1904, quoted in Sacks 1992, p. 286) (282) – it has now been confirmed through magnetoencephalographic imaging that such wave excitation spreading across the striate cortex is "a quantitative and measurable fact" that "may actually be visualized during the course of migraine aura", mescaline hallucinations, and similar acute pathological conditions (Sacks 1992, pp. 287–288). He admits in the revised edition of the book that science needs a "radically new principle or theory" in order to fully understand this type of complex neuronal functioning and organization. In this regard, Sacks believes that Ilya Prigogine's breakthroughs in irreversible thermodynamics might one day be applied to biology and to neuroscience more specifically. It is a hope inspired by Prigogine himself who, Sacks claims, "reminds us that nature 'thinks' in non-integrable differential equations, 'thinks' in terns of chaos and self-organization, 'thinks' in terms of non-linear dynamical systems. 'The universe,' Prigogine says, 'is like a giant brain.' " (Sacks 1992, p. 297). Sacks, like Michaux before him, also hopes that advances in brain imaging technology will one day confirm not only the general neuronal wave diffusion during acute hallucinations, but will be able to illustrate precisely and in real time that the form and movement constants seen in such hallucinations are indeed mapped on the striate cortex. "This imaging would provide an objective 'photograph' of migraine processes, where hallucination can only provide a subjective one" (Sacks 1992, p. 296). Francisco Varela's work on autopoiesis can be seen, in the biological domain, as offering a scientific model comparable to what Prigogine has done in physical chemistry. Furthermore, in his later work, Varela began to develop a method he calls "neurophenomenology" that fully addresses this last hope and concern of Oliver Sacks, namely, that we need to find an adequate connection between "objective" and "subjective" analyses of hallucinatory experience. The premise of neurophenomenology is that no purely third-person model would ever be sufficient to overcome the so-called "hard problem" of consciousness and that neuroscience must be expanded to include methodologically rigorous first-person investigations of experience. He claims that "disciplined first-person accounts should be an integral element of the validation of a neurobiological proposal, and not merely coincidental or heuristic information … not a convenient stop on our way to a real explanation, but an active participant in its own right" (Varela 1996, p. 344). For Varela, the most promising methodological models for developing such first-person investigations include phenomenological *praxis*, broadly construed, and Buddhist meditation techniques.

This project of neurophenomenology provides a framework under which Sacks' and Michaux's research can be held together in a way that, to a large extent, mutually reinforces each other. With Sacks' research in mind, we could retrospectively say that Michaux's mescaline drawings and writings present with startling sobriety and with as much objective distance as possible – given the violent waves of force that pulsed his entire being – what he calls the domain of the pre-gestural. After ten years of meticulous and, as Margit Rowell says, almost meditative investigation, he comes to describe this as a "bristling" domain of inner neural movements that has a significance beyond mere personal hallucination and, in fact, "reveals" something fundamental about the workings of the human brain. Remarkably, Sacks' neuroscientific research into the phenomena of migraine aura suggests that there is more to this claim than the naive musing of a poet in search of artificial paradises.

References

Bacon, F. (1987). *The Brutality of Fact: Interviews with Francis Bacon* (ed. by D. Sylvester). London: Thames & Hudson.

Bressloff, P., Cowan, J., Golubitsky, M., Thomas, P., & Wiener, M. (2002). What Geometric Visual Hallucinations tell us about the Visual Cortex. *Neural Computation*, 14, 473–491.

Cytowic, R., & Eagleman, D. (2009). *Wednesday is Indigo Blue*. Cambridge, Massachusetts: MIT Press.

de Ajuriaguerra, J. (1964). *Contribution à la connaissance des psychoses toxiques: Expériences et découvertes du poète Henri Michaux*. Basel: Sandoz.

de Mèredieu, F. (1994). *Histoire matérielle et immatérielle de l'art moderne*. Paris: Bordas.

Epstein, J. (1921). Le phénomène littéraire. *L'esprit nouveau, 8*(11/12), 859.

Klüver, H. (1966). *Mescal and Mechanisms of Hallucinations*. Chicago: University of Chicago Press.

Michaux, H. (1963). *Light Through Darkness* (transl. by H. Chevalier). New York: Orion Press.

Michaux, H. (1974). *The Major Ordeals of the Mind & the Countless Minor Ones* (transl. by R. Howard). New York: Harcourt Brace.

Michaux, H. (1976). *Peace in the Breaking Flood* (transl. by M. Fineberg). Consigny: Embers.

Michaux, H. (1998). *Oeuvres Complètes I* (ed. by R. Bellour). Paris: Gallimard.

Michaux, H. (2000). *Emergences/Resurgences* (transl. by R. Sieburth). New York: The Drawing Center.

Michaux, H. (2000). To Draw the Flow of Time. In C. de Zegher (Ed.), *Untitled Passages* (pp. 7–9). New York: The Drawing Center.

Michaux, H. (2001). *Oeuvres Complètes II* (ed. by R. Bellour). Paris: Gallimard.

Michaux, H. (2002). *Miserable Miracle* (transl. by L. Varèse & A. Moschovakis). New York: New York Review Books.

Michaux, H. (2006). *Stroke by Stroke* (transl. by R. Sieburth). New York: Archipelago Books.

Rowell, M. (1972). *La peinture, le geste, l'action: existentialisme en peinture.* Paris: Klincksieck.

Sacks, O. (1992). *Migraine: Revised and Expanded.* Berkeley: University of California Press.

Siegel, R. (1977). Hallucinations. *Scientific American*, 237(4) (October), 132–140.

Spira, A. (Ed.). (1999). *Henri Michaux.* London: Whitechapel Gallery.

Varela, F. (1996). Neurophenomenology: A Methodological Remedy for the Hard Problem. *Journal of Consciousness Studies, 3*(4), 330–349.

Moving without moving

A first-person experiential phenomenological approach

Natalie Depraz
Université de Rouen

1. Introduction

My first "move" when hearing the title of the present collective volume on the motor dimension of imagination was one of perplexity and curiosity: "imaginative inner moving" is an expression that is in itself an oxymoron: what does it mean to move in imagination or *inward*? At first sight, moving involves a bodily behaviour, which is external and visible for others. If an inner move is to be found, it implies that I might move while remaining motionless seen from the outside. Hence the title of my chapter: "moving without moving", or "moving from within" to quote the title of Francisco Varela's *The View from Within*, a special issue of *Journal of Consciousness Studies* he edited with Jonathan Shear in 1999.

In the third book of his *Physics*, Aristotle (1983) identifies four kinds of movement (*kinesis*), which all refer to an objective modification that is observable from outside, be it a change/alteration (*alloiosis*), an increase/decrease (*auxitou/phthitou*), a generation (*genesis*) or a local transfer (*phtora*), even if the fourth meaning of *kinesis* only, the local transfer, corresponds to a mechanical objectified move. The first three, in contrast, all include a lived inner component: the living bodily being, while altering/changing, growing and generating is both inward *and* outward moving. Actually, the phenomenological approach (mainly Edmund Husserl and Maurice Merleau-Ponty) will apply to the fourth meaning of *kinesis*, the local transfer (*phtora*), such a double-sided understanding of move, both objective and subjective, which was limited to the first three ones by the Greek philosopher of movement. Indeed the challenge of phenomenology is to understand *kinesis* as such (whatever it is) as both lived and worldly, in the same way as my body is at the same time *Körper* and *Leib*, object and subject, depending on the stress I put on each mode of being and depending on the process I stress: subjectivation or objectivation, increasing my feeling of my bodily tensions and plasticity (like in sport, in instrument playing) or focussing on my bodily resistances and hindrances (in the case of illness, of being paralysed).[1]

With phenomenology we gain a more encompassing view of bodily movement: the *inner* dimension is an intrinsic component of movement in the sense of a lived movement. Move is not only a move from outside, an outer move, as we stated first, starting from what phenomenologists call the "natural attitude" (or the physicalist behaviourist attitude). Here "inner" equates "lived". However such a statement opens the way for a question: what would be a move that would be only "inner"? Is this phenomenologically possible? Does not phenomenology claim the integration of inner and outer experience, of move "from within" and "from outside"? Does the contention of an inner move call for some limitations of the phenomenological approach, or for some new steps within it? In the following I will therefore try to answer the question to what extent it is phenomenologically possible to "move without moving".

2. Two contrasted third-person philosophical phenomenological accounts of the "inner move"

To start with I recall two different pheno-philosophical accounts, which both broach the issue of "inner move". Even if Husserl's account of kinaesthetic experience is inaugural and crucial I focus here on two later phenomenological analyses which tackled this issue more directly, either through a stress on motricity or through the innovating concept of self-affection.

2.1 Merleau-Ponty: From kinaesthesia to motricity

Merleau-Ponty's critical stance against Husserl leads him to favour the multimodal and synaesthetic movement of the living being. He therefore considers Husserl's stress on the kinaesthetic perceptive intentional activity of the subject as too much linear-directed and vision-led. Hence Merleau-Ponty's development of a view on embodied perception that is embedded into movement and action-oriented.

1. For more on these limit-processes, see N. Depraz, *Lucidité du corps,* Dordrecht: Kluwer 2001.

In his courses at the Collège de France,[2] recently worked out by Stefan Kristensen for the years 1952–1953 for example,[3] it is clear that there is no movement without a field of perception and a bodily involvement, as was stated nicely by Jan Patochka (1995, p. 18): "Movement presupposes that there be a direct coincidence of the subjective and the objective, which is only possible because something corporeal (Körperliches) submits itself to our subjective 'I can' or 'I do'." As such, movement operates at the interface between inner and outer, interior and exterior. When you observe the way an external movement is produced, it is the result of a certain inner function of my organic organisation. For example, if I observe a bird flying in the sky, the only thing that is observable in myself — in the retina — is the "successive activation of distinct regions" (Merleau-Ponty 1968, p. 65). However, such an inner move is unconscious in the sense of a cognitive unconscious: it occurs in my brain or my retina but I have no subjective access to it. Therefore Merleau-Ponty suggests making a distinction between such an "objective" inner move and my actual subjective perception of movement. Here "inner" means either neurodynamic unconscious (it occurs in me without me) or subjective conscious in the sense of "lived", even if this is not a reflexive consciousness. Merleau-Ponty refuses to dissociate what is physical and what is lived and suggests integrating both dimensions within the process of an emerging meaning of being. When I move my hand, there is a global experience at work: a local transfer (an objective external move), a neurological process (an objective inner move), a subjective lived move (I am preconsciously involved as a feeling subject) and also an expressive move towards myself or others, something which may allow to equate move and gesture here.[4]

Movement is the main characteristic of the phenomenal field for Merleau-Ponty, with ceaseless exchanges between ground and forms. The dynamics

2. M. Merleau-Ponty, *Résumés de cours*, Paris, Gallimard 1968, pp. 11–21: "Le monde sensible et le monde de l'expression".

3. For what follows, see Stefan Kristensen "Maurice Merleau-Ponty, une esthétique du mouvement", *Archives de Philosophie* 1/2006 (Tome 69), pp. 123–146. www.cairn.info/revue-archives-de-philosophie-2006-1-page-123.htm

4. Cf. Merleau-Ponty 1968, p. 70: "If left and right side move apart at the same speed, then the left side comes back to the same speed as the 'head' continues to move forward slowly, and we get a figure that swims, i.e. propelled from the back. Thus the phenomenon cannot be analysed as 'global displacement + internal movement'." Our translation of "Si côté droit et gauche s'écartent à la même vitesse, puis le côté gauche revient à la même vitesse pendant que la 'tête' continue de progresser lentement, on obtient une figure qui nage, *i.e.* propulsée par l'arrière. Ainsi le phénomène ne peut être analysé comme 'déplacement global + mouvement interne'."

therefore operates spontaneously, without the deliberate intervention of a rational wilful subject: it means that it generates from itself the expression of a meaning like a dynamics of self-organisation. If it is not the movement of an individual subject any longer (local, wilful or pre-conscious), it means that these different dynamics within the perceptive field that operate *per se* anonymously as an immanent configuration of meaning characteristic of the dynamics of being itself (Merleau-Ponty 1968, pp. 70–72, p. 84).

2.2 Michel Henry and self-affection

Contrary to Merleau-Ponty who ends up identifying movement and being, and inner move and the immanent dynamics of the perceptive field, the philosopher of life equates inner move and self-affection. It means that for Michel Henry an inner move is something that is highly and radically subjective. His whole thrust lies in a general critical stance against the objective physical body, which is unable to feel anything: life can only be experienced and felt ("éprouvée") from inside. In that respect, sensitivity is highly and exclusively interior. From his first book *Phénoménologie et philosophie du corps* (1965) to *Incarnation* (2000) Henry's leading thread amounts to describing the lived bodily experience as inner affective force, having its own immanent dynamics and not depending on any external event whatever.

> (…) the affective, 'impressional' character of the impression [which] is therefore nothing which we must confine ourselves to in order to see its facticity, its arrival of which we don't know how it happens, or where it comes from, or wherein it is: it refers to its innermost possibility, to its belonging to the flesh, and to the pathetic self-revelation of the latter in life." (Henry 2000, p. 90, our translation)[5]

Besides, such an affective inner move has little to do with a kinaesthetic transfer of my body embedded in space; it refers much more to a kind of growth and to a generation of my bodily resistance and drive. In *Incarnation*, the explicit discussion with Merleau-Ponty shows quite clearly how Henry parts with him with regard to considering movement as lived mechanical *phtora* and in contrast resonates with the early Aristotelian understanding of *auxitou/phthitou* and *genesis*. Henry does not consider move as the interface between subjective and objective dimensions of

5. Our translation of " (…) le caractère affectif, 'impressionnel' de l'impression [qui] n'est donc rien dont on doive se borner à constater la facticité, sa venue on ne sait comment, on ne sait d'où, dans on ne sait quoi: il renvoie à sa possibilité la plus intérieure, à son appartenance à une chair, à l'auto-révélation pathétique de celle-ci dans la vie."

my body but as a more archaic affective undivided experience situated beneath the distinction of subjective and objective, and which he calls "life".[6]

To recapitulate, the Henryian inner move is affective and self-generating whereas the Merleau-Pontian inner move is ontological and expressive-gestural. Both agree with the immanent component of inner move, but they understand it in a diametrically opposed way. For Merleau-Ponty, immanence means a worldly and fleshy being, whereas for Henry it refers to a passive radical self-revelation of myself.

3. Two first-person experiential phenomenological accounts of "inner move"

3.1 From a third-person to a first-person approach

Since Merleau-Ponty and Michel Henry both claim the necessity to experience movement from within, that is, from the point of view of a lived or affective experience, it might seem strange to identify their phenomenological approach with a third-person approach. Indeed a third approach is usually defined as an objective scientific one, which does not take the lived experience of a subject into account but only what is observable from outside as a behaviour or what can be registered directly from the brain without the subject being aware of it. Actually I agree with such an understanding: those approaches cannot do justice to any "inner move" but only to an objective physical movement.

However I would like to extend the meaning of the third-person approach to the phenomenological philosophical accounts (which I will call now "phenophilosophical") and make a distinction within phenomenology between them and a first-person experiential phenomenology.[7] Of course the two practical frameworks to which I appeal below may be dealt with from a third-person point of view (either scientific or philosophical, extracting categories of such lived experiences) but I have the feeling that an experiential first-person approach will be more fitting in order to describe the kind of inner move that is at play in such practices. Of course it does not exclude (on the contrary) appealing to scientific or philosophical third-person accounts in order to indicate other aspects of the

6. For more on this matter, see F. Martins, "L'autre: le corps vivant", in *Michel Henry: pensée de la vie et culture contemporaine,* Paris, Beauchesne 2006, pp. 74–75.

7. On this matter, see N. Depraz, *Lire Husserl en phénoménologue: Idées directrices pour une phénoménologie (I).* Paris: PUF, 2008, and *Edmund Husserl: une phénoménologie expérientielle.* Paris: Atlande 2009.

experience which will enrich it, either confirming or questioning it. It could be the project of a further inquiry and indeed in my third concluding part I will give some clues of such a co-generative comparison with the phenophilosophical categories I underlined in the first part.

Now I would like to move towards two different practical settings (sitting meditation and manual fasciatherapy) where the experience of "moving inward" is clearly identified because of its structural dissociation from any external move, be it my looking at a moving object or my self-movement. Indeed, both settings are *structured* by the externally motionless posture of the subject. Both focus on the thematic exploration of what is going on within my lived body while remaining still. In short, no visible movement is going on. The concrete methodological hypothesis is the following: when I am observing persons or things moving (talking in the underground, a car in the street while I am crossing the road) or when I am moving myself while achieving a certain activity (walking quickly in order to get my train to Rouen), my attention is immersed into such outer movements and it is more difficult for me to become simultaneously aware of what is going on in my lived body. So – following here the general move of *On becoming aware* (N. Depraz, F.J. Varela & P. Vermersch 2003)[8] – I will apply the method of the *épochè* to movement, bracketing every external move and redirecting my attention to the observation of "inner moves".

3.2 Meditation: Moving while remaining still

To begin with I will quote a first-person description of a particular moment of sitting meditation I experienced and was able to describe thanks to a self-elicitation technics I got built into thanks to Pierre Vermersch and Claire Petitmengin. Then I will comment on it with regard to the experience of inner move.

The following segments of description are extracted from a "verbatim" which was first published as the core of an article entitled: "The failing of meaning. A few steps into a 'first-person' phenomenological practice".[9]

Dechen Chölin, May 2000. First meditation retreat with the Sakyong: intense meditation time (10 hours a day).

8. French text: *A l'épreuve de l'expérience : pour une pratique phénoménologique*, Bucharest, Zeta Books 2011.

9. N. Depraz, "The failing of meaning. A few steps into a 'first person' phenomenological practice", C. Petitmengin (Ed.), *Journal of Consciousness Studies, Special Issue, First-person Methodologies: the legacy of Francisco Varela* 2009, pp. 90–117.

1. A talk each afternoon. The Sakyong is teaching, he lets us see the nine stages in shamatha. He lets us feel and see the inner path with the space of mind, I am going into it with him, living it with him.
2. His way of talking comes back again to me, a modality of speech which is at once smooth, light, and slow. Yes, he speaks slowly but without ever repeating himself. He leaves some time between his utterances, but not much, for you never feel any gap, you never feel you are waiting for the following utterance. You always feel related to him and at the same time, what he says inhabits you: he takes his time in order for you to have what he says resonate in yourself.
3. I am following his track while he brings me from the first stage to the second one, then to the third one, each time, I am saying to myself: yes, that's it, I know that, that's what I am living.

   [...]
8. The words of the Sakyong while I am related to his talking: the "same village". He talks about his relationship with Trungpa; I am looking at him, I am making notes, I am intensively focussing towards his speaking presence, an invisible thread is linking me to him. He only speaks for me; he speaks of it: stage 1: he places my body; stage 2: he places my breath, he helps me link myself to my breath. I am going through the stages exactly while he "speaks them". I am doing what he says to do and I do it at the very moment when he says it: it provides me with an inner experiential texture of "dense presence". I don't do it afterwards, I even do it a little bit just before, I know what he is talking about. He recreates within myself something I know quite well, he furnishes it with a specific thickness; stage 3: he places my thoughts upon my breath; he places the dis-synchronicity, the unsteadiness, the to and fro moves, the fluctuations: presence, non-presence.
9. I prepared myself to experience what he now speaks about: observing the arising thoughts, seeing them fade away, not be aware when I am not there any longer, becoming aware of it too late, observing thoughts again, feeling that I am elsewhere, feeling frustrated because I failed again to grasp the arising thought, because I was not able to welcome it without grasping it. I have been going through all these thoughts again and again for hours. His speech therefore comes to me as just ripe fruit that only waits for being plucked.
10. He talks about me. Great feeling of familiarity.
11. Then he talks of the "observer" (*sheshin*), who is both inside/outside, and then, I have the feeling that I enter an unknown space, something new, which attracts but does not fit into my lived experiences.
12. Somehow, I know it quite well such an enigmatic *sheshin*. At the very moment when he mentions it, I try to identify it within my lived experience. I am endeavouring to approximate it – such a magical word and experience – within

> my well-known familiar experiences and words; he also calls it an "observer"; I know very well it is not exactly the right word. Of course I can also name it thus, which means that it grasps a fragment of my lived experience. I try to catch it that way, which I feel that it is definitely not the right word. The word "*sheshin*" is beating in my head in a compulsive manner, in an almost panicking way, like an empty space that the word does not fill out, and it even seems as if the wording still increases the gap, still makes it more open (wide-open, gaping: "*béant*"). A kind of opening of something abyssal, which is related to a radical lack of experiencing. My own experience of *sheshin* appears to me blurred, fragmented, scattered, confusion-laden, I sometimes half-see it as the very temporal quality of my being always too late to what arises in myself as thoughts-events: again, I am structurally late to what I am present, the move of my becoming conscious is always too late. I just become aware (too late) that I have been there when the thought arose.

What strikes me while re-reading such a description (and re-living the very living experiential texture of it) is the great mobility of my mind and the multifarious events that are occurring within this very short moment (about 2 minutes) of sitting meditation. Here "inner move" is not only a concept or an expression any longer. It *becomes* the dynamic experience of numerous thoughts crossing each other and permeating each other in my mind, which is experienced as an inner mobile space. Here thoughts themselves are not unbodily mental Cartesian occurrences but very tangible forces endowed with a power of growth and transformation of what I am becoming (in the lines of William James and Gilles Deleuze). In short my whole mind-body is an intersection of multifarious moves which are inner concrete dynamic thoughts, as physical as they are mental.

All this inner mobile activity occurs while I am sitting motionless: the embodied texture and dynamics of my thoughts emerge as a flow of vivid images. My physical body as such is very little focused on, I might feel some pressure of my hands, hear somebody cough next to me, but I decide (it is part of the meditative technics) not to focus on it, as little as I focus on what is occurring in myself. The thing is that the motionless physical posture operates as a leaning point that opens up the possibility to become aware (more than during daily moving activities) of the moves of my mind.

3.3 Manual fasciatherapy: Experiencing one's inner moves thanks to the other's hand-move

The second practice I want to focus on – manual fasciatherapy – also relies on a motionless bodily posture as a methodological practical condition for experimenting what is going on within myself. But contrary to sitting meditation the exploration focuses on the inner moves proper to the *physical* lived body. Such a manual technics is, moreover, intrinsically intersubjective: I am guided in my exploration of the very materiality of my body by a fasciatherapist, that is, somebody who was built up in psycho-motricity, physiotherapy and more precisely here in "somato-psychopedagogy".[10] Quite concretely the fasciatherapist practices hand-pressure at different parts of my body, he or she touches me in a very firm way with his or her both hands and makes me feel my material body from within, in a way that you usually don't feel. It is as if he or she was "touching me from within" while he or she remains external to me, and I also experience within myself genuine moves while remaining objectively motionless.

But instead of describing in a third-person way what occurs in such an experience of "inner move" (the expression "mouvement interne" was created by Danis Bois, who founded in the seventies this branch of fasciatherapy called somatopsychopedagogy), let us read my first-person description of such an experience (about 40 minutes).[11] What follows is not a "verbatim" like in the meditation description but two self-elicitation descriptions on the go: the first one (1) was written just after the experience, on the evening of the same day (30 minutes),[12] (2) the second two days later (20 minutes):[13]

1. Eve suggests to 'treat' me (me 'traiter') first without saying anything, just to see what I feel while she is touching me.

I lay down, put my glasses off and close my eyes.

She begins to practice a pressure at the level of my thorax, from downward to upward, following a vertical movement. I feel quite quickly that I slide down, like in a sledge, and that I come back upward. There is an instant where I stand still, motionless point, then I come back upward.

Then she practices side-pressures at the same level, that makes me shift on the side, left, then right, like in a merry-go-round.

10. On this matter, see for example E. Berger, *La somato-psychopédagogie, ou comment se former à l'intelligence du corps*. Paris: Editions Points d'appui 2007, and "Praticiens-chercheurs du Sensible: vers une redéfinition de la posture d'implication" (pp. 167–190), in *Sujet sensible et renouvellement du moi. Les apports de la fasciathérapie et de la somato-psychopédagogie*, D. Bois, M.-Ch. Josso & M. Humpich (eds.). Paris, Editions Points d'appui.

11. First meeting of "sensory introspection", Friday, April, 9th, 2010 at Eve's home (11.50 a.m. to 12.30 a.m.).

12. April, 10th, 6 p.m.-6: 30 p.m.

13. April, 11th, 6 p.m.-6: 36 p.m.

Then she practices a pressure with both hands at the level of the clavicles, then at the level of the neck and cervicals. I feel less flexibility at this level, more tension. I feel some resistance, some degrees where it moves, I feel myself resisting, I let it go, it stops and comes back.

Afterwards, she puts her hands on my back and I feel that I fall down into the mattress, as if I was on a air-cushion that wimps out; I feel myself letting it gradually go, I fall down step by step lower and deeper inside my body. I also feel a small ache, feeble and quick, at the level of the left scapula.

Then she practices a pressure at the back of my skull with both hands and here, I feel that my head enlarges, deepens, on the back of it, I say to myself: these are the visual areas, could there be effects on my visual activity?

Then she tells me: I am also going to touch you at the level of the legs and the feet, just to go through your whole body. I open my eyes one moment, but prefer to close them quickly in order to keep the sensation of the enlarged volume of my body.

First the legs, where I feel that I become bigger so as to become like a log of nearly one meter long, same movement of expansion, stop and come back; then the ankles, finally the feet, which I feel as dissociated from me, as if they floated far away from me.

2. My self-instruction for this second self-elicitation is to read once more my first description and to contact again my inner bodily experience.

«I feel quite quickly.» What do I feel just before ? Eve hands' pressure on me, on my breast. I wonder if I am without tension. I wonder if Eve feels my heart beat, if it is regular. Then my thoughts fade away. I begin to move quickly like in a corridor that dives down and I have the sensation to go down very quickly and very far. Then I think of a slightly inclined tunnel. The going up again, beyond the stop-moment where I feel my body balanced and quiet, rather steady, is far less vertiginous, more spontaneous.

«that makes me shift»: such a movement is far more subtle, more uncomfortable also. I feel that parts of my body gradually are 'lift off', part of my skin, of my flesh, and the whole does not come together, some bits separate…

«more tension»: something resists. I feel tensed, I feel my precarity, I feel that the bits that separate are all a bit mechanical, I think of it and it blocks me, so that Eve's hand pressure stops in turn.

«an air-cushion that wimps out»: I feel at ease again, I feel some pleasure again to feel again the first sensation of openness and of growth I felt at the very beginning. I enjoy this moment of lightness and growth of my body beneath myself.

«my head enlarges, deepens…» One inner commentary comes back to me. I think of my mummy, of her dead body on the 31th of last December, of her lost bodily flexibility, of her increased rigidity, of this body that had to be 'broken' in order to give it its shape back when it was prepared, of the violence of such a manipulation.

«I open my eyes». I see Eve standing before me at the level of my feet, her eyes closed. I feel my left leg quite strongly when she practices a hand pressure on it, which resists more than my right leg.

«as if they floated far away from me.» I see my feet come off myself. I recall then the image of a Buñuel's film where cut feet are seen on the ground.

The most striking element of such an experience for me was the sensation of a growing body within myself: I felt my different bodily parts as Eve touched them as being far bigger than I knew, I had the sensation of bodily amplitude; moreover, I had a couple of times the feeling of a sudden acceleration of my body moving from downward to upward, or quickly falling down; also I had several sensations of forces within my body that were driving me towards some directions, and again, a strong feeling of flow and coming back.

Now, all these movements happened in myself while remaining still, laying down without moving. During the experience I had some images in mind, not only associations (like thinking of my mother's dead body), but embodied images that described precisely the felt moves: the "sledge" (toboggan), "the merry-go-round" (manège).

4. Crossing third-person and first-person phenomenological approaches: Emergent subcategories of "inner move"

In this conclusive part I bring together in a schematic table the a priori categorial results of the pheno-philosophical inquiries of the first part (Merleau-Ponty and Michel Henry) and the a posteriori experiential categories from both first-person practices. The idea is to show through it how both may generate and constrain each other and thus help inventing a more complex platform for inner move bodily experience.

While doing so I am relying on Varela's methodological suggesting of co-generativity and applying it to the cross-perspectives within phenomenology between philosophy and psychological self-elicitation. Such a table sketches a comparison between conceptual a priori and experiential categories. For lack of space and time, I won't go here into the cross-evaluation of the categories of both type one through the other, and allow myself to keep it for another later contribution.

Categories	Experiential field	Modality of inner move	Self-other	Texture of mobility
Merleau-Ponty	being	expression-gestural	non-individuated world relationship	pulsional flesh
Michel Henry	affection	self-revelation	individuated radical subject	growing inner force
Meditation	mind	flowing and interruptions	inner subjective	multiplicity of multilayered flowing thought moves
Manual therapy	body	growing, accelerating	intersubjective interaction	multidirectional circular and multifocused bodily moves

What can be said for the time being as a conclusive word is the following: it is striking to see when comparing a priori philosophical categories and experiential emergent ones that the plurality of moves and their complex directionality are described through the latter categories while the apriori ones focus on one sole kind of move (drive or growing force). Clearly the experiential practices enriched our descriptive abilities by refining the experience and its description. On the other side, the philosophical categories offer fruitful tools in order to discriminate between different kinds of inner moves, linear and directional, growing and generating, which could not be considered as such if we had only to do with experiential first-person descriptions. As mentioned above, I leave the fuller categories comparison for another time-space and invite the reader to carry on on her own if she likes to.

References

Aristote (1983). *Physique: I–IV,* vol. 1 (trad. par H. Carteron). Paris: Les Belles Lettres.

Berger, E. (2007). *La somato-psychopédagogie, ou comment se former à l'intelligence du corps.* Paris: Editions Points d'appui.

Berger, E. (2009). Praticiens-chercheurs du Sensible: vers une redéfinition de la posture d'implication. In D. Bois, M.-Ch. Josso, & M. Humpich (Eds.), *Sujet sensible et renouvellement du moi. Les apports de la fasciathérapie et de la somato-psychopédagogie* (pp. 167–190). Paris: Editions Points d'appui.

Depraz, N. (2001). *Lucidité du corps.* Dordrecht: Kluwer.

Depraz, N., Varela, F.J., & Vermersch, P. (2003). *On becoming aware: a pragmatics of experiencing.* Amsterdam/Philadelphia: John Benjamins Publishing Company (French text (2011). *A l'épreuve de l'expérience : pour une pratique phénoménologique.* Bucharest: Zeta Books).

Depraz, N. (2008). *Lire Husserl en phénoménologue: Idées directrices pour une phénoménologie (I).* Paris: PUF.

Depraz, N. (2009). *Edmund Husserl: une phénoménologie expérientielle.* Paris: Atlande.

Depraz, N. (2009). The failing of meaning. A few steps into a 'first person' phenomenological practice. *Journal of Consciousness Studies, Special Issue, First-person Methodologies: the legacy of Francisco Varela* (ed. by C. Petitmengin), *16*(10–12), 90–117.

Henry, M. (1965). *Phénoménologie et philosophie du corps* (Collection Epiméthée). Paris: PUF.

Henry, M. (2000). *Incarnation, Une philosophie de la chair.* Paris: Seuil.

Kristensen, S. (2006). Maurice Merleau-Ponty, une esthétique du mouvement. *Archives de Philosophie,* 1(69), 123–146. Available at www.cairn.info/revue-archives-de-philosophie-2006-1-page-123.htm (accessed October 2012).

Martins, F. (2006). L'autre: le corps vivant. In J.-F. Lavigne (Ed.), *Michel Henry: pensée de la vie et culture contemporaine* (pp. 67–79). Paris: Beauchesne.

Merleau-Ponty, M. (1968). *Résumés de cours – Collège de France 1952–1960.* Paris: Gallimard (English translation by John O'Neill (1970). *Themes from the Lectures at the Collège de France, 1952–1960.* Evanston: Northwestern University Press).

Patochka, J. (1995). *Qu'est-ce que la phénoménologie?* Grenoble: J. Millon.

Varela, F., & Shear, J. (Eds.). (1999). *The View from Within, First person approaches to the study of consciousness,* special issue of *Journal of Consciousness Studies, 6* (2–3).

The "I cannot, but it can" of aesthetic perception

Erica Harris
Hoger Instituut voor Wijsbegeerte, Katholieke Universiteit Leuven

"Where is the painting?", Maurice Merleau-Ponty asks in *Eye and mind* (1964a, p. 23, my translation). The "where" of a painting, he answers, is a "neither/nor": "The animals painted on the walls of Lascaux are not there in the same way as are the fissures and limestone formations. Nor are they *elsewhere*" (Merleau-Ponty 1996, p. 126). Aesthetic space is thus somewhat unfamiliar: while he holds that it is perceptual in nature, it is clearly unlike the space of one's habitual involvement (Merleau-Ponty 1964a, p. 23). This is also true for the 'objects' that inhabit aesthetic space: the women in Paul Cézanne's painting of *The bathers* are not given to me in the same way on the canvas as the strangers I encounter as I walk through the park on the way to work. The tension between the way that I perceive an artwork and the way that I perceive habitual objects is perhaps most evident in the museum. The artwork is presented to me, in contrast to the wall upon which it hangs, as a kind of window that opens onto another space beyond the gallery walls. The painting is somehow both at home in the museum and a stranger to it. Merleau-Ponty seeks to maintain this unfamiliar quality of images while at the same time doing away with the traditional phenomenological dichotomy between imagination and perception. According to him, painting is not somewhere beyond or outside of the familiar world, nor is it independent of the artistic material out of which it is made. The painting appears amongst everyday perceptual objects and is only properly understood in relation to them. In what sense, then does the painting not entirely fit into perceptual surroundings? In this chapter, I will explore the enigma of painting from the point of view of bodily movement in aesthetic space. I suggest that the particular aura of strangeness that characterizes the painting is a function of the body's relation to it. The body cannot engage with the painting in the same way that it does with everyday objects, I argue, because the painting is a purely visual object that does not offer itself as something that can be explored by my body as a synaesthetic whole.

In this chapter, I develop and discuss the tension between the lived body, understood as a potentiality for movement, and aesthetic perception. I begin by considering the definition of the body as "I can" from Merleau-Ponty's

Phenomenology of Perception, and then apply it to the realm of imagination and the perception of paintings more specifically. The tension between body and image, I argue, is present in both figurative and non-figurative artwork, although it is more difficult to detect and account for in the former. I then consider the question of whether or not the motor tension between artwork and body entails the separation between perception and imagination that Merleau-Ponty sought so desperately to avoid throughout his career. I argue that it does not, but that it does necessitate a shift from the "I can" to the "it can" of anonymous movement that is accompanied by a feeling of paralysis or limitation.

1. The personal body and its spatiality: I can

Merleau-Ponty is best known for arguing for the primacy of perception and the embodiment of consciousness. His philosophy, like Edmund Husserl's before him, begins, as he believes all theory must, with a description of our most fundamental way of being-in-the-world: perceptual engagement. The subject who perceives, Merleau-Ponty explains, is embodied: it perceives in and through its hands, eyes, ears, and nose. For this reason, it is literally *in* the world and not beyond it, as most transcendental phenomenologists suggest. Merleau-Ponty famously describes the lived body in terms of its special kind of self-awareness: the body schema. The body schema, Merleau-Ponty explains, is an "undivided possession" of one's body; a special kind of non-theoretical knowledge that my body has of its parts and their intimate inter-relations (Merleau-Ponty 1996: 98). Merleau-Ponty uses the term "tacit" to distinguish the body's self-knowledge from the self-consciousness of transcendental phenomenology and Sartrian existentialism. Tacit awareness is, unlike the latter, not fully transparent to itself; it is and remains a mystery to reflective cognition. This means that it is a "knowledge" that can never be made theoretically explicit (Merleau-Ponty 1945, p. 116). Merleau-Ponty defines the body schema in three steps in the chapter entitled "The spatiality of one's own body and motility" of *Phenomenology of Perception*. He begins with the most rudimentary – and also the most misguided – explanation of the body's self-awareness. According to this model, the body learns or acquires a sense of itself as a meaningful whole by way of habituation and association. This account is akin to the description of the mirror stage in developmental psychology. Over time, the child assembles a picture of itself on the basis of its experience of the way that its body works (Merleau-Ponty 1945, p. 99). This account is rejected in favour of an understanding of the lived body as a form or Gestalt. This second definition stresses the primordiality of bodily unity. The sense of my body as a whole is now something that I possess from the outset, rather than something that is achieved over time. To say that the body is a Gestalt is to say that it is a whole whose parts cannot be thought of independently of it (Merleau-Ponty 1945, p. 100). My body is thus a dynamic organism: hands have their particular function only in relation to the way that my arms, torso, head and legs are organized. If this organization were to change, as pathological cases attest, then my hands would function differently (Merleau-Ponty 1942, p. 70). Ultimately, however, Merleau-Ponty argues that this definition of the body schema is also wanting since it fails to account for the body's special position in the world. He insists that the body is only properly described as a *projective* Gestalt (1945, p. 129). On this level, the body is not only aware of its inner structure, but also maps this self-awareness onto its surroundings. In this way, the world shows up to it as a milieu of possible interaction; objects – like apples – appear, on this basis, as things that *I can* pick up, eat, throw, or draw (Merleau-Ponty 1945, p. 160).

To say that one must understand the body in terms of *I can* is to emphasize two things: first, that my body is egoic – "I" – and second, that it is practically oriented. These two moments of the body schema are deeply intertwined: only something that is able to distinguish between itself and its surroundings is able to act in a goal-oriented manner. If I had no sense – or only a very vague one – of the boundaries between myself and the objects in front of me, I would have no basis upon which to operate. This is the lesson at the heart of structuralism: things must be well-ordered in order to function practically. Without the clear distinction between what is "me" and what is "not me", my perception would be too hazy or chaotic to allow for purposeful behaviour. This is why, in the early chapters of the *Phenomenology of perception*, Merleau-Ponty speaks of it as a "possession" or "personal core" at the heart of experience (Merleau-Ponty 1996, p. 155).

I distinguish between my body and the objects that surround it on the basis of the particular way in which the former is given to me. In *Phenomenology of Perception*, Merleau-Ponty speaks of the body schema as the "darkness in the theatre" or the "background" that allows the perceptual scene or 'foreground' to show up (Merleau-Ponty 1996, p. 102). In his later, ontological works, he designates this distinction in terms of inner and outer sense, which he takes over from Husserl's *Ideas II*. The body, he explains, lives from the 'inside' what it attributes to the 'outside' (Merleau-Ponty 1964, p. 24). This is to say that the body senses things in two ways. When I touch the keyboard in front of me, I feel its smoothness inside my fingers as well as on the surface of the keys. The latter is experienced as a property of the thing it perceives while the former is a perception of my own body. Husserl calls this second kind of feeling 'sensing' (Husserl 1989, p. 152). Inner touch sensations are, according to him, the means through which I am aware of my body and its limitations (Husserl 1989, p. 157). Without them, he argues, I would have no sense of myself as being 'this' or 'here' (Husserl 1989, p. 158).

The body as *I can* perceives the world through the lens of its Gestalt. The process of perception, or filtration, ought, according to Merleau-Ponty to be understood as a process of communication. The model for this communication is a question-answer dynamic. A situation or object asks the body to find its 'proper place' with respect to it (Merleau-Ponty 1945, p. 305). This is a motor request: the body is asked to find and adopt an optimal stance from which to perceive its interlocutor. Perception, therefore, is structured around the quest for equilibrium between the body and its environment, an equilibrium in which the body's sense of itself is compatible with the way that the objects around it appear. Equilibrium is thus characterized by the notion of "habitation". The world, when properly perceived, is one that the lived body *inhabits,* an environment in which the body belongs. In equilibrium, the lived-subject experiences the world as a well-delineated, stable space filled with determinate objects that it can then explore and use to achieve its goals.

Although Merleau-Ponty's understanding of the body-world relation matures throughout his career, this understanding of *I can* as pole of perceptual orientation still haunts *Eye and Mind*:

> All my changes of place figure on principle in a corner of my landscape; they are carried over onto the map of the visible. Everything I see is on principle within my reach, at least within reach of my sight, and is marked upon the map of the 'I can'. (Merleau-Ponty 1993, p. 124)

He seems, then, to want to preserve the role of the practical body schema in artwork. Is the body that participates in painting really the same as the one that is characterized by the *I can* of the projective Gestalt as this passage seems to suggest? Is the body that the painter "lends to the world" (Merleau-Ponty 1964a, p. 16), to use Merleau-Ponty's words, in order to create art the one that I call "mine"? This is the main question that I will consider in this chapter.

2. Introducing the *I cannot*

Of the many features that make a painting unlike other perceptual objects, one seemingly obvious one is that the painting depicts a place where I cannot go, objects that I cannot touch, smell, or hear, and people with whom I cannot speak. This is not to say that the body has no motor-engagement with the artwork whatsoever. On the contrary, it positions itself with respect to the painting, as it would in the case of any perceptual object, in order to perceive it "optimally" *as an artwork.* What I perceive in the painting, however, is present to me only as a spectacle. As Robert Sokolowski explains in *Phenomenology of the human person*:

"I do not picture myself doing anything in the landscape I see hanging on the wall; I am there simply as a viewer, not as a simulated agent" (Sokolowski 2008, p. 142). This is the case even if the painting is of a place that I could visit or a person whom I know. Even though I may travel to France to see the Mont St. Victoire on my next holiday, I will nevertheless have the sense that the mountain in the picture is beyond my reach. The "real" mountain, therefore, is experienced differently than its image: it is something that I could climb or walk around to see from a different angle. The pictorial mountain, however, is positioned in a space that I see but cannot explore. I cannot *do* anything with this mountain other than see it as it is painted.

Part of the reason for this feeling of limitation has to do with the way that the painting seems to cut itself off from all non-visual sensations. In *Eye and mind*, Merleau-Ponty claims, echoing Clement Greenberg's argument in his pamphlet on modernist painting, that the painter's only task is to explore the enigma of vision (Merleau-Ponty 1964a, p. 26). If painting truly comes into its own as, according to Greenberg, it does in modernism, it must isolate its proper domain – vision – from those that it shares with others, such as texture or depth (1960, p. 2). Thus, Merleau-Ponty speaks of painting as a "voracious vision" with the power to both do away with the reference to other senses and to give "visible existence to what profane vision believes to be invisible" (Merleau-Ponty 1993, p. 127). Exclusively *visual* entities, like paintings, break with Merleau-Ponty's holistic description of sensation. In normal perception, senses are synaesthetic: they, like the parts of my body, entail one another. When I see a carpet, for example, I immediately have a sense of what it would feel like to walk barefoot on it, what it would sound like if I were to shake the dust out of it, or what it would smell like if I were to place my face next to it. According to Merleau-Ponty, this overlapping provides our merely visual perceptions with "depth" or sense (Merleau-Ponty 1945, p. 265). If the goal of painting, however, is to consider vision in isolation, then, in doing so, it modifies the way that our bodies normally perceive. Painting, in being cut off from my other senses, is thus experienced as being cut off from the body as a multi-sensory whole. This purely visual space is thus radically different from the perceptual space that is polarized by the body schema; it is a bodily enigma.

Nevertheless, one may object: many painted objects and the spaces to which they belong are understood in terms of the whole body. When describing *Landscape with the Fall of Icarus*, for example, I say that, in the bottom right-hand corner of the painting, Icarus has fallen into the water and is thrashing his feet in the air as he drowns. The sense I have of "right", "feet", "falling" and "thrashing" are grounded in my awareness of my body and what it can do. In what way, then does the example of painting challenge Merleau-Ponty's notion of "I can"?

According to David Freedberg and Vittorio Gallese, painted images do, in fact, stimulate goal-oriented bodily responses. Their article "Motion, emotion and empathy in esthetic experience" applies new neurological findings to the perception of the work of art in order to explain why spectators often have "a sense of inward imitation of the observed actions of others in pictures" (2007, p. 197). They base their argument on the discovery of mirror and canonical neurons in macaques and human beings. These neurons, according to Gallese and Freedberg, are responsible for the pre-cognitive understanding of others' behaviour. More precisely, they account for how humans immediately, yet tacitly, perceive others and even objects in terms of their own possibilities of action. This, they argue, is in line with Merleau-Ponty's phenomenological description of the body schema as the cornerstone of perceptual experience (Freedberg & Gallese 2007, p. 198). Brain imaging reveals that "the same neurons discharge when an action is observed as when it is executed" (Freedberg & Gallese 2007, p. 200). This is the case even when the action is observed partially or only intended. They hypothesize that the brain processes the artwork in much the same way that it perceives objects and other subjects: in terms of what the body can do (ibid).

There are, however, two important limitations to Freedberg and Gallese's argument. The first is one that they acknowledge in the concluding remarks of their essay: there is a difference in degree between the way that the brain responds to artwork and the way that it responds to real life actions (Freedberg & Gallese 2007, p. 202). Is the way that the body normally perceives simply in the background, informing the sense that the painted object appears, or is the painted object *really given* just like any other? The answer to this question, they admit, is beyond the scope of their research. The second and most important limitation is that their theory seems to have a different application to representative and non-representative art. They explain that the brain responds to either the motor cues present in what the depicted object or the stylistic motor cues left by the artist in aesthetic material, such as paint thickness and brush strokes (Freedberg & Gallese 2007, p. 199). Some types of painting are more likely to evoke one type of reaction than the other. Gallese and Freedberg imply that the brain only responds to the represented object in the painting when the latter are presented as 'manipulable' (Freedberg & Gallese 2007, p. 200). This means that the body seems to only understand the objects in the painting in terms of its own possibilities for movement when those objects are discrete and/or when they resemble the objects of our everyday perception. This is why they illustrate their claim by appealing to still-life artwork (Freedberg & Gallese 2007, p. 201). When the observer perceives a "non-representative" painting (i.e. a painting that is not concerned with "copying" everyday visual perception), Gallese and Freedberg speak instead of the way that she internally "mirrors" the artist's movement that is suggested by the traces of his gestures in the aesthetic material (Freedberg & Gallese 2007, p. 202). This description then leaves aside the difficult phenomenon that I am considering in this paper: the body's response to the aesthetic object that it does not recognise as "manipulable".

Even if my body is somehow involved in perceiving artworks and in giving them their sense, I argue, its role is different from the one it has in everyday perception. What is blatantly different in these two situations is the way that the whole body is able to cast its projects onto objects. Even if my intention were to enjoy a walk along the coast, the pathway that I see in *Icarus* would never appear to me as *a road I could walk*. While I may use my body's awareness of itself, its parts, and its habits or previous experiences to "understand" the painting, therefore, the space before me on the canvas is never given as one in which I could accomplish my goals.

This description of the visual image does more than challenge the scope of the body schema; it also seems to run counter to Merleau-Ponty's account of imagination. According to him, the "absence" of the painted object before me in the painting is no different than the absence that permeates our habitual engagement with things (Colonna 2003, p. 111). Since there are no adequate perceptions of things, namely, no "God's eye view" of objects, he argues that every sensation, like every object, hints at – and acquires a meaning in relation to – what is not "intuitively present" (i.e. the sides of the objects that I cannot see, the way that an object that I only perceive visually would feel if I touched it, etc.) (Steeves 2004, p. 48). Imagination, according to Merleau-Ponty, is just the term for this "invisible depth" underneath the surface of the objects that I see and touch that gives them their meaning (Merleau-Ponty 1964a, p. 24). It is, therefore, not radically distinct from perception. The visual sensations that I achieve with the painting, therefore, have horizons just as other perceptual objects do.

The most obvious explanation for my experience of bodily limitation with respect to the painting is that the latter is two-dimensional. Without depth, there is literally nowhere for something three-dimensional – like my body – to go. What is more, two-dimensional space, and the objects within it, has no hidden aspects: there is nothing *more* to see of a two-dimensional thing than the surface it presents to the observer. Contrary to theorists like Greenberg, who describe painting primarily in terms of its flatness (1993[1960]), Merleau-Ponty argues that every sliver of perceptual being – even surfaces that we naively believe to be two-dimensional – have depth (1964a, pp. 74–75). Two-dimensionality, Merleau-Ponty argues, is actually an abstraction of the third dimension and cannot be understood independently of it (1964a, p. 65). This "third dimension", however, ought not to be understood simply in spatial terms. "Depth" is a trope in Merleau-Ponty's discourse that denotes possibility in general, not simply the possibility of movement. The depth of the painting's flat surface, I argue, is a limited version of the one that we encounter in perception. It is a purely visual depth and, as such, does not present possibilities to my body as a whole. For this reason, my body, which grasps itself as more than just visible, is limited with respect to its engagement with it.

The body's role in aesthetic experience seems to be more akin to its pathological functioning. In *Phenomenology of Perception*, Merleau-Ponty addresses the case of a wounded war veteran, Schneider, whose brain injuries prevent him from being able to perform abstract movements such as pointing to the parts of his own body. Merleau-Ponty explains that his failure is due to his inability to place himself in a fictive situation (1945, p. 157). Schneider cannot turn his attention away from the actual demands of his spatial surroundings; he cannot "project" new aims onto the world. Aesthetic space, I argue, is "dead" for the subject-body in the same way as virtual space is dead for Schneider. Objects in both realms no longer "speak" to the subjects who address them: "the [patient's] intentions are [not] immediately reflected in the perceptual field, polarizing it, or placing their seal upon it, or setting up in it, effortlessly, a wave of significance" (Merleau-Ponty 1996, p. 151). Our inability to inhabit aesthetic space, unlike Schneider's, is essential rather than contingent. My inability to see the painted object from a different angle or to apprehend it as a possible object of practical engagement is not related to any injury I might have suffered. Aesthetic space is, rather, a universal limitation to the projective quality of the body schema.

3. The *I cannot* and non-representational art

Why, then, does Merleau-Ponty overlook this fact in his works on aesthetics? I wager that is because of the kinds of artwork that he considers. Our body's inability to inhabit purely visual space is more or less covered over in figurative and representational painting. This style of artwork strives to mimic the well-organized perceptual space of our habitual engagement with the world. It, therefore, invites us to grasp the objects that it depicts in terms of the *I can*, to which Gallese and Freedberg's article attests. I see the room depicted in Diego Velázquez' *Las Meninas* as one that can be entered and explored; I empathize with the young, blonde girl in the centre of the picture who is probably being told to remain still while her portrait is being painted; I can almost hear the dog breathing and smell its fur (Merleau-Ponty 1966, p. 26). I am able to do this because the objects painted by Velázquez are discrete or "manipulable" and resemble the objects with which I am perceptually familiar. They are a reflection of my world. This reflection, however, is importantly incomplete; it is merely visual and, therefore, not the kind of thing with which the body is able to engage with as a whole. For this reason, the painting is a mirror through which the embodied subject, unlike Alice in Lewis Carroll's famous story, cannot pass unscathed. This is why one can sympathize with Jean-Paul Sartre when he says of the painting:

> We do not enter and we do not leave. On the scene, in miniature, there are people who are like us and who mime a sacred drama, but, as violent as the tumult may be, it remains in the box and hits up against its walls without breaking them [...] Entirely absorbed by the event that impels them, they ignore us; as for us, we would not touch them even if we would scratch the canvas with our nails
> (Sartre 1981, pp. 184–185, my translation)[1]

While I may grasp *Las Meninas* in terms of what my body is able to do in the perceptual world, I do not experience it as a place of possible interaction. The painted space, then, unlike what Merleau-Ponty's discussion of imagination suggests, is not simply a horizon like others. It is not a place that invites me like the space on the other side of the wall. It is not open to exploration; it is a place where my body, as a whole, cannot go.

Painted space is, therefore, *unlike* all perceptual forms of bodily constraint. My inability to move in painted space or to engage with the objects in it is unlike my inability to jump four feet in the air from a standing position, or my inability to take off into flight like the pigeons in the city square. In other words, it is not a *failure of my body's power*, nor is it a specifically *human* shortcoming. My body, after all, does have some sense of what it would be like to jump high into the air, and, although it is not the kind of body that can fly, it can and does understand the bird's flight in a bodily way. What is more, and perhaps most significant, is that, these mundane experiences of *I cannot* occur within the familiar world of engagement. The sense of *I can* that I have in this context is not *omnipotence*; it is just the sense that, *in principle*, I can encounter and somehow engage with everything that falls within the range of my senses. As Merleau-Ponty explains: "everything I see is on principle within my reach" (Merleau-Ponty 1993, p. 124). The painted space, however is *in principle not within my grasp*. This is because it is paradoxical: it is a space that is not really a space and contains objects and people that are not really objects and people. It is not an "I cannot right now, but I could if I had trained or if I had been made differently", it is an "I never could".

1. "[...] on n'y entre point, on n'en sort pas. Sur la scène en miniature, il y a des gens pareils à nous qui miment un drame sacré mais, si fort que soit le tumulte, il reste dans la boîte et se cogne aux parois sans les briser [...]. Tout absorbés par l'événement qui les a suscités, ils nous ignorent: quant à nous, dûssions-nous grater la toile avec nos ongles, nous ne les toucherons pas (Sartre 1981, pp. 184–185).

The dimension of *I cannot* in aesthetic experience is more evident in non-representational art. The lived body is unable to project its particular, functional aims onto what is depicted on such canvases because what is there is not yet a space, properly speaking. This is more obvious the less the artwork tries to resemble perceptual reality. Abstract painting, for example, does not depict familiar, perceptual wholes. The body has no coherent sense of what it can do with respect to Jackson Pollock's *One*, for example. The painting is, therefore, another kind of object – one with which the body must have a different kind of relation. I will describe this different relation in the final section of this chapter.

4. A non-dualistic solution to the problem of the *I cannot*

In spite of Merleau-Ponty's arguments about the perceptual-imaginative couple, our discovery of the *I cannot* in aesthetic experience inclines us to differentiate between the way that the body engages with the painting as a physical thing in the familiar world of our engagement that is our *home*, and the imaginative space of the painting that is *unheim* to it. Would this be tantamount to reintroducing the distinction that Husserl and Sartre make between the "physical image" and the "image object" (Husserl 2005, p. 20)? According to Sartre and Husserl, due to its material substrate, the painting is both a "physical image" – a perceptual object like the wall on which it hangs – and an "image-object" – a mountain or a spring surrounded by bathers. It is, however, never *both of these objects at once* when I engage with it (Sartre 1940, p. 213). According to them, consciousness can only intend one kind of object at a time: it either apprehends the painting as a physical thing – paint and canvas – or it apprehends the "image" (i.e. the picture as such). On this understanding, the perceptual intention negates the imaginative one instead of implying it as Merleau-Ponty would like. By stressing the incompossibility of the way that consciousness – or in our case, the body – relates to the image and the object, one runs the risk of introducing rifts within experience that lead to dualism.

In order to avoid this undesirable outcome, Merleau-Ponty must redefine the body beyond the projective *I can*. Instead of locating the difference between the way that one engages with perceptual and aesthetic space in an irreconcilable schism between perceptual and imaginative acts, Merleau-Ponty can appeal to a fluidity within the body itself. The body need not only grasp itself in terms of its practical and egoic engagement with the world; it also has the power to organize itself into different kinds of wholes. The body that perceives in a habitual, everyday context is unified by its sense of its possibilities for practical action; the body that perceives the artwork, I argue, is organized according to a different principle:

transitivity. This principle, borrowed from one of Merleau-Ponty's lecture courses on child psychology at the Sorbonne, denotes the trans-personal unity between the lived body and what it perceives. The transitive body has not yet succeeded in demarcating its boundaries and is, therefore, an *indeterminate* whole. Such a body does feel alienated by the artwork because its sense of self is malleable; it is, therefore, better able to adapt itself to the artwork's particular demands. This solution avoids dualism since it is the same body that achieves both types of organization: the transitive body is always there beneath the surface of the practical body. This means that Merleau-Ponty does not have to abandon the body schema he presents in *Phenomenology of Perception* in the face of my aesthetic objection. Instead, he must simply acknowledge the limitations of defining the body in terms of its projective capacity.

Merleau-Ponty begins to scratch the surface of the body's relation to the artwork beyond the scope of intentional projection in *Eye and Mind* and *Cézanne's Doubt*, where he considers what I believe is a middle ground between representational and abstract art. According to Merleau-Ponty, Cézanne's artistic goal was to depict the "feverish genesis" of objects in perception (Merleau-Ponty 1993, p. 128). This means that he sought to visually reveal how we, through bodily communication with our surroundings, come to see objects in the first place (Merleau-Ponty 1964a, p. 69). Non-representational painting like Cézanne's, which does not strive to copy objects as they are given in everyday perception, harnesses the magical power that vision has to make seen what was otherwise invisible. It teaches us how to see things before they properly become things before our eyes (Merleau-Ponty 1964a, p. 69). The object of Cézanne's painting, therefore, is not properly an object at all as we normally experience it; it is an expression of the *il y a* (*there is*) before the *qu'est-ce qu'il y a* (*what there is*) (Merleau-Ponty 1964a, p. 12). The question of the body's potential for movement with respect to it is effectively suspended since the objects in question and their spatial location are only germinating. Since the space of the aesthetic object is not yet fully constituted in post-impressionistic painting, it is experienced as a kind of "nowhere" that the habitual subject-body cannot yet meaningfully navigate.

What kind of bodily organization corresponds to the *il y a* of Cézanne's painting? I argue that it must be a body that is organized in the same way as its object: a body "in the making". That is to say, a body that is, like the apple or the mountain on the canvas, on the way to becoming a familiar, meaningful whole. This argument is based on Merleau-Ponty's claims in his 1963 course at the Sorbonne on the child's relation to the other. The central argument of his lecture is that there is always a correspondence between the way that the world is perceived and the sense that the body has of its boundaries and its possibilities (Merleau-Ponty 1963, p. 12). As a child develops, he argues, he develops a sense of his body as subjective. This means that it comes to an understanding of itself as a demarcated whole defined by the body schema (Merleau-Ponty 1963, p. 29). This organization of the body, however, is not the most original one. Prior to grasping itself as a unique, goal-oriented whole, the child lives in what Merleau-Ponty calls a situation of confusion or unity with others and the world. This is what explains certain aspects of infantile behaviour. A baby will, for example, cry when its mother leaves the room even when it is neither in pain nor in need of any particular physical attention. Merleau-Ponty explains that this is because the baby does not yet experience a gap or separation between himself and the other. The baby cries in his mother's absence because he feels himself to be incomplete without her (Merleau-Ponty 1963, p. 29). The baby's body is, therefore, not something that is properly his own: he shares it with others. The child acquires a sense of his body as a subjective whole primarily through the process of mirror recognition (Merleau-Ponty 1963, p. 25). By recognising himself in the mirror and, by extension, through pairing with others, the child acquires a visual sense of his body's boundaries. Put differently: he comes to know himself as a Gestalt or form that is distinguished from – but related to – others.

The body schema as described in *Phenomenology of Perception* is, according to this argument, a modification of a more original sense of bodily unity. This means, therefore, that there are bodily experiences that precede and exceed one's sense of *I can*. The body schema is, furthermore, a transient modification: it is not a permanent possession. Merleau-Ponty insists that the practical body continues to harbour the germs for its dissolution into the more primordial sense of transitive unity (Merleau-Ponty 1963, p. 25). This is particularly evident in limit experiences such as love. Accepting to love or be loved," Merleau-Ponty explains, "is accepting to also exercise an influence, to decide for another to a certain extent. Loving is inevitably to enter into a situation of indistinction with the other" (1963, p. 59, my translation). The body, therefore, constantly shifts between two different forms of organization: one that I call "mine", and another that is shared.

The distinction between these two different forms of bodily organization helps to clarify what Merleau-Ponty refers to as the "anonymous body" in *Phenomenology of Perception*. In the chapter entitled "Sense experience", he reiterates the account of perception as a process of communication between world and body that I have already explained. He adds to this, however, that one experiences the body that is involved in the process of bringing perception about as a "one" rather than an "I". Objects in the world solicit me to perceive them in a certain way and my body responds by giving itself over to them, letting them fill it up and guide its action (Merleau-Ponty 1945, p. 248). This process is achieved by a body that seems to act independently of me and whose movements are essentially mysterious. This is why he says that

> Every perception takes place in an atmosphere of generality and is presented to us anonymously. I cannot say that I see the blue of the sky in the sense in which I say that I understand a book or again in which I decide to devote my life to mathematics. My perception, even when seen from the inside, expresses a given situation: I can see blue because I am *sensitive* to colours, whereas personal acts create a situation: I am a mathematician because I have decided to be one. So, if I wanted to render precisely the perceptual experience, I ought to say that *one* perceives in me, and not that I perceive. Every sensation carries within it the germ of a dream of depersonalization such as we experience in that quasi-stupor to which we are reduced when we really try to live at the level of sensation. … I am no more aware of being the true subject of my sensation than of my birth or my death (Merleau-Ponty 1945, p. 250)

The anonymous level of perceptual experience underlies the one where I cast my net of projects onto the world; the body that corresponds to it is a reorganization of the projective bodily Gestalt that I call "mine". I am only able to organize the world in light of my goals once there is a network of perceivable and functional objects around me. This network is first brought about by a body that, from my personal point of view, is beyond the realm of what *I* am familiar with. The body that I call "mine", the one that realises my projects, my *I* can, comes about, as Merleau-Ponty argues that objects do in *Eye and Mind*, through a mysterious process of communication between a body that does not yet belong to anyone and a world of not-yet-objects.

The anonymous body is characterized by "*it* can" rather than "*I* can". Like the lived body, it "just knows" how to act, but it is not yet a fully formed or well delineated "something". As such, it is paradoxical: it is both distinct from and the same as the pre-objective environment with which it communicates. Since its boundaries are obscure, it can never really be *mine*.

The encounter of the subject-body with the *it can* is an experience of motor limitation. The *it can* is the former's hidden, inner threshold that, when manifest, threatens to swallow the "I" into its folds. The experience of the *it can* is a reversion to a more primordial, unified sense of the body. It is also, however, the temporary death of the "I" who cannot retain its singular form and function within it (Merleau-Ponty 1945, p. 250). As such, it also entails the loss of the ego-body's motor projects and, most importantly, its sense of ownership over its acts. "I" *cannot* make or cross the bridge into anonymity; only that other part of me, the "it", can.

The pre-personal body and the pre-objective world are normally never experienced as such. They are rather the conditions of possibility of what Merleau-Ponty called perception at the beginning of the *Phenomenology of Perception*. For the most part, this pre-personal moment of the perceptual process is invisible or "lived through" as one sees through eyeglasses into a sharper world. Because it is the living ground of the experience of both my body and the objects that I perceive, however, it is always present and has the potential to be disclosed for what it is. The *it can* leaks into the familiar perception "home" in abnormal or limit experiences. It is evoked, for instance, in Merleau-Ponty's example of the warped glasses in *Phenomenology of Perception*. Participants in a scientific experiment were made to wear disorientating glasses for a period of days. At first, when they put the glasses on, the world seemed completely distorted: objects were not where they seemed to be and the subjects did not know how to engage with them. Over time, they learned how to re-organize their perceptual field into a meaningful realm of possible interaction (Merleau-Ponty 1945, pp. 282–283). This is an experience of the *it can*: the loss of the world and the efficacy of the body followed by the mysterious rebirth of order and meaning. Love is another limit experience that dissolves the boundaries of my projective Gestalt and plunges me into the *it can*.

The most protracted encounter with the pre-personal and pre-objective, however, happens in aesthetics. The body that creates artwork is, according to Merleau-Ponty, the *it can*, or the passive body, rather than the *I can*. The artist does not accomplish the painting by following the blueprints of an existential project, as one does in the case of becoming a philosopher, for example. Instead, he relinquishes his mastery over the situation as well as his hands and eyes and "discovers" the painting as if by chance (Menasé 2003, p. 34, p. 38). The painting is a project that is accomplished in and through the artist's person by "he knows not who" (Menasé 2003, pp. 10–11). The creator in question, however, is not truly foreign to the lived body, it is merely foreign to the "I" who is attached to it. The personal perspective is, however, our most familiar way of relating to our bodies and the world. When artists speak of the creative process, therefore, they speak from out of the "I". From this point of view, it seems to them as though their creative movement actually emanates from the things they perceive (Merleau-Ponty 1964a, p. 31), or as if some mysterious spirit, "the muse", spoke through them.

The "it can" is also the body that *perceives* the painting. The artistic product, at least in its non-representational form, is the visual depiction of the pre-objective world to which the "it can" corresponds. The painting, therefore, extends the pre-objective world into the familiar world of every day perception. It solicits the lived body, as would any other object in one's environment, to take up a certain position with respect to it, to "see according to it" as Merleau-Ponty says (Bernet 2003, p. 95). The proper interlocutor for the pre-object, however, is the *it can*. The painting, therefore, demands that the body give up its "I" and dissolve back into its foundational pre-being. This process begins with the experience of *I cannot*.

The body's transition from *I can* to *I cannot* to *it can* is fairly clear in the case of the perception of abstract artwork or non-representative like Cézanne's.

Its application to figurative painting is, however, more difficult to discern. For this reason, the philosopher is often tempted to overlook its ubiquitous role in aesthetic experience. Although I preserve a sense of *I can* when I perceive paintings like those by Velázquez in the sense that I understand the imaginary objects depicted in them in terms of the objects of my habitual, goal-oriented behaviour, I know that they are nevertheless beyond my reach. This phenomenological description of aesthetic experience led us to discover the *I cannot* as a structural limitation of the body schema. I then addressed the implications of the body's experience of aesthetic objects and determined that the *I cannot* does not entail a strict, Sartrian, dualism between perception and imagination. Instead, I appealed to Merleau-Ponty's later work on child development to develop a more complex notion of the body. Along this path, I argued that the body has two fundamental modes of organization, the subjective *I can* and the anonymous *it can*. The body oscillates between these two different types of organization. The *it can body* is, however, often overlooked as it only tends to surface in limit experiences that are then superseded by the projective bodily Gestalt. Even painting that is characterized by the *I cannot* succeeds in covering over the limitations of the subjective *project-body*. The bodily limitations of aesthetic perception, however, usher us into a new and deeper understanding of subjectivity, functionality, and meaning as achievements arising out of an anonymous, confused, and potentially chaotic ground. The phenomenology of painting, therefore, accomplishes the task that Merleau-Ponty believes all good philosophy should: it re-thinks the definitions of "subject" and "object" by blurring the boundaries between the body and the world (Merleau-Ponty 1964b, p. 170). In so doing, it challenges the modern sense of ownership that I have over my body, its power to move, and its artistic creations.

References

Bernet, R. (2003). Gaze, drive, and body in Lacan and Merleau-Ponty. In J. Corveleyn, & P. Moyaert (Eds.), *Psychosis: Phenomenological and Psychoanalytical Approaches* (pp. 89–103). Leuven: Leuven University Press.

Colonna, F. (2003). Merleau-Ponty penseur de l'imaginaire. In R. Barbaras (Ed.), *Chiasmi International Vol 5: Le Reel et L'imaginaire* (pp. 111–144). Paris: Vrin.

Freedberg, D., & Gallese, V. (2007). Motion, emotion and empathy in esthetic experience. *Trends in Cognitive Science*, 11(5), 197–203.

Greenberg, C. (1993 [1960]). Modernist painting. In J. O'Brian (Ed.), *Clement Greenberg: The Collected Essays and Criticism, Volume 4*. Chicago/London: The University of Chicago Press (cf. also http://www.sharecom.ca/greenberg/modernism.html, last access 4 June, 2012).

Husserl, E. (1989). *Ideas Pertaining to a Pure Phenomenology and to a Phenomenological Philosophy, second book* (transl. by R. Rojcewicz, & A. Schuwer). Dordrecht. Kluwer Academic.

Husserl, E. (2005). *Phantasy, Image Consciousness, and Memory* (transl. by J.B. Brough). Dordrecht: Springer.

Menasé, St. (2003). *Passivité et création*. Paris: PUF.

Merleau-Ponty, M. (1942). *La Structure du Comportement*. Paris: Quadrige/PUF.

Merleau-Ponty, M. (1945). *Phénoménologie de la Perception*. Paris: Gallimard.

Merleau-Ponty, M. (1963). *Les Relations avec Autrui Chez L'enfant*. Paris: Centre de Documentation Universitaire de la Sorbonne.

Merleau-Ponty, M. (1964a). *L'oeil et L'esprit*. Paris: Gallimard.

Merleau-Ponty, M. (1964b). *Le visible et l'invisible*. Paris: Gallimard.

Merleau-Ponty, M. (1966). Le Doute de Cézanne. In *Sens et Non-sens* (pp. 15–44). Paris: Editions Nagel.

Merleau-Ponty, M. (1993). Eye and mind. In G. A. Johnson (Ed.), *The Merleau-Ponty Aesthetics Reader* (pp. 121–149). Evanston: Northwestern University Press.

Merleau-Ponty, M. (1996). *Phenomenology of Perception* (transl. by C. Smith). London: Routledge.

Sartre, J.-P. (1940). *L'imaginaire: Psychologie Phénoménologique de L'imagination*. Paris: Gallimard.

Sartre, J.-P. (1981). Saint Marc et son double (Le séquestré de Venise) (inédit). *Obliques, 24/25*, 171–202.

Sokolowski, R. (2008). *Phenomenology of the Human Person*. Cambridge: Cambridge University Press.

Steves, J.B. (2004). *Imagining Bodies: Merleau-Ponty's Philosophy of Imagination*. Pittsburgh: Duquesne University Press.

Name index

Subject index